ASSESSMENT AND THERAPY

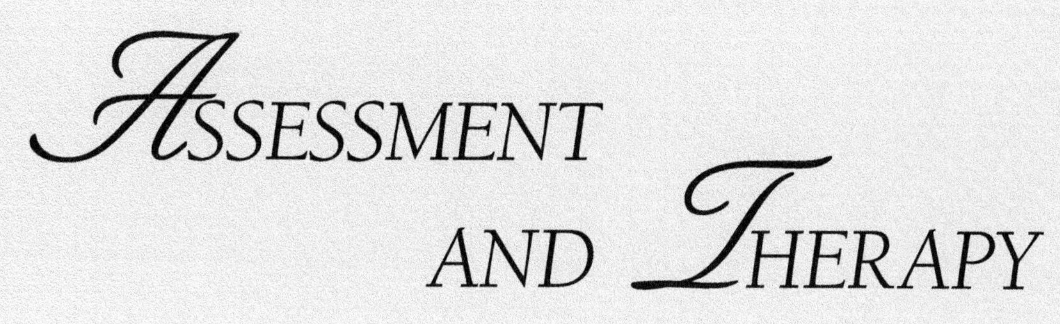

Assessment and Therapy

Specialty Articles from the Encyclopedia of Mental Health

Editor-in-Chief

HOWARD S. FRIEDMAN

Department of Psychology
University of California, Riverside

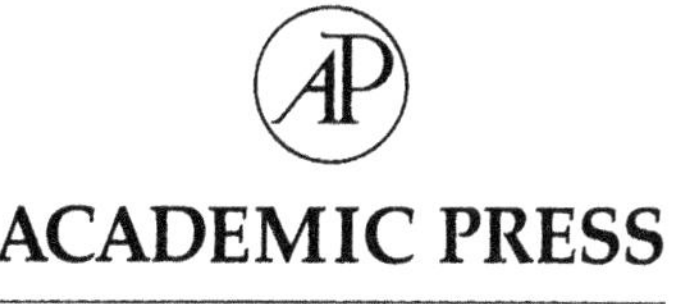

ACADEMIC PRESS

A Harcourt Science and Technology Company

SAN DIEGO   SAN FRANCISCO   NEW YORK   BOSTON   LONDON   SYDNEY   TOKYO

This book is printed on acid-free paper. 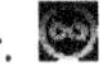

Compilation copyright © 2001 by ACADEMIC PRESS

All Rights Reserved.
No part of this publication may be reproduced or transmitted in any form or by any means, electronic or mechanical, including photocopy, recording, or any information storage and retrieval system, without permission in writing from the publisher.

Requests for permission to make copies of any part of the work should be mailed to:
Permissions Department, Harcourt Inc., 6277 Sea Harbor Drive,
Orlando, Florida 32887-6777

Academic Press
A Harcourt Science and Technology Company
525 B Street, Suite 1900, San Diego, California 92101-4495, USA
http://www.academicpress.com

Academic Press
Harcourt Place, 32 Jamestown Road, London NW1 7BY, UK
http://www.academicpress.com

Library of Congress Catalog Card Number: 2001088681

International Standard Book Number: 0-12-267806-0 (Paperback)

Printed and bound by CPI Group (UK) Ltd, Croydon, CR0 4YY

Transferred to Digital Print 2011

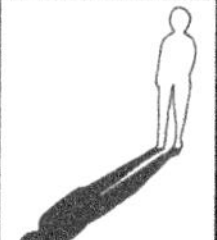

Contents

About the Editor-in-Chief

HOWARD S. FRIEDMAN is Distinguished Professor of Psychology at the University of California, Riverside. He also holds an adjunct appointment as Clinical Professor at the University of California, San Diego Medical School. Dr. Friedman attended Yale University, graduating magna cum laude with honors in psychology. He was awarded a National Science Foundation graduate fellowship at Harvard University, where he received his Ph.D.

Professor Friedman is a thrice-elected Fellow of the American Psychological Association and an elected Fellow of the Society of Behavioral Medicine and the American Association for the Advancement of Science (AAAS). Friedman is author of many influential scientific articles in leading journals and was named a "most-cited psychologist" by the publishers of the Social Science Citation Index. His books include two textbooks, *Health Psychology* and *Personality;* three edited scholarly volumes; and the authored comprehensive analysis titled *The Self-Healing Personality.* Dr. Friedman's research centers around the relations of mental and physical health, with a special focus on expressive style. He has taught undergraduates, graduate students, medical students, and postdocs.

Professor Friedman has received the career Outstanding Contributions to Health Psychology Award from the Health Psychology Division of the American Psychological Association. He also received the Distinguished Teaching Award from the University of California, Riverside, and the Outstanding Teacher Award from the Western Psychological Association.

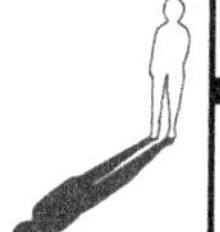

Preface

A number of scientific and intellectual trends have converged to change our understanding of mental health. Conceptions of mental health and mental disorders have broadened significantly to take into account new knowledge about the genetic, biological, developmental, social, societal, and cultural nature of human beings. Our award-winning *Encyclopedia of Mental Health* was the first to bring together these emerging trends in one resource, and now the contributions primarily relevant to assessment and to the mental disorders are being made more accessible to those who desire a more concise and focused reference work.

What are these mental health trends affecting our understanding of the disorders? First, our understanding has moved well beyond the artificial nature–nurture dichotomy. We know more and more about the biological underpinnings of mental states and behavior, but we also better understand how these biological tendencies unfold in a family, social, and cultural environment. Second, we have moved beyond the old "mental" versus "physical" ("mind versus body") dichotomies. To a greater extent than previously imagined, there is a strong reciprocal relation between our health and activity and our cognitions, moods, and mental well-being. Third, the experts increasingly recognize the complementary importance of prevention and treatment. A simple model of treating mental "disease" is often ultimately futile without associated prevention efforts, yet prevention cannot sensibly ignore the need for efficacious treatments. Fourth, we now emphasize primary mental health promotion—the structural, environmental, family, and cultural context of mental health. Fifth, the best scholars now recognize meaningful variations across ages, genders, cultures, families, and societies. That is, to understand fully and improve significantly a person's mental health, we need to know not only about that person's biological and personal makeup, but also about his or her age, family, work, and position in society.

CONTENTS

This volume on mental disorders thus encompasses various levels of analysis, from the molecular and biological, through the social and family, to the cultural. We have therefore included coverage of key topics not traditionally found in such a reference work. We of course include topics such as clinical assessment, psychoanalysis, brain neuroimaging, and family therapy. But we also examine couples therapy, support groups, and assessment of mental health in older adults. Also of note is that methodological issues receive attention throughout, including important chapters on nontraditional approaches to classifying mental disorders, and on standards of psychotherapy.

Stress is increasingly recognized as a complex interaction of the person, the environment, the social support structure, and the culture. Thus, many of our articles deal with the mental health aspects of such topics as coping with stress, as well as social support and community mental health.

Aside from the striking breakthroughs at the genetic and molecular levels, perhaps the greatest current interest is in the family and developmental context for mental health and mental impairment. We include a truly exceptional discussion of various relevant issues, including expert articles on childhood abuse, couples therapy, domestic violence therapy, and family therapy. Such articles should certainly be of value to anyone involved with the mental health of children and families.

Finally, we have not neglected those fascinating topics usually would not be considered psychiatric pathology but seem integral to understanding therapy. For example, take a look at the article "Hypnosis and the Psychological Unconscious."

DISTINGUISHED SCHOLARS

With the assistance of the outstanding editorial board, we have secured contributions by the most distinguished scholars and practitioners. Many are founders of their fields, and they are justly famous. But some contributors represent the brilliant new generation of mental health scholars. I have encouraged the contributors to write about what is most important. We thus have a reference work that is rooted in the present and looking toward the future, rather than bogged down in obsolete notions and topics. Emphasis has been placed on clarity and accessibility.

Howard S. Friedman

How to Use This Reference

Assessment and Therapy is intended for use by students, research professionals, and practicing clinicians. Each article serves as a comprehensive overview of a given area, providing both breadth of coverage for students and depth of coverage for research and clinical professionals. We have designed this reference with the following features for maximum accessibility for all readers.

Articles are arranged alphabetically by subject. Because the reader's topic of interest may be listed under a broader article title, we encourage use of the Index for access to a subject area, rather than use of the Table of Contents alone. Because a topic of study in mental health is often applicable to more than one article, the Index provides a complete listing of where a subject is covered and in what context.

Each article contains an outline, a glossary, cross-references, and a bibliography. The outline allows a quick scan of the major areas discussed within each article. The glossary contains terms that may be unfamiliar to the reader, with each term defined *in the context of its use in that article*. Thus, a term may appear in the glossary for another article defined in a slightly different manner or with a subtle nuance specific to that article. For clarity, we have allowed these differences in definition to remain so that the terms are defined relative to the context of the particular article.

The articles have been cross-referenced to other related articles. Cross-references are found at the first or predominant mention of a subject area covered elsewhere. Cross-references will always appear at the end of a paragraph. Where multiple cross-references apply to a single paragraph, the cross-references are listed in alphabetical order. We encourage readers to use the cross-references to locate other articles that will provide more detailed information about a subject.

The Bibliography lists recent secondary sources to aid the reader in locating more detailed or technical information. Review articles and research articles that are considered of primary importance to the understanding of a given subject area are also listed. Bibliographies are not intended to provide a full reference listing of all material covered in the context of a given article, but are provided as guides to further reading.

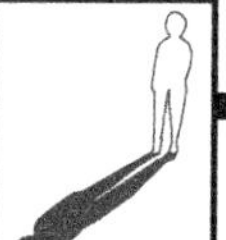

Assessment of Mental Health in Older Adults

Carolyn M. Aldwin and Michael R. Levenson
University of California, Davis

Age Effects Statistical relationships due solely to the effect of chronological age.
Cohort Effects Statistical relationships due primarily to the effect of year of birth, for example, having lived through a particular historical era at a specific age.
Discriminant Validity The degree to which an assessment discriminates between groups and/or shows differential patterns of correlations with different outcomes, for example, the personality trait of hostility should predict anger and resentment better than anxiety or depression.
Ecological Validity How well an assessment applies to or reflects the experience of the particular sample under study.
Internal Reliability The cross-item consistency of a scale, that is, whether all items in the scale assess the same construct.
Period Effects Statistical relationships due primarily to time of measurement effects.
Predictive Validity The degree to which an assessment predicts an outcome of some sort, generally behavior (e.g., self-reported symptoms).
Sequential Analyses Statistical analyses which contrast age, cohort, and period effects.

ASSESSMENT OF MENTAL HEALTH processes in the elderly can be particularly challenging, in part due to the fact that many assessment instruments were developed on younger populations and may not provide as accurate a picture in older populations, who vary greatly in their levels of cognitive, sensory, and motor abilities. In addition, many physical and mental illnesses in late life can present similar symptoms, and differentiating between the two is the focus of much of the assessment research in late life. Finally, the elderly may be less likely to disclose certain types of problems, and thus special techniques may be necessary to assess sources of psychological distress, including substance abuse and life events. However, less is known about what constitutes positive mental health in late life.

I. HETEROGENEITY IN OLDER POPULATIONS

A. Age Influences on Validity and Reliability

As a developmental stage, late life encompasses more than 45 years, from roughly ages 65 to 110. Not surprisingly, there is an extraordinary amount of hetero-

Copyright © 1998 by Academic Press.
All rights of reproduction in any form reserved.

geneity in this population. Some elders are physically and cognitively very healthy; others develop disabling chronic illnesses quite early on. Thus, it is often very difficult to make generalizations about "the elderly." Not surprisingly, gerontologists have subdivided this developmental stage into three groups: the young-old, whose ages range from 65 to 79; the old-old (80–99); and the oldest-old, or centenarians. Others differentiate between optimal aging, in which there is little decrement or even improvement in some functions; normal aging, in which there are some decrements for which the elderly can readily compensate to maintain adequate psychosocial functioning; and impaired aging, marked by declines in physical and cognitive function.

Thus, it is very important to understand the position along these continua of the elder or sample of elders to be assessed. In general, in the United States, the young-old are relatively healthy and it is likely that assessment techniques used in younger populations are quite adequate for this population. Indeed, if one attempts to use instruments developed for impaired elders in the ordinary young-old population, one rapidly runs into ceiling effects—nearly all elders will score in the top range, rendering criteria for predictive and discriminant validity nearly useless. In other words, if there is no variance on an instrument, it cannot be used to correlate with other measures or to distinguish between groups.

In contrast, for frail elders, who are more likely to be in the old-old age group, the use of standard instruments may pose a problem in both the reliability and validity of the data. Cognitively impaired elders may become confused when confronted with typical Likert scaling, and dichotomously scaled instruments may have more reliability and validity. (We have found that even elders in good condition generally dislike and mistrust the Procrustean bed of fixed response formats, and often need to be cajoled into translating their phenomenological experience into admittedly arbitrary numbers.) In addition, frail elders may have poor attention spans, requiring the administration of brief forms of standard instruments and/or multiple testing sessions over several days. Although elders in general respond as accurately on surveys as younger populations, it is unlikely that cognitively impaired elders can do so, and interviews are more likely to yield valid information.

Elders with visual impairments may have difficulty in reading questionnaires, requiring the use of larger fonts. In addition, we have found that scantron sheets which use relatively pale type faces with poor contrast (e.g., lavender script on cream-colored paper) are contraindicated with elders who have acuity problems.

Individuals with motor impairments, such as tremors associated with Parkinson's disease or severe arthritis in the hands or wrists, may have difficulty in filling out questionnaires, and will require longer periods of time to complete them. For elders with severe forms of these illnesses, scantron forms are virtually impossible. Some researchers have switched to computer presentations of instruments which can aid in overcoming such sensory and motor deficits.

In general, we have found that frail elders do best in interviews in which the required responses to questions are available in both verbal and visual forms. If Likert scales are necessary for some instruments, then response cards, written in large fonts, which elders can hold and point to responses, are very helpful. Given that cognitively impaired elders often have difficulty in switching tasks, changing response cards is a good way of signaling that one task is done and that attention needs to be refocused on another.

However, interviews conducted in home settings may pose a special problem in assessing the elderly. In our experience, it is very difficult to interview just one member of an elderly dyad, especially in long-term married couples. Such couples may learn to compensate for memory problems by consulting with each other, and typically the non-target spouse will respond to questions, making accurate assessment of the target individual problematic. Thus, we have found it necessary to physically separate couples, either by giving the non-target elder an instrument to complete in another room, or by using pairs of interviewers to conduct simultaneous interviews, again in separate rooms.

B. Cohort Influences on Validity

Gerontologists distinguish among age, cohort, and period effects. In general, age effects are those which are solely due to an individual's chronological age, cohort effects refer to historical impacts reflected in a person's birth year or events experienced by a group of peers (e.g., the Depression), and period effects refer to larger social influences at the time of measurement. Neither cross-sectional nor longitudinal designs can adequately differentiate among these three types of effects, and only sequential designs, which follow multiple cohorts over different periods, can adequately differentiate these three types of effects. For any given effect to be accurately attributed to age, one must demonstrate that individuals of a given age are more likely to exhibit a particular response, regardless of what cohort they are in or the year in which they are assessed.

Age, cohort, and period effects also have implications for the validity of assessment instruments. For example, the validity of instruments used in older populations may be affected by cohort differences in language use and expression, a problem that has received relatively little attention in the assessment literature. One must be sensitive to whether the language used in any particular inventory is appropriate to the population under study. Indeed, the language used in older instruments is often more relevant to that used by older cohorts. For example, in the MMPI, there were several items which reflected older word usage (such as playing "drop the handkerchief"). While the revised MMPI (MMPI-2) has eliminated anachronistic items, in 1991 Butcher and his colleagues found that nearly all of the age differences in the MMPI-2 still reflected either differing health statuses or cohort differences in language and experience (e.g., the use of marijuana was much less likely to be endorsed by older groups).

Many instruments commonly in use in psychology were developed on student populations, and, as such, may have poor ecological validity for the elderly. For example, a mastery or control instrument may include items about perceived fairness of grading practices or juggling work versus parenting roles. Certainly, any instruments used to assess mental health in the elderly must be sensitive to items that are more relevant to student or young adult experiences.

Less obvious sources of poor ecological validity may lie in cohort differences in reporting style. The current cohort of elders may be less willing to reveal emotional distress and/or use different terminology to refer these states. Older men in particular may be less comfortable in identifying stressors than younger men.

The possibility of response bias in the elderly has some interesting implications for the relative validity of diagnostic techniques. There is surprisingly little research available comparing the validity of self-report versus observer ratings in the elderly for specific illnesses. In general, observer ratings are thought to be more objective than self-report inventories, although there may be age-related biases in observer ratings, reflecting stereotypical biases about elders as more impaired, irascible, and so on.

A further problem is that clinical interviews often yield categorical classification, for example, full-blown depression versus none. To the extent that elders, even in clinical interviews, under-report symptoms, then such procedures may underestimate the existence of problems. For example, in 1992 Koenig and Blazer reviewed studies showing that the prevalence of major depression in the elderly, based upon clinical interviews, was about 1% (which is rather less than that reported for younger populations), but some 20% or more of older samples reported problems with negative affect on self-rated inventories, a figure much more comparable to younger samples. This is not to say that different criteria or cutoff points on standardized clinical assessment tools necessarily need to be developed, but rather that much more research is needed into this issue.

II. DIFFERENTIATING BETWEEN MENTAL AND PHYSICAL HEALTH PROBLEMS

Perhaps the issue which has received the most attention in the literature concerns the differentiation between mental and physical health. Many mental health scales include physical symptoms, which may be relatively uncommon in younger populations and indicative of psychological distress. However, in older populations, with their greater incidence of chronic health problems, such instruments may yield very high rates of false positives. Further, mental health problems often have physiological concomitants, and physical health problems can affect psychological states. Obviously, identifying the primary source of the symptoms is crucial in determining treatment options, although sometimes the only way in which to determine the precise etiology for a particular illness is to test different treatments. However, there are critical issues in differentiating anxiety, depression, and psychoses from a variety of physical health problems.

A. Differentiating Depression and Anxiety from Physical Health Problems

Self-report inventories of depression typically include many somatic complaints, such as fatigue, headaches, back and neck pain, constipation, and sleep disturbances. While in younger individuals these types of complaints may be indicative of depression, such symptoms are very common among the elderly. Thus, this inclusion of physical health symptoms in psychological assessment instruments may lead to Type I errors. On the other hand, there is some indication that depression in the elderly may be presented in terms of physical symptoms, and a relatively high proportion of medical visits to general practitioners by the elderly may be due to depression manifesting in physical complaints. Thus, screening for recent life events and/or changes in living conditions (see below) may be an important way for clinicians to determine whether bereavement or social isolation may be important factors underlying such visits.

On the other hand, many illnesses common to the elderly, as well as prescribed medications, may have concomitant symptoms of depression and anxiety. For example, elders are at increased risk for hypothyroidism, cardiovascular disease, and chronic obstructive pulmonary disorder, which may cause fatigue, sleep disturbances, and negative affect. Other disorders, such as myocardial infarctions, vitamin deficiencies, anemia, pneumonia, and hyper- and hypothyroidism, may present with symptoms of anxiety. Further, many medications commonly prescribed in the elderly, such as antihypertensives, may also create symptoms of depression. Thus, physical, mental, and social health are often tightly intertwined in the elderly, and multipronged assessment techniques may be necessary to adequately establish the etiology of symptoms of depression and anxiety in the elderly.

B. Differentiating Depression from Dementia

Some depressive symptoms mimic cognitive impairment, especially in the elderly. In particular, psychomotor retardation and memory lapses in the elderly are usually attributed to dementing processes, but actually may reflect depression. Pseudodementias can result from a wide variety of disorders, including nutritional deficiencies, prescribed medications, alcohol and substance abuse, and surgical procedures. Thus, assessment of the occurrence of problems of this type may be an important component in elders presenting with cognitive impairment. In turn, dementia is often associated with difficulty concentrating, loss of energy, and psychomotor slowing, even in the absence of depression. A number of different screening inventories have been developed to differentiate between these types of disorders.

In 1992, Newman and Sweet identified a number of different features which may distinguish depression from dementia. Depression often has a rapid onset while dementia often has a gradual one. In addition, there may be differences in both patient and familial awareness of the problems, with recognition greater in depression-related cognitive impairment than in problems related to dementia. Patients who are depressed may be able to provide greater detail about their impairment and to manifest subjective distress, while dementing patients may have vague, nonspecific complaints and may be more likely to conceal cognitive deficits. Depressed patients typically show poor motivation and give up easily on tasks, while dementing patients may struggle with tasks.

In addition, there are a number of differences between the two groups in both cognitive testing and neurological examination. For example, depressed patients typically have problems with both recent and long-term memory, and report poorer concentration than actual knowledge testing, whereas dementia patients typically have much worse recent than long-term memory deficits and general knowledge is worse than concentration skills. Finally, depressive patients typically demonstrate no problems with specific neurological testing, while dementing patients typically present with dyspraxias and agnosias, and show abnormal CAT scans, with increased ventricular size. In addition, the administration of antidepressive medications may be one way to distinguish depression-related pseudodementias from true dementias resulting from neurological disorders.

C. Distinguishing Schizophrenia from Dementia

While the onset of schizophrenia typically occurs in adolescence or young adulthood, schizophrenia may also occur in late life. Schizophrenia with a late life onset is often called paraphrenia, and may occur in individuals who have a history of eccentricity and are socially isolated. However, dementia can also produce hallucinations and delusions, and thus, like depression, it is important to distinguish between the two conditions.

Given that late-life onset of schizophrenia is relatively rare, very few systematic studies have been conducted. However, neuropsychological assessment studies have been done, and, in many cases, it is possible to rule out dementing processes.

D. Assessment of Behavioral Disorders

Particularly disturbing concomitants of the cognitive and affective disorders prevalent in late life are behavioral disturbances. These disturbances, including wandering, sleep disruptions, verbal and physical aggression, and hallucinations and delusions, may have serious impacts on the quality of life for both elderly individuals and their caretakers. Patients who exhibit such behaviors may be labeled as "problems" by nursing home staff and then regularly given psychotropic medication to control their behavior, which can result in a variety of adverse physical, cognitive, and affective side effects. While there have been regulatory efforts to decrease the use of psychotropic medications in nursing homes, paradoxically, this regulation can result in increased use, as nurses are given less discretion and physicians must prescribe the use of such drugs on a regular basis.

In 1994, Teri and Logsdon reviewed the variety of scales which have been developed fairly recently to assess behavioral disturbances. These typically are observational measures, and may be administered by researchers, clinicians, nurses, or caregivers. A major purpose of these scales is to quantify the frequency and severity of such disturbances to devise appropriate treatment strategies. Detailing the exact pattern of aggressive and disruptive behavior may result in a more objective picture of the actual problems created by such patients, facilitate behavioral intervention, and result in less reliance on psychotropic medications.

III. ASSESSING FACTORS AFFECTING MENTAL AND PHYSICAL HEALTH

There are a variety of factors which can affect physical and mental health in late life. In terms of behavioral factors, alcohol and substance abuse, as well as stress, are two of the most important ones.

A. Assessing Alcohol and Substance Abuse in the Elderly

In the late 1960s Cahalan and his associates developed a survey assessment instrument for alcohol consumption and problems. It assessed alcohol consumption using three different scales: (1) the usual number of drinks of beer, wine, and distilled spirits consumed "nowadays," as reported in drinks per day, week, month, or year; (2) the number of drinks of beer, wine and distilled spirits consumed the day before completing the questionnaire; and (3) the regularity of alcohol consumption on specific days of the week. For example, a respondent may indicate that, in a typical week, he or she drinks one glass of wine during the evenings and two drinks each on Friday and Saturday night. Thus, this individual, on average, drinks nine drinks a week, which then usually is translated into drinks per year.

Independently of consumption, respondents indicate the frequency (e.g., never, once per week, month, or year) of experiencing alcohol problems. These items assess the frequency with which alcohol affects physical, psychological, or social functioning. In general, convictions for drunk driving and alcohol-related traffic accidents are weighted more heavily than other types of problems. Although they reflect some components of a *DSM-IV* diagnosis of alcoholism, they do not permit such a diagnosis, which requires the use of a diagnostic interview.

The shortest and simplest self report of alcohol abuse is the four-item CAGE instrument, in which a positive response to two or more of the items suggests alcohol abuse. The items assess feeling that one should drink less, being annoyed by others' criticizing one's drinking, feeling guilty about drinking, and drinking in the morning. The items have good face validity, yet this instrument does not appear to be sensitive in older populations. The Michigan Alcoholism Screening Test (MAST) for older adults is a much longer (24-item) instrument that has been validated on the hospitalized elderly but may not be practical for screening outside hospitalized populations. It should be noted that other versions of the MAST have not been equally valid in all populations tested.

The use of self-report surveys of alcohol consumption and problems may prove difficult, especially with the elderly. However, for the general population, Midanik concluded in 1988 that "the validity of self-reports is not an either/or phenomenon." There is no "gold" standard against which to compare self-reports, only a variety of "lead" standards such as collateral reports, diaries, official records, laboratory tests, or interviews. All of these methods assess overlapping but nonisomorphic aspects of an individual's alcohol use. Sobell and Sobell noted in 1990 that the relevant issue is the extent of discrepancy among sources of information that are being used to investigate a given research question. The latter observation may be especially relevant for the elderly.

Tobacco, alcohol, and prescription drugs (usually anxiolytics) are the most abused drugs in the elderly. Indeed, alcohol consumption both reduces thiamine uptake and interacts with prescription drug use, a fact that is further complicated by the reduced capacity of elderly persons for clearing such drugs. Thus, use of both types of substances may carry a risk for health problems that increases with age. Moreover, the elderly may not recognize that their relatively nonproblematic levels of consumption at younger ages may cause problems in later life.

While drinking has been shown to decline with age, this may not be a reliable predictor of future trends since recent research has shown that changes in drinking patterns appear to be more closely associated with period rather than age effects. These considerations may render assessment of risk for problem drinking (with its attendant drug interactions) more difficult in the elderly.

In 1997, Atkinson argued that the relatively low reported rates of alcoholism in those over the age of 60 (no more than 2% in men and less than 1% in women) may underestimate the actual prevalence of problems) largely due to a failure to accurately report consumption and problems in surveys. The "discrepancy problem" may be more pertinent among the elderly than in younger populations. Thus, there may be special difficulties with self-report in the elderly, with a problem/reported problem ratio perhaps increasing with age. This is further complicated by cohort effects, with younger cohorts more willing to acknowledge problems than older ones, if such cohort differences are maintained in later life.

Excluding daily blood alcohol level testing, there are several reasonable supplements to self-report in the elderly. First, there is a pattern of cognitive deterioration associated with alcohol abuse in the elderly that is distinct from that associated with senile dementias such as Alzheimer's and even Korsakoff's Syndrome (which involves irreversible brain damage due to long-term severe alcohol abuse). This pattern is summarized in *DSM-IV* as involving deficits in memory, language, motor functions, object recognition (without organic motor or sensory impairment), and abstract thinking and planning. Evidence has supported this diagnostic approach with an additional strong finding that name-finding was almost completely spared in alcohol-related dementias, in contrast to Alzheimer's Disease, in which dysnomia is pronounced.

Second, and perhaps most helpful, are in-home assessments. In addition to standard consumption interviews and listing the prescriptions and home remedies that the elderly use, other data and relatively unobtrusive observations can be employed. These include a history of falls, grooming, odors present in the house (also, obviously, useful for an assessment of tobacco use), bruises at the level of furniture, tremors, incontinence, and many others (many of which could be associated with non-alcohol-related dementias or depression). Naturally, such an assessment would require considerable training and would obviously be available only for that minority of the elderly who receive home care from outside agencies.

Unfortunately, there is no good way of assessing the dependence on prescription tranquilizers (principally benzodiazepines) in the elderly unless withdrawal symptoms, such as extreme anxiety and irritability, occur since dependence is not typically associated with dose increase. Such dependence is more frequent among elderly women than men. Signs of toxicity from long-term use are easily mistaken for other disorders of the elderly, such as memory loss and other cognitive impairments, as well as problems with mobility. It is likely that alcohol and drug abuse may reflect the levels of stress in elders' lives.

B. Assessing Stress and Coping in Late Life

There are several different ways of assessing stress, including traumatic events, life events, chronic role strain, and daily stressors or hassles. In the last decade, it has rapidly become apparent that both type and frequency of stressors change with age. While early studies suggested that the number of stressful life events decrease with age, perusal of the types of events typically found on early life event scales reveal that many are far more relevant to younger populations than to older ones (e.g., marriage, divorce, changing jobs, imprisonment). Several instruments are now available that assess life events that are more relevant to older populations such as caretaking for spouse and parents, institutionalization of parent or spouse, death of a child, child's divorce, problems with grandchildren, and the like. These instruments are less likely to show a decrease in stressful life events with age.

However, the number of daily stressors does decrease with age, most probably due to the decline in the number of social roles. For example, most older adults have relinquished active parenting and work roles, the source of the majority of hassles in mid-life. While there is a concomitant increase in the number of hassles associated with both health problems and avocations in retirement, for most older adults, these typically do not generate as many hassles as do work and childrearing roles.

In part, this may be due to changes in the nature of stress in late life. Stress in earlier life is more likely to be episodic in nature, such as children's crises or problems at work, whereas stressors in late life may be more likely to be chronic, for example, managing chronic illnesses or caregiving for an ill spouse. If chronic problems are successfully managed, they may not be perceived as "problems" per se. An 80-year-old with multiple health problems may well assert that he or she has had no problems in the past week, despite obvious impairments requiring careful management. Thus, among the old-old, interviews may be better assessments of stress than self-report instruments.

However, the decrease in stress reporting may also be due to age-related changes in the way individuals cope. In some ways, older people are better copers, in that they are less likely to use escapist strategies such as alcohol, drugs, or wishful thinking—or perhaps individuals who survive until late life are less likely to use escapist strategies. However, the old-old may be more likely to use denial as a coping strategy. Denial of the severity of health problems, for example, may be a palliative strategy, as long as appropriate instrumental actions are taken, such as adhering to a medical regimen. However, the old-old are often reluctant to admit problems for fear that they will be institutionalized, with all that entails, including separation from spouse and loved ones and the loss of control. Thus, they may deny and/or hide problems, even those which could be adequately treated in the home, which can lead to worse problems, greatly increasing the risk of institutionalization. Thus, accurate assessment of problems in the elderly are crucial to both their treatment and may permit successful home treatment and forestall institutionalization. [*See* Coping with Stress.]

IV. ASSESSING POSITIVE MENTAL HEALTH

Mental health is not simply the absence of symptoms, but entails positive functioning as well. Unfortunately, positive mental health has received less attention in the elderly, with the possible exception of one of its dimensions, life satisfaction.

Despite the widespread dissemination of Erikson's theory of ego development in adulthood, only a handful of scales have been developed to assess generativity and ego integrity. The most extensive scale development on positive mental health in late life has been done by Ryff and her colleagues in the 1980s. They developed measures of complexity, generativity, integrity, and interiority, as well those that assess self-acceptance, positive relations with others, autonomy, environmental mastery, purpose in life, and personal growth. Although Ryff's scales are correlated with the Big Five personality factors (neuroticism, extraversion, openness to experience, conscientiousness, and agreeableness), they correlate independently with positive affect, suggesting that they assess more than just the standard personality dimensions. It remains to be seen whether these scales will enjoy widespread use as indicators of positive mental health in the elderly.

V. SUMMARY

In summary, assessing mental health in the elderly requires attention to a number of factors, including the age and functional ability of the elder and whether or not the instrument used has adequate reliability and validity for older populations. While elders may be more or less accurate at reporting symptoms as younger groups, the crucial assessment issue appears to be differentiating between possible sources of the problems. Further, more research needs to be done in assessing positive mental health in the elderly.

BIBLIOGRAPHY

Aldwin, C. (1994). *Stress, coping, and development: An integrative approach.* New York: Guilford.

Atkinson, R. M. (1997). Alcohol and drug abuse in the elderly. In R. Jacoby & C. Oppenheimer (Eds.), *Psychiatry in the elderly* (2nd ed., pp. 661–688). Oxford: Oxford University Press.

Garland, J. (1997). Psychological assessment and treatment. In R. Jacoby & C. Oppenheimer (Eds.), *Psychiatry in the elderly* (2nd ed., pp. 246–256). Oxford: Oxford University Press.

Howard, R., & Levy, R. (1997). Late-onset schizophrenia, late paraphrenia, and paranoid states of late life. In R. Jacoby & C. Oppenheimer (Eds.), *Psychiatry in the elderly* (2nd ed., pp. 617–631). Oxford: Oxford University Press.

Newman, P. J., & Sweet, J. J. (1992). Depressive disorders. In A. E. Puente & C. R. Reynolds (Eds.), *Handbook of neuropsychological assessment: A biopsychosocial perspective* (pp. 263–308). New York: Plenum.

Pachana, N. A., Gallagher-Thompson, D., & Thompson, L. W. (1994). Assessment of depression. In M. P. Lawton & J. A. Teresi (Eds.), *Annual Review of Gerontology and Geriatrics, Vol. 14* (pp. 234–256). New York: Springer.

Rabins, P. V. (1992). Schizophrenia and psychotic states. In J. E. Birren, R. Bruce Sloane, & G. D. Cohen (Eds.), *Handbook of mental health and aging* (2nd. ed., pp. 464–479). San Diego: Academic Press.

Ritchie, K. (1997). The development and use of instruments for the psychological assessment of older patients. In R. Jacoby & C. Oppenheimer (Eds.), *Psychiatry in the elderly* (2nd ed., pp. 232–245). Oxford: Oxford University Press.

Ryff, C. D., & Essex, M. J. (1991). Psychological well-being in adulthood and old age: Descriptive markers and explanatory processes. In K. W. Schaie (Ed.), *Annual Review of Gerontological and Geriatrics, II,* 144–171. New York: Springer.

Sheikh, J. I. (1992). Anxiety and its disorders in old age. In J. E. Birren, R. B. Sloane, & G. D. Cohen (Eds.), *Handbook of Mental Health and Aging* (2nd ed., pp. 410–432). San Diego, CA: Academic Press.

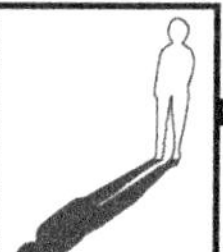

Behavior Therapy

Maxie C. Maultsby, Jr.
Howard University, College of Medicine

Mariusz Wirga
Howard University, College of Medicine

Behavior The things organisms do. There are two types: (1) *overt behavior*—observable by other people; (2) *covert behavior*—observable only by the behaving people themselves, for example, thoughts, emotional feelings, and so on.

Cognitive-Emotive Dissonance The most important stage in new learning, characterized by these two features: (1) it occurs when people first begin thinking and acting in their new, correct ways for their behavioral goal but (2) they are having the uncomfortable emotional feelings that they have when they believe they are behaving incorrectly: People usually describe this experience with "This doesn't feel right," or "This feels wrong to me." A common example of this event is: an American driver "feeling wrong" while driving correctly on the left side of the street in England. This is an unavoidable experience in psychotherapeutic or any type of change in a personal habit. In psychotherapy it is the stage of maximal therapeutic resistance. If cognitive-emotive dissonance is poorly handled in psychotherapy, patient/clients are likely to drop out or become noncompliant.

Conditioning The process of learning in which an innate behavioral response to a learned or innate stimulus becomes a new behavioral response to a formerly neutral stimulus, after that neutral stimulus has been paired a sufficient number of times with the original, learned or innate stimulus. There are two major types of conditioning: (1) Classical (Pavlovian or respondent) conditioning wherein the behavioral response being learned is an innate response for a neutral stimulus such as salivating to the sound of a bell. (2) Operant (Skinnerian or instrumental) conditioning wherein the behavior being learned is new for the subject.

Discrimination The process wherein a subject reacts appropriately to only one, of two or more similar, but different stimuli.

Drive A force that activates or impels people or animals to make a behavioral response. In behavioristic terms, drives are the results of physiologic deprivations, such as of food and water, or the result of pain or some other unpleasant stimulus.

Emotive Imagery The mental process of visualizing real or imaged events so vividly that the person reacts with the most logical emotional and/or physical response for the meaning that those mental pictures have for that person. In behavior therapy, emotive imagery is called mental practice.

Extinction The process wherein the frequency of a learned response to a conditioned stimulus decreases and ultimately disappears, due to lack of reinforcement.

Magic An imaginary but empirically nonexistent power that can exempt real events from the rule of nature that an event occurs only after its essentials for existing have been met.

Magical Thinking Thinking that describes only nonempirical illusions of realities or reality.

Copyright © 1998 by Academic Press.
All rights of reproduction in any form reserved.

Punishment Any undesirable consequence of the subject's behavioral response in a specific situation that decreases (ideally to zero) the probability of that response occurring in similar future situations.

Reinforcement A process of increasing the probability (ideally to 100%) that a specific behavior will be repeated in similar future situations. The two classes are: positive and negative. (1) *Positive reinforcement* occurs when a subject receives or experiences a personally pleasant event, that is, a reward as the consequence of its specific, immediately preceding behavior. The object or experience received is a *positive reinforcer* for the behavior that preceded it. (2) *Negative reinforcement* occurs when a subject receives an unpleasant stimulus that results in a behavioral response that terminates or removes that stimulus. The unpleasant stimulus for the behavior that terminated it is a *negative reinforcer*. The unpleasant simulus is called an *aversive stimulus*. The event of termination or removal of an aversive stimulus is a positive reinforcer—also called a *secondary reinforcer*—for the behavior that immediately preceded that terminating event.

Response and Stimulus Generalization The process wherein a neutral stimulus that is similar to, but different from, a conditioned stimulus elicits the same responses that the original or conditioned stimulus elicits, without having been previously paired with either. Generalization of response is the process wherein the same response is learned to different stimuli.

Stimulus A sensory event that elicits a response from a subject. The two types of stimuli are: (1) Innate or unconditioned stimuli, which elicit only natural or innate responses from a subject such as salivation when exposed to food, and (2) learned or conditioned stimuli, which elicit the responses that innate or learned stimuli elicit, but only after having been paired several times with the real or conditioned stimulus when they elicit their normal target responses.

There are varying opinions about the best way to define **BEHAVIOR THERAPY.** However, most health professionals accept Eysenck's definition: Behavior therapy is the attempt to alter human behavior and emotions in a beneficial way according to the laws of *modern learning theory*. There is only one problem with that definition: There is no generally recognized comprehensive learning theory of human behavior. Consequently, from a phenomenological view point, behavior therapy has the following three objective appearances. First, behavior therapy is a general field of health improvement that deals with learned, undesirable emotional and physical behavioral responses. But these undesirable responses have been practiced so much that they have become personal habits. However, the people who have these undesirable habits believe that they have little or no satisfactory control over them. That is why these habits are often the main behavioral barriers to personally satisfying lives for their owners. Second, as a field of health improvement, behavior therapy consists of a diverse collection of many different behavioral (as opposed to medicinal) regimens. Each regimen has a name and is proclaimed to be based on laws of the yet-to-be-identified modern learning theory. Without a comprehensive unifying learning theory however, behavior therapy will not soon become the genuine health science discipline that it is incorrectly assumed to already be.

Third, the behavior therapy field has a generally unrecognized or generally ignored crisis of disunity. It is quite similar to (if not the same as) the crisis of disunity that Staats recently (1990) described in psychology, the "surrogate mother" of behavior therapy. But unlike the rigidly divided field of psychology, behavior therapy has reached the threshold of identifying one unifying learning theory of human behavior that will enable it to immediately become a genuine health science discipline.

I. EARLY HISTORICAL ROOTS OF BEHAVIOR THERAPY

Attempts to help people solve behavioral problems, with maneuvers similar to those used in today's behavior therapy have a long history. Pliny the Elder, in first-century Rome tried to cure alcohol abuse by putting putrid spiders in the drinking glasses of alcohol abusers. Today that maneuver would be called *aversive conditioning*. The eighteenth-century "Wild Boy of Averyron" was taught spoken language with maneuvers that today would be called *modeling, prompting, positive reinforcement,* and/or *withholding of positive reinforcers*. A nineteenth-century equivalent of today's prison warden, Alexander Maconchi, used what today would be called a *point system* or a *token economy* as the main basis for getting inmates of a

Royal British penal colony to obey the prison rules. In the same century a French physician treated a case of obsessional thoughts with maneuvers that today would be called *thought stoppage* and/or *reciprocal inhibition*. Still, as a field of health improvement, behavior therapy is less than fifty years old.

The direct history of behavior therapy is inextricably interwoven with the history of psychology, which was its surrogate mother. Psychology resulted from the intellectual revolution of a group of scientifically minded European philosophers. They abandoned philosophy and started psychology, the science of the structure of the mind and consciousness. From their research focus came the name or their school of psychology: Structuralism. Their main research technique was structured, personal introspection. Their goal was to make psychology a "pure" natural science, on an equal "footing" with the other natural sciences. They were the first experimental psychologists; but they showed no interest in investigating human behavioral health problems.

Wilhelm Wundt started the structuralistic psychology in Germany. After training with him, Edward R. Titchener brought structuralism to America in the late nineteenth century. Passive, structured introspection of one's own mind, however, proved to be unproductive. Envy of the natural scientists soon developed among American psychologists, because unlike psychologists, the natural scientists had concrete, objectively observable constructs. Those constructs could be manipulated with satisfying predictable and reportable results. Those results could be recognized and objectively replicated, and they could produce honors and recognition for the scientists who discovered them. The charismatic Cattell, of the psychology laboratory at the prestigious Columbia University, continually made this boast. The research in his laboratory was as independent of introspection as was in the research in physics or zoology. The rapidly increasing general professional interest in doing that type of research led to the first American psychological rebellion, which occurred early in the twentieth century.

A. The Results of That Rebellion

The main result was the production of three new schools of American psychology: *Gestalt, Behavioralism, and Functionalism*. Each school had these two goals: (1) to effectively eliminate the other schools, by making their school synonymous with American psychology, plus (2) to put American psychology on as firm a scientific basis as were the natural sciences.

However, there still was no stated interest in treating behavioral health problems. That was probably due to this reality: At that time, people were usually thought of as belonging to one of only four groups: (1) normal people, that is people in everyday life situations; (2) insane people, such as inmates of those foreboding stone fortresses called insane asylums or "nut houses"; (3) criminals, such as inmates of prisons or jails; and (4) medically ill people, such as patients of physicians. There was no recognized need then for a health field devoted to behavioral health improvement.

The Functionalists seemed to have been the most well organized of the three new psychological schools. In addition, they had decided to switch their research focus from passively observing the subjective structure of a passive mind, to observing the contents of active minds at work in every day life. That interest might have led to a later psychotherapeutic focus. However, neither the Functionalist nor the other two schools attracted much attention. That was probably due largely to the aggressively attacking and rejecting stance the behaviorists took toward the other schools of psychology. The behaviorists were led by the charismatic, proselytizing behavioral psychologist named John B. Watson. He had become a strong enthusiast of the idea of making Pavlovian conditioning the basis for behavioral psychology.

II. IMPORTANT BEHAVIORISTS AND THEIR CONTRIBUTIONS

A. Ivan P. Pavlov and Classical Conditioning

Ivan P. Pavlov (1849–1936), the Russian physician and physiologist, and 1904 Nobel Prize laureate, serendipitously discovered *classical* or *respondent conditioning* in the late nineteenth century. Here is the standard procedure for producing it. First, select a neutral stimulus and an animal (human or nonhuman), for example, a dog. Animals often respond with a startle response to unusual stimuli. So, it is important to make sure that a selected stimulus is really neutral, that is, one the animal normally ignores. Common neutral stimuli used for conditioning are a light or the sound of a bell or buzzer. To ensure that it is neutral for the selected animal, the stimulus is repeatedly presented to the animal until it is consistently ignored. That maneuver is called *stimulus habituation,* or *adaptation.*

Next, select an innate, or *unconditioned stimulus*—that is, anything to which the dog has an innate response is appropriate. Common examples are food for the salivation response or electric shock for the escape response. Then, a bell or buzzer is sounded a second or two before giving the hungry dog food or before giving a satiated dog an electric shock. After several such pairings of those two stimuli, the hungry dog will salivate and the satiated dog will run away from the sound of the bell or buzzer alone. That event indicates that classical conditioning of the unconditioned stimulus' response to be a response to the formerly neutral stimulus has occurred. Then the same response will occur in response to either stimulus.

I. Drawbacks of Early Pavlovian Conditioning Theory

There were three major drawbacks in early Pavlovian Conditioning Theory: (1) Except for salivation and fear, Pavlovians ignored the other autonomic nervous system responses. That fact severely limited the variety of learned behaviors that they could study. (2) It could not explain in empirically accurate ways active and passive escape or avoidance behaviors and some of the behavioral results of punishment. Yet, those learned behaviors and the consequences of punishment are as important for survival and enjoyable living as are approach behaviors. (3) The technical aspects of Pavlovian conditioning were much more complex than those of the main competing learning theory: namely, Thorndike's reward-based, trial and error, learning-by-doing theory of behavior. Largely because of Watson's inflexible commitment to it, Pavlovian conditioning became one of the two main focuses of the behaviorists.

B. John B. Watson and Radical Behaviorism

Starting in the second decade of the twentieth century, John B. Watson (1878–1958) led American behaviorists in continual rebellion against the other schools of psychology. The behaviorists' canons were: (1) Behaviorism, a term coined by Watson, maintains that the concept of consciousness is merely an undefinable replacement of the religious concept of soul and therefore completely rejects it. (2) Behaviorism is a clean break with all of the current theories and traditional psychological terminology that do not describe directly observable responses. (3) Behavior is best explained in terms of reward and punishment learning or in terms of Pavlovian conditioning of the stimulus-response (S-R) reflexes of the subject's nervous system. Watson even believed that human language learning was best explained on the basis of spinal reflexes. On that point, Watson was more of a reflexologist than a behaviorist.

Watson was not the first one to see the positive scientific potential of focusing on Pavlov's conditioned reflexes. In his 1890 book, *Principles of Psychology,* William James wrote a chapter titled *"The Functions of the Brain."* There he described the case history of a child who had become afraid to touch a candle after having been burned by one. James' description of the child's presumed brain activity revealed a conceptual grasp of some such phenomenon as conditioning. Also, in his 1896 psychological article, *"The Reflex Arch Concept in Psychology,"* John Dewey stated his dissatisfaction about the lack of a unifying theory in psychology. He also stated his belief that Pavlov's concept of the reflex arch came closest to meeting the unifying need of psychology than any other current concept. But unlike Pavlov, who believed that activity of cerebral reflexes was important in behavioral learning, Watson rejected all reflex action that was higher in the nervous system than the spinal reflex.

Watson is best remembered for the 1920 case study of Little Albert that he and Rosalie Rayner did. They conditioned that 11-month-old infant to have an irrational fear response to furry animals. As the unconditioned stimulus they used the infantile startle response to an unexpected loud noise. That was the first confirmation of Pavlov's theory in America, using a human subject.

Little Albert spontaneously *generalized* his fear response to furry animals to other furry objects, for example, to furry articles of clothing. But he did not exhibit fear in response to nonfurry objects of clothing. It remains a mystery why that observation of *stimulus discrimination* did not lead Watson to make this insight: Little Albert could not have made the above stimulus discrimination without possessing the faculty of consciousness. Still, Watson and Rayner's work made it seem logical to assume that irrational fears could probably be eliminated by induced extinction. So with Watson's encouragement, Mary Cover Jones, one of his graduate students, successfully investigated that possibility.

To induce fear extinction, Jones subjected abnormally fearful children to a combination of behavioral conditioning maneuvers. The two most effective ones were *social imitation* (now called *modeling*) and what she called *direct conditioning*, which, 30 years later Wolpe called *counterconditioning* and *reciprocal inhibition*. For direct conditioning, Jones would gradually present to irrationally fearful children their feared object, while they were enjoying their favorite food. The effectiveness of this maneuver depended upon Jones making sure that the children always experienced stronger pleasant sensations from eating than fearful ones in response to the gradually presented, feared animal or object. For modeling, Jones would have the fearful child watch and join peers, fearlessly playing with the feared animal or object.

Watson did more to popularize behaviorism as an area of scientific study than any of his contemporary behaviorists. Still Watson's positive influence on behaviorism came more from his excellent public speaking and writing skills than from his research. Consequently, his admirer, Herrmsteim, made this summary statement in his introduction to the posthumous edition of Watson's book, *Comparative Psychology:* "Watson's importance to behavioral psychology was more sociological than substantive."

C. Edward L. Thorndike: Reward Learning Theory

Edward L. Thorndike (1874–1949), was the most influential non-Pavlovian American behaviorist in the first three decades of the twentieth century. His popular 1898 book, *Animal Intelligence,* made him one of the earliest internationally renowned American psychologists. However, his subsequent work had a lasting effect on American psychology mainly because it was the professional "springboard" for the research of B. F. Skinner. Skinner was Thorndike's most famous and productive student.

Thorndike's theory was: When, by trial and error, hungry or thirsty rats behave in ways that result in them receiving food or water, the tendency to have that behavior in similar future situations is increased. Conversely, if a specific behavioral habit-reflex of a rat is punished enough with an electric shock, the tendency to have that behavior is decreased and or extinguished. Or, an untrained rat will quickly learn avoidance behavior in response to those shocks.

Thorndike used a puzzle box—later called the Skinner box—in which trial and error, *reward-based learning research* was done using food- or water-deprived rats. The rats were rewarded with food or water immediately after making the appropriate behavioral responses in the experimental conditions. Thorndike also used satiated rats, to which he gave an electric shock immediately after inappropriate behavioral responses.

Unlike Pavlov, Thorndike had no interest in neuronal reflexes. For Thorndike (and later for Skinner) the stimulus-response (S-R) reflex was merely the statistical correlation of specific responses with immediately following rewards and/or punishments. Although Thorndike and Pavlov had different concepts of the behavioral stimulus-response (S-R) reflex, both theories seemed to explain approach behavior equally well. Unfortunately, each theory was equally incapable of explaining avoidance learning and some of the effects of punishment on learning in a way that accurately fit the human experience of them.

D. Burrhus F. Skinner and Operant Conditioning

Burrhus F. Skinner (1904–1990), extended, modified and perfected Thorndike's reward learning theory as *operant conditioning.* In Skinner's 1953 book with Lindsley and Solomon, the term *behavior therapy* was introduced into the psychology literature. Skinner however, had worked with nonhuman animals; so that term may have been used in reference to the past work of Mary Cover Jones. It may also have referred to the exciting new, non-Freudian hypothesis of Joseph Wolpe that neurotic fears are learned and can be efficiently treated with behavioral treatments.

Like Watson, Skinner was committed to *radical behaviorism.* He too rejected traditional psychology and all of its concepts that implied what he called *mentalism.* That meant any concept that reflected a belief in cause/effect relationships between mental entities or activities and learned behavior. In the 1966 edition of his 1928 book, *The Behavior of Organisms,* Skinner still labeled the belief that emotions are important factors in behavior a "mental fiction." He agreed with William James' assertion that "people are sorry because they cry," or that "people are afraid because they tremble." In addition, they both believed it is incorrect, or at least unscientific, to think that people cry because they are sorry or tremble because they are afraid.

To my knowledge, James' assertion has no clinical application. But, believing in that assertion is a common cause of clinical problems. For example, people who believe they are their behavior often get clinically depressed when they believe that one or two undesirable personal actions "magically change them as human beings." Such students often get depressed and quit school after 1 or 2 days of seriously thinking that they are complete failures because they failed to get the grades that they wanted. However, such thoughts and emotions cannot be directly observed; so, according to Skinnerians, to be "scientific," psychotherapists must ignore those important factors when they treat such depressions or try to get those students to stay in school. Next is the logic of their often futile treatments.

Skinner maintained that emotions are not behavioral responses; instead they are states of reflex strength, similar to drives. According to Skinner, the virtue of understanding emotions that way is that behavioral scientists can ignore them "whenever that concept loses its convenience." However, as we shall see below, Mowrer's research revealed that Skinner's ideas about emotions do not make logical sense, even for nonhuman animals. That fact is all the more interesting because Skinner's research subjects were almost all nonhuman animals—usually rats and pigeons. However, to Skinner's credit, he never advised the extrapolation of his animal research findings to human beings. As late as 1960, he warned that whether or not extrapolation of his research discoveries to people is justified cannot yet be decided. The behavioristic psychologists who introduced operant conditioning into behavior therapy were justifiably impressed by Skinner's research. But, they either did not know or ignored that nonhuman brains cannot and therefore do not process sensory input the same way that human brains process it. Therefore, even in the same stimulus situations, it is still naive to expect humans to respond exactly the way rats or pigeons respond.

1. Skinner's Most Positive and Most Negative Influences on Behavior Therapy

Probably Skinner's most positive influence on behavior therapy was his research about how different *schedules of reinforcements* significantly influence the speed of learning new behavioral habits and their resistance to extinctions. For example a fixed 1:1 ratio of an immediate reward or reinforcement for each appropriate response produces the fastest acquisition of new habits for a given, constant drive level. But those habits are most susceptible to rapid extinction if the response/reinforcer ratio increases or the reinforcers cease to appear.

If behavior therapists are skilled in managing relevant reinforcement intervals and ratios, their cooperative patients/clients will maintain high levels of motivation for therapeutic change. Also, in the world of paid work, if managers are skilled in varying reinforcement intervals and ratios, employees will maintain high morale and productivity with minimal or no increases in company budgets. *Contingency management* is the name of such goal-oriented changes in reinforcement schedules and ratios.

The sustained, high productivity that the 1:1 ratio produces is the main reason some employers prefer a piecework pay schedule over an hourly or other fixed interval pay schedule that is independent of behavioral response rate. Within the limits of a constant drive state, a variable ratio and/or variable interval reinforcement schedule produces behavioral habits that are most resistant to extinction. For example, the gambler continues to bet despite losses because reinforcement—payoff—may occur any time.

Probably the most negative influence Skinner had on behavior therapy was his empirically unjustified defense of his unreliable definition of behavior. He maintained that behavior is only what one organism observes another organism doing. Because Skinner studied nonhuman animals, he had no logical reason to be concerned about a human test of empirical common sense. Had Skinner had this concern, he might have defined behavior in a way that has a greater than 50% chance of being correct, in any specific instance.

For example, with personal observation alone, a behavior *X* (1) may be *X* and may be correctly observed and labeled as *X;* (2) a non-*X* behavior may appear not to be behavior *X* and be correctly observed and labeled as not being behavior *X;* but (3) behavior *X* may appear to be some other behavior, for example, *Z* and may be incorrectly observed and incorrectly labeled as behavior *Z;* (4) behavior *Z* can appear to be behavior *X* and be observed as, and incorrectly labeled as behavior *X*. A 50% error possibility is insufficient for scientific conclusions. Also,

Skinner's definition of behavior leads to unsuspected magical thinking.

For example, in the textbook *Contemporary Behavior Therapy* by Spiegler and Guevremont, this statement appears: "The behaviorist's model for behavior is: "People are what they do." In reality, though, only by magic can making a stupid mistake convert a human being into a stupid person, or swimming like a fish convert a human being into a fish. That is not just a matter of semantics; when one wants to describe behavior in clinically useful, scientific terms, it is all semantics. When scientists ignore that fact, they sometimes use unsuspected magical thinking to describe empirically valid research findings. As a result they misinterpret their data and formulate useless treatment procedures. That is why Mowrer's research was so important for the development of today's comprehensive behavior therapy.

E. O. Hobart Mowrer and Two-Factor Learning

More than the research and writings of any other single pioneer, behavioral psychologist, those of O. Hobart Mower made contemporary, comprehensive behavior therapy possible. He believed that to be clinically useful, any explanation of human behavior has to pass the human test of empirical common sense. Consequently, Mowrer was intrigued by this paradox: Watson was accepted as the quintessential empirical scientist. Yet the basis for Watson's behaviorist revolution against then-contemporary American psychology was mainly his unchecked belief about the concept of consciousness. He believed that consciousness is an undefinable, meaningless substitute for the ancient concept of soul.

But what if Watson had plugged Little Albert's ears (thereby eliminating his sound consciousness) prior to making the sudden loud noises to condition him to be afraid of furry objects)? That would have been the simple first step in a scientific check of his assumption. But he did not take it. The authors believe that if he had taken that simple step, instead of rejecting the concept of consciousness he might have operationally defined it (and its opposite state of being) in clinically useful terms.

Another observation that intrigued Mowrer was this: When he analyzed the research of the Skinnerians on avoidance behavior, he found their research was carefully done and their data were valid. Their theoretical explanations of that excellent data, however, involved presumably unsuspected but definite magical thinking. That unsuspected magical thinking obscured the invalidity of the basic Skinnerian assumption that directly observable behavior itself is the only factor worthy of scientific study.

That view is called the one-factor stimulus-response (S-R) model of learned behavior. The following common conditioning experiment reveals the serious limitation of that assumption. Take, for example, a dog that has been conditioned with strong electric shocks to run away in response to the sound of a formerly neutral buzzer, which had been sounded within 2 seconds of those shocks. After four consecutive running responses occurred before the electric shock could be administered, the shocks were permanently stopped. Why then does this dog continue running away from the sound of the buzzer?

Here is the Skinnerian answer. The painful electric shock is an unconditioned aversive stimulus. The unconditioned drive states of pain and fear result from painful aversive stimuli. The dog's running responses terminated the dog's pain, and the fear that accompanied the sound or the buzzer. That freedom from those two intense stimuli is a powerful, positive reinforcer of the terminating running responses at the sound of the buzzer. But, according to Skinner, the fear (not being directly observable) could and should be ignored. The only factors worthy of scientific study were the directly observable running responses, the observable buzzer sounds and the strong, unconditioned, electric shocks.

By occurring within 2 seconds of the dog being shocked, that buzzer sound acquired an aversive property "in its own right." That acquired aversive property made the buzzer sound capable of eliciting the same running responses that the unconditioned stimulus (i.e., the electric shock) elicits. That is why the buzzer sound was then called a conditioned or secondary aversive stimulus. Also, each of the dog's running responses ended with the dog receiving the above powerful, positive reinforcements for running. That fixed 1:1 response/reinforcer schedule is the most powerful way to produce a behavioral habit and to maintain it.

That Skinnerian explanation is logical and believable; but it's also magical. Therefore, it can not pass the human test of empirical common sense. The magical component is the statement: "that buzzer sound acquired an aversive property in its own right." The empirical answer to the following question, however, reveals that that could have happened only if magic existed. What would happen if the first dog and a second, unshocked dog were to be exposed together to that buzzer sound, with its assumed "acquired aversive quality"? Unless some magical power protected the second dog, both dogs would experience and run from the "aversive quality" of the buzzer sound. In reality, though, only the first dog would run. The second dog would ignore the buzzer sound. Since magic does not exist, the only empirical explanation is that the buzzer sound had not acquired an aversive quality. Next is the evidence that supports that fact.

What would happen if the previously shocked dog were prevented from running from the buzzer sound and that dog was never shocked again? That first dog's running response would quickly extinguish and the dog would begin to ignore the buzzer, as the second, unshocked dog would have done from the beginning. Only by nonexistent magic could failure to run from a buzzer sound remove an empirically existing aversive quality of that sound. Since the concept of magic is incompatible with a scientific explanation of an event, this scientific conclusion seems obvious: The buzzer sound never acquired and never had any aversive quality.

But, it could be asked, if having been paired with electric shocks did not result in that originally neutral buzzer sound acquiring an aversive quality "in its own right," why did the first dog continue to run from it? Next is Mowrer's nonmagical, Two-Factor Learning Theory explanation of the above events and the empirically objective answer to that question.

First, it is an empirical fact that: (1) Dogs have an innate autonomic nervous system response called salivation, which is a conditionable response to associated, external sensory entities. Dogs also have autonomic nervous system responses called emotivities, which are both conditionable to associated, sensory entities and are a part of every physical behavioral response to these sensory entities. Mowrer's Two-Factor Learning Theory describes those facts this way: Stimulus, emotive response, Observable Response, or S-er-OR.

With the above shocked dog, the sensory entities were the buzzer sound, the painful electric shock, and the emotive response, called fear. Just as hunger is an unconditioned drive for behavioral responses that terminate it, pain, via any aversive stimulus, is an unconditioned drive for behavioral responses that terminate it and its associated sensory entities. In the case of pain, the reducing and terminating behavioral response was the dog's act of running away.

The brains of normal mammals are genetically structured to include emotive responses of the autonomic nervous system in their processing of all sensory data. The innate emotive response of the autonomic nervous system to pain is fear. Fear is also an unconditioned drive for behavioral responses that terminate it. By the dog hearing a buzzer sound immediately before receiving the unconditioned pain of an electric shock, an involuntary, mental, mnemonic association resulted in that dog's brain between these sensory events: the buzzer sound, the immediately following painful electric shock, and the fear that normally accompanies pain. So, instead of the buzzer sound acquiring "an aversive property in its own right," it merely became a learned mnemonic sign or cue that fearfully alerted the dog that a painful shock was an immediately possibility.

After such a sign or cue learning experience, this happens: When the dog perceives the same or similar, future mnemonic signs or cues, part of the biolectrical component of that sensory entity stimulates its autonomic nervous system to the possibility that a fearful pain seems likely to occur. The learned buzzer cue instantly (i.e., with the speed of electricity) elicits fear, which is a drive for the old running response that had formerly protected that dog from the past electric shocks that had quickly followed past buzzer sounds. That running response still results in the same two, powerful, positive reinforcers described above.

Now, recall the second, unshocked dog mentioned earlier. Having "never been shocked," that second dog would not have learned that the buzzer sound had been associated with a painful electrical shock. Therefore, that second dog would ignore the buzzer sound, even though the first dog would continue to run from it. But, the buzzer sound itself never would have acquired any aversive property. Instead, the first dog's autonomic nervous system would have just become conditioned to instantly produce survival-related fear as a second stimulus to the pain of the electric shock as a drive for running at the perception of the learned mnemonic cue for the possibility of another electric shock.

Here is the final major difficulty that is created by assuming that the buzzer sound had acquired an aversive quality "in its own right." That assumption makes it difficult, if not impossible, to explain in a nonmagical way how natural extinction of the dog's running response occurs after the shocks permanently stop. However, Mowrer's nonmagical, Two-Factor Learning Theory easily explains it in an empirically scientific way.

An unconditioned pain drive for running occurs only when the peripheral pain fibers of the sensory area of the dog's brain are stimulated. At the same time that occurs, the dog's autonomic nervous system produces a fear drive for running away from the electric shock. Via involuntary, mnemonic association with any immediately preceding, neutral stimulus (in this case, a buzzer sound) that stimulus can become a conditioned (i.e., learned) sign or cue for the fear component of the total escape response. Afterwards, the mere perception of that sign or cue is a mnemonic stimulus for the dog's autonomic nervous system to produce that old fear drive for running.

The intensity of such fear tends to parallel the intensity of the unconditioned pain drive that precedes it. The intensity of that fear also parallels the strength of the total positive reinforcing power of the freedom from pain and fear, which reinforces the running response that terminates the fear and prevents the painful shock. Therefore, when the shocks stop, at least half of the most powerful positive reinforcement for running also instantly stops.

The physical distress and fatigue from intense running is itself an unconditioned pain event. But that discomfort, in comparison to the pain of an electric shock, is and remains trivial and ignored until the shocks stop. Then, the only drive for running is the rapidly decreasing, unsupplemented fear, cued by the buzzer sound. Now, the initially ignored physical distress and fatigue of intense running rapidly become progressively stronger punishments for continued running responses. That fact causes the decreasing, unsupplemented fear drive for running to gradually extinguish and the dog's running to stop.

In analogous ways Mowrer's Two-Factor Learning Theory also explains why and how any specific sensory stimuli (which a human or nonhuman animal mnemonically associates in appropriate sequence with painful or pleasant events) can become learned signs or cues for learned behaviors that are associated with those events. But, that explanation applies only to animals that have first had the appropriate mnemonic sign learning experience.

Humans, however, can and often do exempt themselves from that naturally occurring behavioral extinction that nonanimals normally experience. Jones' research on excessively fearful children was probably the first to reveal that fact. She noted that when re-exposure to the unconditioned aversive stimulus stopped, her human subjects' conditioned fears sometimes failed to extinguish. This indicated that nonhuman brains do not work exactly like human brains work. Modern human research on the neuro-psychophysiology of language indicates that the above difference in brain functions is probably due to these facts: Humans are the only known animals that have the faculties of self-talk (i.e., thinking about their own thinking). Humans are also the only known animals that can imagine or re-create at will mental, emotional, and physical virtual realities, independently of current or past empirical life events. That is how and why people's imagined events can be as powerful emotional and physical stimuli for habit learning as corresponding empirical life events are, or can be.

That unique human ability seems to best explain the following fact: Pavlov did not report a single dog that ever tried to eat the bell used in its conditioning experiences. Yet, humans often incorrectly call themselves and others names (such as "jackass" or "mouse") that do not refer to any real human things; then without realizing it, they condition themselves to react emotionally and physically to themselves (and to those others) as if they really are the nonexistent things to which their incorrect names refer. (See the Mouse Lady case example in the book *Rational Behavior Therapy.*) That universally popular human habit seems to be an important mental mechanism in many cases of self-mutilation and unprovoked hate crimes.

I. Mowrer's Most Important Contributions to a Unified Field of Behavior Therapy

1. Mowrer's firmly supported Two-Factor Learning Theory made this fact obvious: If consciousness and emotions had not already existed, equivalent con-

cepts would have had to be invented to serve their essential survival functions.

2. Empirical evidence that classical or respondent conditioning is the only type. In addition, during the conditioning process, the former "neutral" stimulus never acquires a new property. Instead, it becomes the subject's new, conditioned sign or cue for associated learned autonomic nervous system responses to that formerly "neutral" stimulus.

3. Empirical evidence that there are two types of behavioral learning: (1) operant or instrumental and (2) sign or cue learning. But they both are byproducts of associated, conditioned impelling emotional drives (e.g., fear, hope, anger, etc.) or other responses controlled by the brain's autonomic nervous system.

4. Empirical evidence that the main survival functions of learned behavioral signs and cues seem to be alerting the concerned subjects to possible positive or negative changes in their current situation and to help them prepare for possibly needed self-protective or other survival related actions.

5. Mowrer demonstrated that Pavlov was correct. Personally understood words are entirely real conditioned stimuli; they substitute for and elicit the same responses that are elicited by the real or imagined stimuli that they represent. Therefore, psychotherapy is word therapy, designed to change the person's internal milieu, that is, to change certain of the person's undesirable, habitual autonomic nervous system responses. That fact makes vicarious learning and extinction of behaviors possible. It also makes therapeutic imagery the main mental mechanisms by which permanent therapeutic improvement occurs.

6. Empirical evidence that via their control over their conscious thoughts, people retain executive-type controlling power over their emotional and physical behavioral responses. That insight enables empirically thinking people to instantly take these two ideally healthy, emotional actions at the same time: First, refuse to believe any longer in the universally popular, but magical and unhealthy "emotional It-monster myth." Second, stop the unsuspected, but still unhealthy emotional self-abuse that believing in that magical emotional myth causes them to experience.

The most easily recognized forms of that unhealthy emotional myth are the frequent, sincere, but irrational thoughts and accusations such as: "It or she/he made or makes me mad, sad, glad," and so on. The empirical reality almost always is: "I made or make me mad, sad, glad, and so on, about it or what she/he is doing or did. If I want to however, I can change my belief about what they did, or are doing and thereby give myself a healthier emotional reaction to it, without using alcohol or other drugs."

III. BEHAVIOR THERAPY AT THE THRESHOLD OF IDEAL UNIFICATION

A scientific discipline cannot exist without a comprehensive, empirically valid, unifying theory. To unify the field of behavioral health improvement, a theory must be based on and/or meet at least five or the following seven sets of empirical facts and criteria.

1. The human brain is a person's main organ of survival, comfort and learned self-control.

2. The theory must make possible clinically useful explanations of both healthy and unhealthy learned behaviors, which are also based on well-established medical facts about relevant normal brain functions.

3. Human cognitive, emotional and physical behaviors interact in this hierarchical way. Coincident with the onset of correct spoken and unspoken human language, the cognitive behaviors (i.e. the brain's mental activities) instantly take executive type, control over human emotional and physical behaviors.

4. To be generally useful, a learning theory of human behavior must explain both healthy and unhealthy learned behaviors in terms of empirical, cause/effect relationships, with the cognitive activities having ultimate control of the emotional and physical behaviors.

5. Unless they are medically or psychiatrically indicated, drugs are to be excluded from the treatments of learned behavioral problems.

6. The maneuvers in behavior therapy must reflect the above-mentioned hierarchical relationships between groups of behaviors.

7. The theory must make possible accurate predictions of treatment outcomes in terms of temporary or permanent replacements of unhealthy cognitive, emotive, and physical habits with personally acceptable, healthy ones.

Space limitations in this article permit only the discussion of pioneers in the behavior therapy field whose conceptual and technical contributions reflect at least five of these seven criteria.

A. Joseph Wolpe and Systematic Desensitization

In the early 1950s, this South African psychiatrist became dissatisfied with the poor therapeutic results he was getting from treating his patients with psychoanalysis. But, at that time there was no credible alternative psychotherapy in South Africa. So, as a psychotherapeutic rebellion, Wolpe combined his medical training with his understanding of behavioral learning theory and made these two important achievements: (1) He created a medically credible, non-Freudian hypothesis of the origin of neurotic fears. (2) He formulated behavioral maneuvers for treating those neurotic fears. Wolpe's behavioral treatment maneuvers were a major contribution to the beginning of behavior therapy as a recognized field of human behavioral research and systematic, mental and emotional health improvement.

Wolpe's most popular treatment maneuver was called *systematic desensitization.* It is a combination of *deep muscular relaxation* and an effective technique of *emotive imagery.* The latter had been formulated and tested by Arnold A. Lazarus, then a psychologist, student/colleague of Wolpe and later a behavior therapist of international acclaim. A typical treatment session is an hour in which patient/clients first self-induce a state of deep muscle relaxation, followed by the therapist verbally pacing them in imagining events on a prepared list of feared objects or events. Starting with the least fearful event, patient/clients are to maintain their initial state of deep muscular relaxation as the therapist verbally paces them up the list to the target fear. If, however, the patient/client becomes noticeably anxious during the session, he or she is to terminate that imagery and focus on reestablishing their former relaxed state before resuming those images.

Wolpe quickly surprised the psychiatric field with his demonstrations of the rapid effectiveness of his behavioral treatment maneuvers. He also reported the largest number of human cases that had ever been successfully treated by one therapist. Prior to Wolpe's report behaviorists had annually reported less that three such successfully treated cases.

B. Albert Ellis and Rational Emotive Therapy

Like Wolpe (but without knowledge of his work), in the mid 1950s an internationally renowned American psychologist named Albert Ellis became discouraged because of his poor therapeutic results using psychoanalysis. Again like Wolpe, as a psychotherapeutic rebellion, Ellis developed a highly effective, authoritatively directive method of psychotherapy called Rational Emotive Therapy. The main stimulus for Ellis' new treatment method was the Greek stoic, emotional canon: "People do not get upset by things, but by the view they take of them."

Ellis saw the great psychotherapeutic relevance to that philosophical observation. So, he converted it into his internationally acclaimed, empirical, *ABC model of human emotions.* That model of human emotions has proven to be one of the most clinically useful psychotherapeutic concepts in the twentieth century. In addition, Ellis' ABC model probably made Rational Emotive Therapy the first comprehensive behavior therapy.

In the ABC model of human emotions: A is the activating event, that is, any event to which the person reacts. B is that person's personal belief about that perception. C is that person's emotional response to that A, the activating event. Ellis's ABC model reveals that people's emotional feelings are not caused by the activating events at A. Their emotional feelings are directly caused by their personal beliefs at B about their A-activating events. Ellis reasoned, therefore, that the drug-free, therapeutic way to help people most quickly behave better physically, or to most quickly feel better emotionally at C, is to get them to adopt "better personal beliefs" at B about their A perceptions.

To Ellis, "better personal beliefs" meant beliefs that seem to be the most logical ones for the person's desired new emotional and physical self-management. Ellis called such beliefs rational, and the contrary ones irrational, beliefs. Logically, therefore, Ellis' technique has always focused on getting people to recognize and eliminate their irrational belief systems. That fact probably made Ellis' technique the first cognitive therapy. In fact, Ellis is now recognized by many mental health professionals as the "father" of the cognitive therapeutic movement in behavioral psychology.

Initially, Ellis gave patients/clients and trainees little or no specific empirical guidelines for recognizing and discovering for themselves if their beliefs were rational. Still, the following two features made his method more rapidly and comprehensively effective than the other then-popular psychotherapies seemed to be. (1) Ellis' method encouraged therapists to be active, objective and firmly directive. (2) It also encouraged the effective use in talk therapy of Pavlovian-type verbal conditioning of more rational beliefs than those that seemed to have caused the patients/clients' problems. That feature enabled therapists to rapidly help patients/clients create the new emotional ABCs that produce and maintain the self-management they desired.

The inclusion of Pavlovian type conditioning in Ellis' method was sufficient for Eysenck to classify Ellis' Rational Emotive Therapy as a behavior therapy. In the 1994 revision of his original 1962 "bible" of Rational Emotive Therapy, entitled *Reason and Emotions in Psychotherapy,* Ellis changed the name of his historic therapeutic technique to Rational Emotive Behavior Therapy.

Of course there is much more to Ellis' therapeutic technique than his ABC model of human emotions. But space limitations do not permit their coverage here. However, those unmentioned features all are logically based on or related to his ABC model of human emotions.

Remarkably similar to Ellis' cognitive orientation is Aaron Beck's cognitive therapy. Beck's technique has been proved to be as effective for treating some depressive disorders as is medication. Beck's method has also proved to be more effective than medication for preventing recurrences of those depressive disorders; it therefore prevents the unhealthy medical side effects of long-term drug treatment. [*See* COGNITIVE THERAPY.]

C. Maxie C. Maultsby, Jr., and Rational Behavior Therapy (RBT)

While still a psychiatric resident, Maxie C. Maultsby, Jr., studied briefly with Joseph Wolpe in 1967 and with Ellis for the following 7 years. At the 1975 Chicago National Conference of Rational Emotive and Behavior Therapists, Maultsby described his unique method of psychotherapy called Rational Behavior Therapy, or RBT. Then RBT was (and probably still is) the only method of psychotherapy that is based on the well-established facts about the mental activities of normal human brains that make learning and behavioral self-management possible. That fact was first noted in print by Arnold M. Ludwig, M.D., in the forward of the book *Rational Behavior Therapy.*

Rational Behavior Therapy is based on the psychosomatic learning theory of normal human behavior. Therefore, it takes the most comprehensive behavioral stance: namely that cognitive emotional and physical actions that have not been genetically determined are learned. Consequently, all three of those learned behavioral groups are the most logical, simultaneous focus of psychotherapy. This psychosomatic, human learning theory is one of the few that is based on the fact that normal human brains are genetically programmed to instantly and automatically give people the most healthy and desirable, or the most unhealthy and undesirable emotional and physical behaviors that are most logical for their beliefs and attitudes. The theory is both culture free and as universally applicable to the various learned human behavioral problems as the germ theory is to the various infections. Finally, this theory fulfills all seven sets of the essential empirical criteria (listed earlier) for being an ideal unifying theory of modern behavior therapy.

1. The Main Unique Therapeutic Constructs and Techniques in Rational Behavior Therapy

First are Maultsby's two theoretical models of habitual emotions: the AbC construct for attitude-triggered, habitual emotions, and the aBC construct for belief-triggered habitual emotions. At the neurobioelectrical level, both constructs are logical extensions of Ellis' ABC model of new or not-yet-habitual human emotions. Their two main clinical values are that the aBC belief construct reveals to patients/clients how they have unwittingly taught themselves much of their emotional problems; they will have done it via vicarious, mental practice. But most important, the aBC construct shows them why and how they can use rational beliefs and the same mental process and rapidly achieve the therapeutic success they desire. The AbC attitude construct readily reveals these two instantly helpful clinical facts: (1) How and why people's own attitudes make them instantly and automatically react in their habitual emotional and physical ways, even without initial conscious thoughts of doing it, and (2) Why it is unhealthy, incorrect, and often emotionally self-abusive to accuse "It" (some external event) or some other person of making oneself (or anyone else) have the emotional feelings one habitually has. With their silent (i.e., unspoken) AbC attitudes, people do that to themselves.

2. The Five Rules for Ideally Healthy and, Therefore, Rational Thinking

1. Rational thinking is based on obvious facts.
2. Rational thinking best helps people protect their lives and health.
3. Rational thinking best helps people achieve their own short-term and long-term goals.
4. Rational thinking best helps people avoid their most unwanted conflicts with other people.
5. Rational thinking best helps people feel emotionally the way they want to feel without using alcohol or other drugs.

For thinking (and therefore any learned behavior) to be rational, it only has to obey at least three of these five rules at the same time. Habitually thinking rationally gives people the best probabilities for being as healthy, successful, and happy as they desire to be. There are almost no life situations that cannot be handled better with ideally healthy and, therefore, rational thinking.

3. Written, Rational Self-Analysis (RSA)

This technique facilitates developing skills in instantly and automatically doing two things: (1) Deciding for oneself when it will probably be healthiest and most personally beneficial to instantly respond with positive, negative, or neutral emotional and/or physical behavioral reactions, and (2) when the opposite responses will be healthiest and most personally beneficial.

4. Rational Emotive Imagery (REI)

This technique enables patients/clients to practice at will their desired new emotional and physical behavioral responses. Thereby they decide how rapidly and successfully they achieve their therapeutic goals.

5. The Five Stages of Therapeutic Emotional and Behavioral Reeducation

Psychotherapy means word therapy, without drugs or other medical treatments. Of course, if patients/clients need medication for some existing medical or psychiatric problem, RBT therapists see that they get it. But without medication or electric shock therapy, all therapeutic change is really therapeutic emotional and behavioral reeducation. It occurs in the following five sequential stages, regardless of the type of psychotherapy being used.

First is intellectual insight, or learning what has to be practiced to achieve therapeutic success. Second is the mental and physical practice of the new therapeutic ideas that are essential for learning the desired new emotional and physical habits. Third is cognitive-emotive dissonance (see the glossary). Fourth is emotional insight; patients/clients have it when they begin to have their desired new emotional and physically responses instantly and automatically in their desired situations. Fifth is new personality trait formation. In this case, patients/clients have their desired new emotional and behavioral reactions as instantly and automatically in their desired situations as they formerly had their undesirable emotional and behavioral reactions.

There is much more to RBT than the listed therapeutic models and techniques. For more in-depth knowledge, please refer to the bibliography.

IV. BEHAVIORAL ASSESSMENT AND THE THERAPEUTIC PROCESS

Behavior therapy is designed for and meant to treat only learned behavioral problems. Sometimes, however, medical problems appear to be a learned behavioral problem; sometimes medical and a learned behavioral problems coexist. Before beginning behavior therapy, therefore, it is important for patients/clients to be evaluated to determine if they (1) have a learned behavioral problem alone, or (2) have one plus an unrelated, medical problem, or (3) have a learned behavior problem as a part of a psychosomatic disorder, or (4) have a medical problem that just appears to have been learned.

Behavioral assessment has three other goals: (1) to define the target behavioral problems; (2) to identify the cognitive habits that are maintaining those behavioral problems; and (3) to make it possible to objectively measure therapeutic progress. To best achieve the latter, behavior therapy focuses on the present manifestations of the target problems. But to ensure the most comprehensive therapeutic results, the therapist gets a detailed personal and medical history. Such historical data are easily obtained using standard personal data forms. For the target problem, however, personal interviews by the therapist are essential.

Important information about the target problem includes the following: When were patient/clients free of their problem? What has been the progression of the problem? What makes it better or worse or temporarily disappear? What desirable or undesirable personal experiences does the problem prevent or cause? What are the patient/clients' beliefs about their problem and what are their expectations for therapy? For the most immediately useful clinical understanding of a patient/client's problem, putting these data in Ellis' ABC models of human emotions is invaluable.

Effective behavior therapy produces weekly therapeutic progress. The popular self-assessment and objective behavioral monitoring forms are usually adequate for this purpose. If weekly therapeutic progress is not happening, reassess the patient/client for overlooked medical or psychiatric problems, or for problems with therapeutic involvement or misunderstanding.

V. BEHAVIORAL MEDICINE

Chronic diseases have replaced acute, infectious diseases as the leading causes of death. Those chronic diseases often have cause/effect behavioral relationships with unhealthy behavioral habits such as cigarette smoking, lack of exercise, poor eating habits, substance abuse, and so on. Those facts are the main reasons behavioral medicine is one of the most clinically valuable, recent byproducts of comprehensive behavior therapy. Behavioral medicine has already demonstrated great clinical value in preventing and treating health problems. For example, in recent decades there has been a significant decrease in the death rate for cardiovascular diseases. That decrease resulted largely from people making healthy changes in their personal habits and learning healthier techniques of emotional distress management. [*See* BEHAVIORAL MEDICINE.]

For more than 25 years oncologist O. Carl Simonton has demonstrated the clinical advantages of treating cancer patients with behavioral techniques. His results have been confirmed in controlled prospective trials by David Spiegel at the UCLA Medical Center, even in patients with metastatic breast cancer. The patients who had received behavioral treatment plus conventional oncological treatment lived twice as long as the patients who had received conventional oncological treatment alone.

Recently, the prominent British psychologists Hans Eysenck and Ronald Grossarth-Maticek developed and reported their behavior technique, called Creative Novation Behavior Therapy. They have been using it to treat patients with cancer and cardiovascular disease. Initial treatment results indicate an additional possible potential for improved disease prevention. Further study and attempts to replicate their favorable results are in progress. However, their work is worthy of note because it is consistent with the excellent research by Robert Ader and Nicolas Cohen on conditioning healthy immune responses. The latter research has produced the newest medical subspecialty: *psychoneuroimmunology*—the descriptive label that was coined by Ader. Modern comprehensive behavior therapies have the characteristics that are needed to help psychoneuroimmunology most quickly realize its great potential for mass general health improvement and disease prevention.

BIBLIOGRAPHY

Ader, R., & Felton, D. (1990). *Psychoneuroimmunology II.* San Diego: Academic Press.

Bandura, A. (1986). *Social foundations of thought and action: A social cognitive theory.* Englewood Cliffs, NJ: Prentice-Hall.

Beck, A. T., Rush, A. J., Shaw, B. F., & Emery, G. (1979). *Cognitive therapy of depression.* New York: Guilford.

Ellis, A. (1994). *Reason and emotion in psychotherapy.* New York: Carol Publishing Group.

Masters, J. C., Burish, T. G., Hollon, S.D., & Rimm, D. C. (1987). *Behavior therapy: Techniques and empirical findings.* San Diego: Harcourt Brace Jovanovich, Inc.

Maultsby, Jr., M. C. (1984). *Rational behavior therapy.* Englewood Cliffs, NJ: Prentice-Hall, Inc. 1984.

Spiegler, M.D., & Guevremont D. C. (1993). *Contemporary behavior therapy.* Monterey, CA: Brooks/Cole Publishing Company.

Staats, A. W. (1990). *Psychology's crisis of disunity.* New York: Praeger Publishing Co.

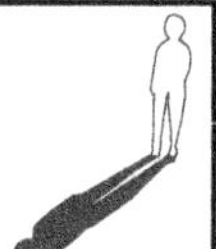

Behavioral Medicine

Robert M. Kaplan and David N. Kerner
University of California, San Diego

Behavioral Epidemiology The study of individual behaviors and habits in relation to health outcomes.

Behavioral Medicine An interdisciplinary field concerned with the development and integration of behavioral and biomedical knowledge and techniques relevant to the understanding of health and illness.

Biopsychosocial Model A conceptualization of health and illness that considers the role of psychological, social, and physical factors in health problems. The model stands in contrast to the traditional biomedical model which focuses only on biological factors.

Cardiovascular Disease Diseases of the heart and circulatory system. These include coronary heart disease, cerebral vascular disease (stroke), and peripheral artery disease.

Cardiovascular Reactivity Changes in blood pressure in response to a stressor. Cardiovascular reactivity may be a risk factor for coronary heart disease.

Chronic Obstructive Pulmonary Disease (COPD) Diseases of airway obstruction in the lungs. COPD, which includes chronic bronchitis, emphysema, and chronic asthma affects about 11% of the adult population in the United States. The diseases are caused by or exacerbated by smoking cigarettes.

Epidemiology The study of the distribution and determinants of disease. Epidemiology seeks to identify the causes of disease in populations and determine risk factors that may be modifiable.

Health Psychology A field of study that encompasses the role of psychology in the promotion and maintenance of health and the prevention and treatment of illness.

Primary Prevention The prevention of a problem before it develops. In primary prevention the preventive effort occurs before any signs or symptoms of a disease have developed.

Psychoneuroimmunology A field of study that examines the effects of stress upon immune function and ultimately upon health and disease process.

Second Prevention Preventive efforts that begin with a population at risk. For example, secondary prevention might involve reduction of blood pressure in order to prevent a heart attack or stroke.

Tertiary Prevention Efforts to prevent an established medical condition from getting worse.

BEHAVIORAL MEDICINE is an emerging specialty. The Society of Behavioral Medicine defines the field as "the interdisciplinary field concerned with the development and integration of behavioral and biomedical science knowledge and techniques relevant to the understanding of health and illness, and the application of this knowledge and these techniques to prevention, diagnosis, treatment and rehabilitation." Several characteristics of this definition are particularly important. First, the definition recognizes the need for collabo-

Copyright © 1998 by Academic Press.
All rights of reproduction in any form reserved.

ration between physicians, biomedical scientists, and behavioral scientists. Efforts of psychologists without medical collaborators, or by physicians without behavioral collaborators, have less potential. Second, the definition stresses the application of behavioral knowledge to problems in physical health. Physical health has not traditionally been within the domain of psychology. Third, the definition excludes the more traditional topics of clinical-abnormal psychology, such as psychosis and neurosis. Although some behavioral medicine specialists study substance abuse, they tend to study traditional psychological problems only insofar as they contribute to physical health. Reflecting the view that mental and physical functioning are closely related, the *biopsychosocial* model of health and illness is endorsed by many practitioners of behavioral medicine. According to this model, health status is determined by multiple factors. The traditional medical model generally views specific biological factors as causing most health problems. Within the biopsychosocial model, psychological factors (thoughts, behaviors, feelings) and social factors are treated as equally important contributors to many health states.

I. DISTINCTIONS BETWEEN HEALTH PSYCHOLOGY, BEHAVIORAL MEDICINE, AND PSYCHOSOMATIC MEDICINE

Health psychology is the umbrella term for a variety of topics related to the interface between psychology and medicine. The Division of Health Psychology of the American Psychological Association defines its specialty as "the aggregate of the specific educational, scientific, and professional contributions of the discipline of psychology, to the promotion and maintenance of health, the prevention and treatment of illness, and the identification of the etiologic and diagnostic correlates of health, illness, and related dysfunction."

The field of behavioral medicine regards the status of medical and behavioral collaborators to be equal, with neither participant taking the dominant role. In contrast to health psychology, which emphasizes work done by psychologists, behavioral medicine emphasizes work that is collaborative between biomedical and behavioral scientists. One distinction between behavioral medicine and health psychology is that behavioral medicine is a collaboration of behavioral and medical scientists to improve health, and health psychology is the unique contribution of psychologists to this process.

II. EXAMPLES OF BASIC RESEARCH IN BEHAVIORAL MEDICINE

Behavioral medicine encompasses a very diverse field of research. It would be impossible to review the entire domain within this short entry. Instead, we will highlight a few key research areas to provide an overview of the kinds of questions with which researchers struggle.

A. Psychoneuroimmunology, Stress, and Health

There exists a long legacy of contradictory and sometimes confused thinking regarding the relationship between mind and body. At one time, the idea that external events and stressful situations could adversely impact health was not accepted by the medical establishment. Those who believed in such a connection could offer no plausible biological mechanism. For such a relationship to be possible, the relationship between the nervous system and the immune system must be understood. These systems are known to interact through two major pathways: the autonomic nervous system and the pituitary-regulated neuroendocrine outflow. A central focus of behavioral medicine research has been to elucidate the nature of the relationship between stress and health status. The field of psychoneuroimmunology (PNI) examines the effects of stress on health and disease processes, primarily as mediated by the immune system. A number of studies have demonstrated that stress may reduce immune system functioning, in both animals and humans.

To understand psychoneuroimmunology, it is important to understand how the immune system works. The immune system is made up of many different structures—cells (lymphocytes), tissues, and organs (e.g., thymus gland, spleen)—that communicate with each other through the bloodstream and lymphatic system. There are two major types of cells, T- and B-lymphocytes. T-cells include helper cells, which tell the immune system to "turn on" in the face of a virus or other invader, and suppressor cells, which tell the system to slow down.

Some PNI researchers ask a basic, but often elusive, question: How does the nervous system interact with the immune system at the cellular level? Recently, they have discovered that lymph nodes (which are made up of lymphocytes) receive neural input from the sympathetic nervous system. (The sympathetic nervous system is also sometimes called the "fight or flight" system.) Other researchers have found that many lymphocytes have special sites that act as receptors for neurotransmitters. Because of these and related discoveries, we now know that the nervous system exerts considerable influence on the activities of the immune system. And the reverse also seems to be true: alterations in immune functioning have been found to affect the activity of neurons in brain areas such as the hypothalamus.

A recent meta-analysis examined the literature on the relationship between stress and immunity in humans. The analysis found that increased stress is reliably associated with higher numbers of circulating white blood cells, and with lower numbers of circulating T- and B-lymphocytes. Increased stress is also linked to decreased levels of immunoglobin, another measure of immune status. Finally, stress was associated with increases in antibodies against the virus that causes herpes.

In one example of a stress immunity study, several immune parameters in 75 first-year medical students were assessed 1 month before final examinations and again at the start of final examinations. Immune cell activity was significantly lower at the (presumably higher stress) time of the examination than it had been a month earlier. In another study, immune status was assessed in 38 married and 38 separated or divorced women. Poor marital quality in the married group and shorter separation time in the second group were associated with poorer functioning on several immune measures.

It is important to note that there are still many unanswered questions about psychoneuroimmunology. Despite the clear relationship between stress and immune status, a solid link between stress and increased rates or duration of disease has been found with much less consistency. One reason for this shortcoming is the relatively low rate of specific poor health outcomes among a healthy population. A few studies have attempted to circumvent this incidence barrier, with some success.

One disease that is relatively easy to study is the common cold. Unlike major diseases such as cancer or heart disease, the common cold can be induced by experimenters with little risk of long-term consequences. In one intriguing study, researchers exposed 357 healthy participants to either a cold virus or a placebo. Higher rates of colds and respiratory infections were associated with higher levels of psychosocial stress.

Other studies of the psychoneuroimmunology of infectious diseases have been conducted, most notably with HIV. Although findings have been mixed, several studies have demonstrated improvement in immune parameters following behavioral or psychological interventions.

Many other issues exist in the study of psychoneuroimmunology. Debate continues, for example, on how best to define stress. Some researchers focus on objective, negative life events such as bereavement, whereas others use self-reported stress levels. Available research indicates that using objective events as the independent variable provides more consistent immunosuppressive results. Other remaining problem areas include achieving a better understanding of the immune effects of specific stressors, the role of stress duration in immune response, and the personal characteristics that make some individuals less susceptible than others to the immune effects of stress.

How people perceive stress, how they cope with stress, and how their social environment affects their reaction to stress may also explain some discrepant findings. In fact, inadequate coping in the face of marked adversity is often part of the definition of stress. According to this argument, stressful events will induce a stress response only if the organism cannot, or believes it cannot, cope with adversity. Thus, an organism's coping attempts may be an important variable in the stress–health relationship. One study found, for example, that stress with academic examinations may be more immunosuppressing among individuals who react with much more anxiety compared with those who do not. One longitudinal study of patients with metastatic breast cancer (in which the cancer has spread beyond the breast tissue) found that long-term survivors appeared to be more able to externalize their negative feelings and psychological distress through the expression of anger, hostility, anxiety, and sadness. Those who survived only a short time tended to be those individuals whose coping styles involved suppression or denial of psychological distress. [*See* Coping with Stress.]

A relationship between suppression of emotion and poor cancer outcome has been noted with enough regularity that some researchers have identified a cancer-prone "Type C" personality that has as a main element exaggerated suppression of negative emotions like anger. In one study of women undergoing breast biopsies, women who were subsequently diagnosed with breast cancer had significantly higher levels of emotion suppression than did women who did not have cancer. Other studies have replicated these results. Because these women already had cancer, however, it was not possible to establish the causal relationship between suppression of emotion and breast cancer.

As the putative link between stress and immune functioning has gained more support, researchers have turned to interventions aimed at ameliorating the detrimental effects of stress. Relaxation training, long used in mental health contexts, was associated in one study with increased immune activity in an elderly population. Other stress control interventions, such as biofeedback and cognitive therapy, have been found in some studies to exert a beneficial influence on immune status. [*See* Biofeedback; Cognitive Therapy; Meditation and the Relaxation Response.]

B. Cardiovascular Reactivity

Because cardiovascular disease is a leading cause of morbidity and mortality, many behavioral medicine researchers study factors that may influence the course of this disease. Many studies focus on the effects of diet and exercise changes on cardiovascular health. Other researchers study a phenomenon known as cardiovascular reactivity. We describe some of this research in the following section.

Not all people respond to stressors in the same way. In general, being exposed to a stressor causes a rise in blood pressure. Some people react to a stressor with a relatively small rise in blood pressure, whereas for others the rise is very large. Behavioral medicine researchers have been interested in the question of whether large blood pressure increases in response to a stressor are risk factors for developing hypertension (high blood pressure), and whether these changes predict heart attack, stroke, and death. Researchers are also attempting to determine whether individual, potentially modifiable factors such as personality are related to this hyperreactivity. Studies examining the predictive power of reactivity have had mixed results. Some studies have found that cardiovascular blood pressure reactivity in childhood predicts the development of hypertension up to 45 years later. Other studies, however, have failed to find any relationship.

Researchers have examined reactivity in adulthood to predict who is most at risk for developing future vascular disease. In one well-known study, researchers attempted to identify risk factors for developing future cardiovascular disease. They found that many factors, such as resting blood pressure, smoking, and cholesterol level, were all predictive of who died from the disease 23 years later. More predictive than those variables, however, was subjects' response to a cold-presser task. The cold-presser task requires subjects to immerse a hand in ice water. Subjects are exposed for a specific time and their blood pressure is recorded. In this study, subjects who had the largest increase in blood pressure in response to the task were most likely to die from cardiovascular disease in the future.

Several factors limit our confidence in reactivity research. Notably, laboratory stressors are not the same as real-world stressors. Therefore, it has been a goal of researchers to measure blood pressure in response to stressors that individuals experience in their daily lives. Recently, the development of ambulatory blood pressure monitors has made it possible to monitor the blood pressure of an individual throughout the day. Participants can keep diaries of stressful events, and researchers can examine how blood pressure varies in response to these stressors. Clinically, this technique could eventually allow for improved risk prediction for at-risk individuals

Researchers are currently attempting to answer several puzzling questions about cardiovascular reactivity. For instance, the physiological mechanism linking hyperreactivity to undesirable health outcomes is not known. Studies have also failed to determine the cause of hyperreactivity. Is it simply a genetic phenomenon? Or are there environmental factors at work? If the cause is environmental, researchers may be able to develop treatments for hyperreactivity. Such interventions have the potential for reducing the number of people who die each year from cardiovascular disease.

C. Personality and Illness

Another major focus of behavioral medicine research is the relationship between personality factors and illness. Interest in this relationship dates back at least to the ancient Greeks, who classified people into one of four basic personality types (phlegmatic, melancholic, sanguine, and choleric); these personalities were presumed to be based on imbalances in bodily fluids, or humors. Early in this century, it was believed that certain diseases, such as hypertension, heart disease, cancer, asthma, ulcerative colitis, and ulcers, were "psychosomatic"—mainly caused by personality. As research data have accumulated, however, it has become clear that the association between personality and illness is much more complex than first believed. Current research examines the impact on health of psychological constructs such as motivation, self-mastery, and self-confidence, as well as the impact of alcohol and substance abuse. Related factors under study include socioeconomic status, gender, and cognitive status.

Since the early 1950s, one major focus of psychosomatic research has been the relationship between the "Type A" personality and cardiovascular disease. Two cardiologists originally described a cluster of characteristics that many of their patients shared. People with Type A personalities were described as highly competitive and achievement oriented. They are also typically in a hurry and impatient; in addition, they are hostile in social interactions.

Major longitudinal studies in the 1960s and 1970s convincingly supported the notion that the Type A personality was a major risk factor for developing cardiovascular disease. In 1981, a panel organized by the National Heart, Lung, and Blood Institute (NHLBI) concluded that Type A behavior was a risk factor for coronary heart disease (CHD). Since that time, however, several large, well-conducted studies (including the long-term follow-up to the original study which found a Type A–heart disease link) have found no association between Type A behavior and heart disease.

Researchers have proposed several possible explanations for the Type A turnabout. These include that (1) the original findings were just a fluke; (2) the assessment of Type A may have changed over time; (3) society may have changed, making the Type A distinction anachronistic; (4) coronary heart disease population distribution has changed (changing patterns of smoking, diet, and physical activity may interact with Type A behavior in unclear ways); or (5) some aspects of Type A behavior are risk factors, but others are not. Many studies have examined this latter possibility.

In one comprehensive meta-analysis examining the effects of psychological and behavioral variables on coronary heart disease, only the anger and hostility components of Type A were found to be significant CHD risk factors. Overall, Type A was unrelated to future disease status. Other studies, using both the Type A Structured Interview and the Cook-Medley Hostility (Ho) Scale of the Minnesota Multiphasic Personality Interview (MMPI), have found that "cynical hostility" is predictive of future coronary disease morbidity and mortality. People who are cynically hostile tend to expect the worst of others and dwell on people's negative characteristics. This personality characteristic, unlike overall Type A behavior, does seem to predict future heart disease.

When considering the Type A and CHD research, it is important to note that the majority of research has been conducted with male subjects. Relatively little attention has been paid to CHD risk factors in women, despite the fact that CHD is the leading cause of death among women, killing more women than men each year. Only recently have researchers begun to examine the personality risk factors for women.

The relationship between hostility and diseases other than CHD has also been examined. A number of studies, for example, have found a link between hostility and all-cause mortality. Only one study, however, has controlled for CHD deaths in the analysis. In that study, MMPI Hostility scores correlated with 20-year, all-cause mortality rates, even when CHD-related mortality was factored out. To date, no studies have linked hostility to other major health outcomes, such as cancer.

Besides hostility, many other personal factors have been examined for their relationship to health. Notably, clinical and nonclinical depression have been related to poor health outcomes among certain disease groups. In one study of CHD and depression, clinical depression assessed in recently hospitalized post-myocardial infarction (MI; or heart attack) patients was associated with a 500% greater likelihood of 6-month mortality. In another study, 4000 hypertensive individuals were followed for 4.5 years. In this group, change in depression level (although not absolute level) predicted future cardiac events like infarctions and surgeries.

Other studies have shown that having an optimistic, rather than pessimistic, attitude may have important health consequences. Similarly, a negatively fatalistic outlook on life and health may be a prognostic indicator of poor future health status. In one 50-month study of 74 male patients with AIDS, increased survival time was significantly associated with low levels of fatalism, which was called "realistic acceptance." Patients who had low scores on a measure of realistic acceptance had median survival times 9 months longer than patients with high levels. When potential confounds were controlled for, such as initial health status and ongoing health behaviors, the effect remained significant.

Similar findings have been obtained with other disease groups. Researchers often use all or part of the Life Orientation Test (LOT) as a measure of optimism and pessimism. In one study, a pessimistic attitude (as measured by LOT) was a significant mortality risk factor for young adults with recurrent cancer. Another study found that high LOT pessimism was associated with greater risk of MI during coronary artery bypass graft (CABG) surgery.

Another area of inquiry regarding personal factors and health involves recovery and adaptation after surgery. Researchers assessed a number of psychosocial variables in a population of 42 leukemia patients about to receive allogeneic bone marrow transplants. (Allogeneic transplants involve bone marrow from donors other than themselves or identical twins.) Participants who had an attitude toward cancer characterized by "anxious preoccupation" had increased mortality compared to nonanxious participants.

Finally, socioeconomic status (SES) has emerged as an important determinant of health status. Several studies have shown a clear gradient between SES and a variety of different indicators of health status. Furthermore, the association is continuous. For example, there are differences in health status between moderately poor people and those who are very poor. On the other end of the spectrum, it appears that there are differences between the very rich and those who are moderately well off. These differences are observed in nearly all cultures, including those with universal access to health care. Thus, health care alone does not seem to explain the association between SES and health status.

III. EXAMPLES OF BEHAVIORAL MEDICINE IN CLINICAL PRACTICE

A. Treatment of Heart Disease

Cardiovascular disease (CVD), which includes coronary heart disease, cerebrovascular disease (strokes), and peripheral artery disease, is the single most common cause of death in the United States. Caused by atherosclerosis, the buildup of fatty plaques along the inner walls of arteries, CVD causes significant disability and is a large source of health care costs. Behavioral medicine specialists have developed a number of interventions to prevent and treat CVD.

One risk factor for CVD is high blood cholesterol, or hypercholesterolemia. The diagnostic criteria for hypercholesterolemia are presented in Table I. The most prominent intervention effort aimed at treating hypercholesterolemia, initiated by the National Heart, Lung, and Blood Institute, is known as the National Cholesterol Education Program (NCEP).

If atherosclerotic buildup increases, the arteries narrow and restrict blood flow. The formation of a clot can completely stop blood flow, causing an MI or cerebral vascular accident (CVA; or stroke). Atherosclerosis is a life-long process, partially controlled by inherited genetic factors such as metabolism. Although humans have no influence over their genes, our physiological factors affecting atherosclerosis include blood cholesterol, blood pressure, and obesity. These physiological factors and CVD risk are partially

Table I National Cholesterol Education Program Guidelines for the Treatment of Hypercholesterolemia

Recommended level	200 mg/dl TC[a]	130 mg/dl LDL
Moderate risk	200–240 mg/dl TC	130–160 mg/dl LDL
High risk	>240 mg/dl TC	>160 mg/dl LDL

[a] TC, total cholesterol; LDL, low-density lipoprotein (i.e., "bad" cholesterol).

influenced by modifiable behaviors, for example, physical activity, diet, and tobacco use. Behavioral medicine practitioners are actively involved in developing effective interventions in these areas, at both the patient and caregiver level.

Regular physical activity may reduce blood pressure by reducing obesity, increasing aerobic fitness, and reducing the blood levels of certain stress-related chemicals such as adrenalin. In individuals who already have hypertension, exercise significantly reduced resting blood pressure in most studies. Other studies have examined the effect of activity interventions on individuals who do not yet have hypertension, but who are at high risk for developing it (e.g., people with "high normal" blood pressure). One such study found that increased physical activity was one factor reducing the risk of future hypertension in this population. Many other studies have found cardiovascular benefits from dietary and smoking interventions.

The benefits from these interventions, although significant, are limited. Atherosclerosis has traditionally been viewed as a unidirectional process. Therefore, behavioral and medical interventions have been aimed at slowing, rather than reversing the sclerotic process. Recently, however, the Lifestyle Heart Trial attempted to reverse atherosclerosis through behavior change. This trial was notable for its comprehensiveness. Patients with severe heart disease were randomly assigned to either a standard-treatment control group or a radical lifestyle change intervention. In the intervention group, participants were introduced to the program through a weekend retreat with their spouses. Then, participants attended 4-hour, biweekly group meetings. They were placed on an extremely low-fat vegetarian diet (fat was limited to 10% of calories, compared with a national average of about 40%). Caffeine use was eliminated, and alcohol was limited to two drinks per day. The group sessions included relaxation and yoga exercises; participants were expected to practice relaxation and meditation for 1 hour each day. Sessions also included exercise and smoking cessation instruction for participants who smoked.

The results of this intensive behavior change program were striking. Participants reduced their fat intake from 31% to 7% of total calories. They increased daily exercise from 11 minutes to 38 minutes per day. They increased their relaxation and meditation time from an average of 5 minutes per day to 82 minutes per day. As a result, participants' total cholesterol levels dropped markedly, often to below 150 mg/dl. Blood pressure also fell. They lost, on average, 22 pounds over the 1-year course of the study. Angina (chest pain) dropped by 91% in the experimental group, whereas it increased by 165% in the control group. Impressively, participants in the experimental group were almost twice as likely as control group members to show actual reductions in arterial blockage.

This study demonstrated that a behavioral intervention that includes daily exercise and relaxation, along with an extremely low-fat diet, can have an impressive impact on the clinical picture of individuals with severe heart disease. Related research focuses on the impact of behavioral interventions on individuals who do not yet have heart disease, but who may develop it in the future.

B. Adaptation to Cancer

Cancer is universally feared. According to the American Cancer Society (ACS), cancer is an umbrella term for a group of diseases "characterized by uncontrolled growth and spread of abnormal cells." Not counting some highly prevalent, rarely fatal forms of skin cancer, the most common cancers are (in order of prevalence) prostate, lung, colon/rectal, and bladder (for men); and breast, colon/rectal, lung, and uterus (for women). For both men and women, lung cancer causes the most deaths. Although it kills far fewer people than CVD, cancer is perceived as more dangerous, destructive, and deadly. In reality, the survival rate for cancer has been climbing steadily throughout this century. Taking a normal life expectancy into consideration, the ACS estimates that 50% of all people diagnosed with cancer will live at least 5 years. Nevertheless, cancer remains the second-leading cause of death and is associated with significant pain and disability.

Because behavioral factors have been implicated in the etiology of many cancers (e.g., smoking, eating a low-fiber diet, sunlight exposure), behavioral scientists have developed a large number of programs designed to help people reduce their cancer risk. In addition, behaviorists have focused on what happens to an individual after a diagnosis of cancer is made. Partly because there are so many types of cancers, the experience of cancer is highly variable. Nevertheless, there are commonalities. Most cancer treatments, such as surgery, radiation, and chemotherapy, are extremely unpleasant. Surgery often requires a great amount of recuperation, sometimes causes new physical problems, and may cause substantial disfigurement. Radiation and chemotherapy often cause significant side effects, including hair loss, sterility, even nausea and vomiting, fatigue, and diarrhea. Anticipatory anxiety, classically conditioned by these treatments, may increase the severity of many of these symptoms. In the long term, cancer patients face problems with physical, psychological, and sexual functioning, as well as family and work difficulties. Many studies have demonstrated that cancer patients exhibit increased rates of depression, and some have demonstrated increased rates of anxiety. Behaviorists working in treatment settings have attempted to help individuals with cancer cope as well as possible with these difficulties.

Health researchers have found that cancer may result in self-concept problems. In addition, one study identified four major sources of stress experienced by people with cancer: (1) loss of meaning, (2) concerns about the physical illness, (3) concerns about medical treatment, and (4) social isolation. Social isolation and reduced social activity have been observed in both children and adults with cancer. Behavioral science practitioners are developing interventions to ameliorate the psychosocial effects of cancer.

Interesting and controversial intervention studies have examined the effect of positive attitude and social support in reducing the physical effects of cancer. According to some psychoneuroimmunology studies, depressed mood may reduce immune functioning. "Wellness communities," startled by Harold Benjamin in Santa Monica, California, promote the idea that depression weakens immune response. They suggest that a positive attitude may likewise enhance it. Stronger immunity, it is argued, will lead to reduced physical manifestations of the disease.

The most well-known study of social support and cancer was undertaken with a group of 86 women diagnosed with metastatic breast cancer. (*Metastatic* means the disease has spread beyond the original organ or tissue site.) The women were randomly assigned to either a standard treatment control group or a group that included weekly support groups. The support groups were led by psychiatrists or social workers who were breast cancer survivors themselves. Women in the support group became highly involved in helping the other participants cope with their cancer symptoms, treatment, and difficulties.

Women assigned to the support groups survived an average of 36.6 months, while those in the control group survived an average of only 18.9 months. Support group members also experienced less anxiety, depression, and pain. This study's impressive results have sparked further research into the role of social support and immune functioning, as well as the role of psychotherapy in reducing the psychosocial difficulties of the cancer experience. The study is now being replicated with a larger group of women.

Another often-cited cancer intervention study examined the effects of a 6-week intervention on patients diagnosed with a deadly form of skin cancer known as malignant melanoma. The intervention included weekly 90-minute sessions focusing on relevant education, problem-solving skills, stress management, and psychological support. Outcome data indicated both short-term and long-term effects of the intervention versus the control group. At short-term (6-week and 6-month) assessments, immune markers were significantly better in the intervention group than in the controls. When studied 6 years later, the intervention group participants had lower mortality rates and fewer recurrences than did participants in the control group.

C. Functioning in Lung Disease

Another example of behavioral medicine practice comes from studies of rehabilitation of patients with chronic obstructive pulmonary disease (COPD), which is a common ailment among smokers. It is currently the fourth leading cause of death in the United States. Chronic bronchitis, emphysema, and chronic asthma are the three diseases most commonly associated with COPD. The common denominator of these disorders is expiratory flow obstruction (difficulty exhaling air) caused by airway narrowing, although the cause of airflow obstruction is different in each. Exposure to cigarette smoke is the primary risk factor for each of these illnesses. There is no cure for COPD.

Chronic obstructive pulmonary disease has a profound effect on functioning and everyday life. Current estimates suggest that COPD affects nearly 11% of the adult population, and that the incidence is increasing, especially among women, reflecting the increase in tobacco use among women in the latter part of this century. Medicines such as bronchodilators, corticosteroids, and antibiotic therapy help symptoms, and long-term oxygen therapy has been shown to be beneficial in patients with severe hypoxemia. However, it is widely recognized that these measures cannot cure COPD. Much of the effort in the management of this condition must be directed toward preventive treatment strategies aimed at improving symptoms, patient functioning, and quality of life.

In one study, 119 COPD patients were randomly assigned to either comprehensive pulmonary rehabilitation or an education control group. Pulmonary rehabilitation consisted of 12 4-hour sessions distributed over an 8-week period. The content of the sessions was education, physical and respiratory care, psychosocial support, and supervised exercise. The education control group attended four 2-hour sessions that were scheduled twice per month, but did not include any individual instruction or exercise training. Topics included medical aspects of COPD, pharmacy use, and breathing techniques. In addition, subjects were interviewed about smoking, life events, and social support. Lectures covered pulmonary medicine, pharmacology, respiratory therapy, and nutrition. Outcome measures included lung function, exercise tolerance (maximum and endurance), perceived breathlessness, perceived fatigue, self-efficacy for walking, depression, and overall health-related quality of life.

In comparison to the educational control group, rehabilitation patients demonstrated a significant increase in exercise endurance (82% vs. 11%), maximal exercise workload (32% vs. 14%), and peak VO_2, a measure of cardiovascular fitness (8% vs. 2%). These changes in exercise performance were associated with significant improvement in symptoms of perceived breathlessness and muscle fatigue during exercise.

Traditional models of medical care are challenged by the growing number of older adults with chronic, progressively worsening illnesses such as COPD. Cognitive–behavioral interventions may help patients adapt to loss of function and, when successfully used in a comprehensive rehabilitation program that includes training in energy conservation and the use of assistive devices, may even help to increase function. As a result, behavioral interventions can improve quality of life for patients with chronic pulmonary disease.

As in our discussion of behavioral medicine research, this section on the practice of behavioral medicine has highlighted some areas of active interest. Behavioral medicine practitioners have developed successful interventions in many other areas, such as diet and physical activity, tobacco use, and pain management.

IV. BEHAVIORAL MEDICINE IN PUBLIC HEALTH

In addition to clinical contributions, behavioral medicine often takes a public health perspective. The public health perspective differs from the clinical viewpoint because of its focus on the community rather than on the individual. In public health, the emphasis is on improving the average health of an entire population rather than on the health of specific patients. Three areas where behavioral medicine intersects with public health are epidemiology, preventive medicine, and health policy.

A. Epidemiology

Epidemiology is the study of the determinants and distribution of disease. Epidemiologists measure disease and then attempt to relate the development of diseases to characteristics of people and the environments in which they live. The word *epidemiology* is derived from Greek. The Greek word *epi* translates to "among," and the Greek word *demos* translates to "people." The stem *ology* means "the study of." *Epidemiology,* then, is the study of what happens among people. For as long as there has been recorded history, people have been interested in what causes disease. It has been obvious, for example, that diseases are not equally distributed within populations of people. Some people are much more at risk for certain problems than are others.

Traditionally, most epidemiologists studied infectious diseases. For example, people who live in close contact are most likely to get similar illnesses or to be "infected" by one another. Ancient doctors also recognized that people who became ill from certain diseases, and who subsequently recovered, seldom got the same disease again. Thus, the notions of communicability of diseases and of immunity were known many years before specific microorganisms and antibodies were understood. Epidemiologic history was made by Sir John Snow who studied cholera in London in the mid-nineteenth century. Cholera is a horrible disease that causes severe diarrhea and eventually kills its victims through dehydration. Snow systematically studied those who developed cholera and those who did not. His detective-like investigation demonstrated that those who obtained their drinking water from a particular source (a well in London) were more likely to develop cholera. Thus, he was able to link a specific environmental factor to the development of the disease, and actions based on this knowledge saved many lives. This occurred many years before the specific organism that causes cholera was identified.

It is common to think of epidemics as major changes in infectious disease rates. For example, we are experiencing a serious epidemic of Acquired Immune Deficiency Syndrome (AIDS). Yet there are other epidemics that are less dramatic. For instance, we are also experiencing a major epidemic of coronary heart disease in the United States. In 1900, heart disease accounted for about 15% of all deaths, whereas infectious diseases, such as influenza and tuberculosis, accounted for nearly one quarter of all deaths. In the 1990s, cardiovascular (heart and circulatory system) diseases caused nearly half of all deaths. The days when infectious diseases were the major killers in the industrialized world appear to be over. AIDS, although rapidly increasing in incidence, still accounts for only about 1% of all deaths. Today, the major challenge is from chronic illnesses. The leading causes of death include heart disease, cancer, stroke, chronic obstructive lung disease, and diabetes. Each of these may be associated with a long period of disability. In addition, personal habits and health behaviors are associated with both the development and the maintenance of these conditions.

It is important to consider the relative importance of different risk factors and different causes of death. Heart disease is clearly the leading cause of death in the United States, with an estimated 733,867 deaths in 1993. Stroke accounted for another 145,551 deaths. Cancer accounted for 496,152 deaths in 1993. Diabetes mellitus accounted for more than 46,833 deaths, and COPD was responsible for 84,344 deaths.

B. Behavioral Epidemiology

We use *behavioral epidemiology* to describe the study of individual behaviors and habits in relation to health outcomes. Wise observers have been aware of the relationship between lifestyle and health for many centuries. This is evidenced by the following statement from Hippocrates in approximately 400 BC:

> *Whoever wishes to investigate medicine properly, should proceed thus: . . . the mode in which the inhabitants live, and what are their pursuits, whether they are fond of drinking and eating to excess, and given to indolence, and are fond of exercise and labor, and not given to excess eating and drinking.*

There were approximately 2,269,000 deaths in the United States in 1993 (latest CDC report). Deaths are accounted for according to major and underlying cause. The traditional biomedical model has emphasized disease-specific causes of death, and pathways to prevention have typically considered risk factors for particular diseases. For example, cigarette smoking is associated with deaths from cancer of the lung. Thus, efforts to reduce lung cancer concentrate on smoking cessation. However, most of the major causes of death are associated with a variety of different risk factors. Furthermore, many risk factors are associated with death from a variety of different causes. For example, tobacco use causes not only lung cancer, but a wide variety of other cancers, as well as heart disease, stroke, and birth complications.

Major nongenetic contributors to mortality were examined in an important analysis in 1993 by McGinnis and Foege. They identified several behaviors that account for large numbers of deaths. A summary of the estimates for actual causes of death in the United States is presented in Table II. Tobacco use is associated with more than 400,000 deaths each year, and diet and activity patterns account for an additional 300,000. These dwarf the number of deaths associated with problems that the public is generally concerned about, such as illicit drug use. The McGinnis and Foege analysis challenged society to think differently about health indicators in the United States. Only a small fraction of the trillion dollars the United States spends annually on health care is devoted to the control of the major factors that cause premature mortality in the United States. Estimates suggest that less than 5% of the total annual health care budget is

Table II Actual Causes of Death—United States, 1990[a]

Factor	Deaths	Percentage
Tobacco	400,000	19
Diet–activity patterns	300,000	14
Alcohol	100,000	5
Microbial agents	90,000	4
Toxic agents	60,000	3
Firearms	35,000	<2
Sexual behavior	30,000	1
Motor vehicles	25,000	1
Illicit use of drugs	20,000	<1
Total	1,060,000	50

[a]Source: McGinnin & Feoge, *JAMA, 270,* 2207–2212, 1993.

devoted to prevention efforts. Because behaviors are the major causes of death and disability, it is clear that behavioral scientists have an important role to play in many areas of public health and clinical medicine.

To underscore the role of behaviors in premature mortality, we consider two examples; tobacco use and physical activity.

1. Tobacco

Cigarette smoking remains the greatest single cause of preventable deaths in contemporary society. The health consequences of tobacco use have been documented in thousands of studies. Although cigarette smoking has declined in the United States and in the United Kingdom in recent years, the worldwide trend is toward increased use of tobacco products. In addition, although adult smoking has declined markedly, smoking among teens is on the rise. It is projected that worldwide there will be 10 million tobacco-related deaths per year by the year 2010. Current estimates suggest that tobacco use in the United States is responsible for 434,000 deaths each year. These include 37,000 deaths from cardiovascular disease resulting from exposure to tobacco smoke in the environment (so-called second-hand smoke). Furthermore, smoking is responsible for poor pregnancy outcomes. Between 17 and 26% of low birth weight deliveries are associated with maternal tobacco use and 5 to 6% of prenatal deaths can be attributed to maternal tobacco use. McGinnis and Foege suggest that about 25,000 deaths in the United States can be attributed to motor vehicle accidents, and about 20,000 deaths can be attributed to illicit drug use. In contrast, deaths associated with tobacco use account for more than 20 times the number associated with drug use, 16 times the number associated with auto crashes, and 15 times the number of homicides.

Financial barriers to treatment for nicotine addiction have been formidable—for the patient and for the provider. Most health insurance plans in the United States, public and private, exclude coverage for tobacco addiction treatments. This helps to explain why only 10 to 15% of the U.S. smokers who have tried to quit have ever received any formal treatment for nicotine addiction, and why low-income and disadvantaged Americans have been least likely to get help. Lack of reimbursement also helps to explain why, even today, only 50% of the nation's smokers report ever having been advised by their doctors to quit smoking.

2. Physical Activity

Research shows that people who are physically active live significantly longer than those who are sedentary. These studies have documented a relationship between physical activity and all-cause mortality, CHD mortality, mortality from diabetes mellitus, and mortality associated with COPD and other lung diseases. In addition to living longer, those who engage in regular physical activity may be better able to perform activities of daily living and enjoy many aspects of life. Furthermore, those who exercise regularly have better insulin sensitivity and less abdominal obesity. Regular exercise has also been shown to improve psychological well-being for those with mood disorders. Successful programs have been developed to promote exercise for the general population. Also, specific interventions have been developed for those diagnosed with particular diseases.

Despite the benefits of exercise, few people will start an exercise program, and many of those who start do not continue to exercise. Some predictors of failure to exercise regularly include being overweight, poor, female, and a smoker. However, the most commonly reported barriers to exercise are lack of time and inaccessibility of facilities.

Studies show that exercise patterns change as people age. Children are active, but physical activity declines substantially by the late teens and early twenties. It appears that Americans are shifting toward less vigorous activity patterns, with walking becoming the most common form of exercise. Physical *inactivity* may be increasing as Americans spend more time watching television or working with computers.

Methods to enhance exercise include environmental manipulation, behavior modification, cognitive–behavior modification, and educational approaches. The behavior modification interventions use principles of learning to increase physical activity. These interventions typically control the contingencies associated with physical activity and reinforce active behaviors. Cognitive–behavior modification interventions are similar to behavior modification approaches. However, they also modify self-defeating thoughts that may turn people off to exercise. Educational interventions attempt to increase activity by teaching people about the benefits of being physically active. Statistical analysis that average results across studies (called meta-analyses) tend to show that interventions based on behavior modification principles produce the largest benefits. Interventions based on health education or health risk appraisal approaches tend not to produce consistent benefits. Cognitive–behavior modification interventions also have produced less consistent results than behavior modification approaches. Interventions that include incentives and social support increase exercise in the short term. Many of the studies show that people have difficultly maintaining their exercise programs over the course of time.

Exercise programs are now common for patients with heart, lung, and blood diseases. Cardiac rehabilitation has become a widely chosen and accepted treatment option for patients with established coronary artery disease. As recently as 1970, post-MI patients were typically hospitalized for 1 month and advised to take total bed rest. Today, the average MI patient is hospitalized for 5 to 7 days and lengths of stay continue to decline. Furthermore, the majority of patients are advised to resume physical activity relatively promptly following an MI. Exercise is the core component of the rehabilitation process. Meta-analyses of controlled studies in rehabilitation have demonstrated 20 to 25% reductions in mortality. Newer studies are beginning to demonstrate improvements in quality of life as well as life duration.

Studies of patients with COPD have also demonstrated benefits associated with exercise. Although studies tend not to show changes in lung functioning, some studies have documented improvements in exercise capacity, performance of activities in daily living, and mood. Studies have not demonstrated improvements in life expectancy.

Although there are few intervention studies, evidence suggests that physical activity also predicts survival for patients with cystic fibrosis. In one study, 83% of patients who had the highest levels of aerobic fitness survived for 8 years in comparison to 58% and 28% of patients in the middle and lowest thirds, respectively, of the distribution for aerobic fitness.

C. Prevention Sciences

Behavioral medicine has a strong commitment to disease prevention. Prevention can be divided into primary and secondary. Primary prevention is the prevention of a problem before it develops. Thus, the primary prevention of heart disease starts with people who have no symptoms or characteristics of the disease and there is intervention to prevent these diseases from becoming established. In secondary prevention, we begin with a population at risk and develop efforts to prevent the condition from becoming worse. Tertiary prevention deals with the treatment of established conditions and is the main focus of clinical medicine. Table III uses the example of high blood pressure to illustrate these three approaches to prevention.

Prevention has different meanings for different

Table III Three Levels of Prevention

Level	When used	Example
Primary	For completely well people	Controlling weight to prevent high blood pressure
Secondary	For people with risks for illness (e.g., high blood pressure)	Using medicine to lower blood pressure
Tertiary	For people with developed disease (e.g., heart disease resulting from high blood pressure)	Rehabilitation to prevent the condition from getting worse

Table IV Examples of Three Types of Prevention Programs

Type of program	Description	Outcomes
Clinical preventive services	Brief counseling, referral, patient education	Difficult to institute; some evidence of success
Community-based preventive services	Changing local patterns of expected behavior, and peer pressure	Difficult to institute; better evidence of success
Social policy for prevention	Taxes, seat belt laws	Better evidence of success

people. Partners for Prevention, a nonprofit organization, emphasizes that there are at least three different components of prevention. These include clinical preventive services, community-based preventive services, and social policies for prevention. Clinical preventive services typically involve medical treatments such as immunization and screening tests. Clinical services may also include counseling and behavioral interventions. Community-based preventive services include public programs to ensure safe air, water, or food supplies, as well as behavioral interventions to change local patterns of diet, exercise, or smoking. Social policies for prevention might involve regulation of environmental exposures or exposure to hazardous materials at the work place. These social approaches also include taxes on alcohol and cigarettes and physical changes to ensure better traffic safety. Examples of these three types of prevention programs are given in Table IV.

D. Health Care Policy

The American Health Care System is perhaps the most complex in the world. The United States represents only about 5% of the world's population, but accounts for about 40% of all health care expenditures worldwide. It is difficult to describe U.S. health care as a "system." Rather, U.S. health care is a patchwork of overlapping systems of public and private insurance, with as many as 40 million persons uninsured for their medical expenses.

It is commonly argued that traditional fee-for-service medicine provides few incentives to offer behavioral medicine and preventive services. Indeed, the higher the rates of medical service utilization the greater the profit. One attractive feature of the current move toward managed care is that there are substantial incentives to prevent illness and to reduce health care utilization. From a public health perspective, managed care organizations have responsibility for a defined population. If they can keep this population healthy by investing in prevention, they may ultimately profit by having reduced costs and higher consumer satisfaction.

There are several reasons why the potential for behavioral and disease prevention has often been overlooked by public-policy makers. Preventive services rarely make headlines or gain the same attention as high technology medical interventions. For example, transplantation of a diseased heart attracts the media and brings adulation from family and friends. A patient who survives such transplantation is thought to have benefited from the miracles of modern medical science and the surgeons are handsomely rewarded. When an illness is prevented, no one is aware that a problem has been avoided. There are no headlines because there is no news, and there are no fees for the experts who helped avoid a catastrophe. The average effect of prevention for any one person may be small, yet preventive services have the potential for a huge impact. As noted in Table II, an estimated 400,000 Americans die prematurely each year as a result of tobacco use. As many as 100,000 people die prematurely each year as a result of unnecessary injuries or illnesses related to alcohol abuse. Substantial numbers of cancer and heart disease deaths may be prevented or at least delayed through lifestyle modification.

Most of the 3 to 5% of the health care dollar used for prevention is devoted to clinical preventive services offered by physicians. For example, the great majority of expenditures on prevention relate to screening for diseases such as breast cancer, cervical cancer, and prostate cancer. The purpose of the prevention service is to detect a disease that already exists and medically treat it so that progression is retarded. The screening tests have become profitable for the providers who offer them and there is growing concern about abuses or profiteering by those who administer tests to people who do not need them. Many behavioral medicine professionals advocate a greater emphasis on prevention programs to change behaviors that are causing the most deaths.

V. SUMMARY

Behavioral medicine is a strong and growing field. It draws its strength from its comprehensive approach and interdisciplinary nature. Rather than retreating to small niches, as is so common in science today, behavioral medicine researchers and clinicians must obtain knowledge from a wide variety of disciplines relevant to their field. A behavioral medicine researcher studying CHD must know about basic cardiac functioning, personality research, and many other seemingly unrelated pieces of information. By the nature of this comprehensive approach, the behavioral medicine specialist, whether she is a nurse practitioner, psychologist, or physician, brings a much needed perspective to the science of health and behavior.

BIBLIOGRAPHY

Kaplan, R. M., Orleans, C. T., Perkins, K. A., & Pierce, J. P. (1995). Marshaling the evidence for greater regulation and control of tobacco products: A call for action. *Annals of Behavioral Medicine, 17*, 3–14.

Kaplan, R. M., Sallis, J. F., & Patterson, T. L. (1993). *Health and human behavior.* New York: McGraw-Hill.

Matarazzo, J. D. (1980). Behavioral health and behavioral medicine: Frontiers for a new health psychology. *American Psychologists, 35*, 807–817.

McGinnis, J. M., & Foege, W. H. (1993). Actual causes of death in the United States. *Journal of the American Medical Association, 270*, 2207–2212.

Peto, R., Lopez, A. D., Boreham, J., Thun, M., & Heath, Jr., C. (1992). Mortality from tobacco in developed countries: Indirect estimation from national vital statistics. *Lancet, 339*(8804), 1268–1278.

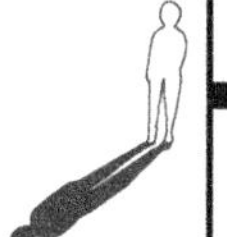

Biofeedback

Elise E. Labbé
University of South Alabama

Autonomic Nervous System The peripheral nervous system that includes neurons outside the bony enclosure of the spinal cord and skull; comprised of the sympathetic nervous system and the parasympathetic nervous system.
Electroencephalograph Instrumentation that monitors brain waves.
Electromyograph Instrumentation that monitors muscle activity.
Operant Conditioning A behavioral principle that states when behavior is reinforced it will increase and when punished or not reinforced will decrease.
Parasympathetic Nervous System Originates in the cranial and sacral regions of the spinal cord and plays a role in conserving energy and is often associated with a relaxed state.
Psychobiology A field of study that considers the interaction of psychological and biological variables in behavior and physical and mental health.
Psychophysiological Disorders Physical disorders in which there are no evident physiological causes and etiological factors may be of a psychological nature. Examples are migraine headache and ulcers.
Self-Regulation The process in which an individual regulates internal physiological responses, as well as emotional, behavioral, and cognitive responses.
Stress Management Psychotherapy focused on helping people cope with stressful events more effectively and reduce anxiety, depression, and sympathetic nervous system responses.
Sympathetic Nervous System Originates within the thoracic and lumbar regions of the spinal cord and is associated with bodily responses that mobilize the organism and is referred to as the "flight or fight" response.

BIOFEEDBACK is a methodology as well as a clinical tool that provides information about an individual's physiological functioning in relation to her cognitive, emotional, and behavioral responses. This article will present a psychobiological approach in discussing the development of biofeedback, theoretical models, types of biofeedback, current research status, and applications of biofeedback.

I. INTRODUCTION TO BIOFEEDBACK

A. Definition of Biofeedback

Biofeedback is any process in which an external device generates information to an individual about his or her physiological responses and that allows the individual to then regulate these responses and receive feedback on changes in the physiological responses. The physiological responses may be any responses that can be measured by an external device. The most common responses measured are muscle tension, heart rate, skin-temperature, and galvanic skin response. The feedback may be in a variety of forms, the most

Copyright © 1998 by Academic Press.
All rights of reproduction in any form reserved.

common being visual and auditory. The feedback may be continuous, intermittent, or provided once a threshold is crossed.

Biofeedback can also be considered a methodology used in studying psychophysiological processes. The methodology includes a baseline measurement of the physiological response(s), then feedback is given to an individual with some sort of instruction to manipulate the physiological response(s). The physiological response is measured during feedback and compared to the baseline measurement. Inferences are then drawn as to the relationship between the physiological response and the individual's response to the biofeedback.

B. Historical Survey of Biofeedback Development

Psychophysiology is the scientific study of the interrelationships between cognitive, emotional, behavioral, and physiological processes. Biofeedback techniques and applications grew out of the research in psychophysiology. Biofeedback research became widespread in the 1960s, when studies reported that a variety of presumable nonvoluntary responses could be brought under operant control. Many studies using electroencephalographic feedback were reported which indicated that alpha brain activity could be brought under voluntary control. As these studies gained the attention of clinicians, soon biofeedback was applied to treating various disorders such as migraine headache and hypertension. The growing body of research on stress also provided support for the use of biofeedback as a research tool as well as a treatment approach. Research on the effects of relaxation, meditation, and hypnosis in producing the relaxation response to counteract the effects of stress provided further support for the concept of self-regulation using biofeedback. Advancing technology provided more efficient, reliable, and sophisticated instrumentation that has allowed for greater in-depth study and validation of applied biofeedback. Researchers also became interested in evaluating the various theories being proposed regarding how and why biofeedback works.

Biofeedback experimentation and methodology represents a major advance in the scientific evaluation of the relationships between behavior, environment, and the regulation of physiological processes. Some historians suggest that it is the single most significant development to occur in the area of psychophysiology. Biofeedback methodology has widened the scope and increased the capability of behavioral models of experimentation and analyses in research on physiological functioning and self-regulation. It has stimulated interest in behavioral models of etiology and treatment of psychophysiological disorders. Biofeedback experimentation has provided evidence for new approaches to the alteration of emotional states and the study of consciousness.

II. THEORETICAL MODELS OF BIOFEEDBACK

Over the years several models have been proposed that attempt to describe what processes and principles allow biofeedback to work. Four of the more popular models will be briefly described: these are the operant conditioning framework, the informational processing model, the skills learning model and the psychobiological model of self-regulation.

A. Operant Conditioning Model

The operant conditioning model is basically atheoretical. This approach emphasizes the use of reinforcement, positive, negative, and punishment, that are made contingent on selected ongoing physiological responses, and the learning that follows the application of reinforcement. Research in this area has focused on a variety of conditioning principles, physiological responses, and human and animal behavior. The emphasis has been on examining similarities and differences between conditioning of skeletal motor and visceral or neural processes within the individual. Systematic exploration of operant techniques has not occurred and there needs to be a more consistent examination on the effects of the environment on physiological regulation. Examples are evaluating the effects of combining different schedules and types of reinforcement with the feedback on a person's ability to learn to change a physiological response.

B. Information Processing Model

In defining biofeedback training, the concept that the individual is "fed" "back" information about biological responses that he or she is not aware of is important. This information provides a sensory analog of the currently occurring physiological responses. Information is provided to the individual at the same instant that the physiological activity is occurring or after a very brief delay. Therefore, some part of the output of a process is now introduced into the input of a process so as to alter the information processing. According to the information processing model, biofeedback stimuli can be conceived of as a symbolic representation of the physiological event, and the individual engages in a response to either reduce or enhance the biofeedback stimuli, resulting in changes in the physiological responses themselves. Research in this area may evaluate different types of feedback stimuli to determine the best display of information. This may include examining the differences between auditory and visual feedback.

C. Theory of Voluntary Control

The theory of voluntary control proposed by Brener emphasizes discrimination and awareness of internal bodily responses and processes. Biofeedback is thought to aid the individual in the learning process and increase awareness of sensations related to physiological responses, or to sensitize the individual to other motor responses as a means of mediating voluntary control over the physiological changes. Thus, emphasis is given to learned physiological control as a form of complex human learning of motor skills.

D. Psychobiological Model

All three of the theories discussed thus far have been supported by some empirical data. There are a number of studies that attempt to isolate and differentiate the effects of the hypothesized variables. At this stage of knowledge, there is no strong empirical evidence to support one viewpoint over another. The psychobiological model integrates these concepts by emphasizing the interrelationships between psychological processes and biological processes. The psychobiological model supports the view that biofeedback helps the self-regulation of the individual's total functioning. The concepts from the information modeling approach provide a way to explain how needed feedback is provided that will allow for better self-regulation. The concepts from the operant approach are used to emphasize the individual differences in effectiveness of various types of feedback and schedules of reinforcement, and the importance of considering environmental influences in self-regulation. Finally, the theory of voluntary control helps explain how individuals can adjust their current motor responses to impact on processes that they are not aware of.

III. THE BIOFEEDBACK LABORATORY

A. Components of the Biofeedback Laboratory

The biofeedback laboratory should be a quiet room free from visual distractions. A recliner chair allows the subject to rest comfortably. The laboratory equipment can vary depending on the goals of the clinician and purposes for which the biofeedback will be used. With the advances in technology, most biofeedback systems are quite compact and attractive. Some of these systems are integrated with a computer screen and will allow for printing of and/or computer display of the feedback. A computer system is advisable so that the results of the biofeedback session can be stored for future reference. Biofeedback instruments monitor physiological responses of interest and allow for measurement of these responses. The instrumentation then presents it in a way that the individual can use and manipulate the information.

Electrodes and transducers convert responses from the skin's surface that are transformed to electrical impulses that go to a preamplifier and then to an amplifier. The amplified signal then drives an output device such as an audio signal or visual display. Electrodes are used to detect electrical currents from one electrode to the next. Transducers come in a variety of forms. A thermistor is one type of transducer used to detect heat. A photoplethysmograph is a transducer used to detect changes in density of the skin as a result of changes in blood volume. And a strain gauge is a transducer that measures mechanical changes, such as the movement of some part of the body.

B. Establishing a Biofeedback Laboratory

A minimum requirement would be to establish a large enough area that could hold a recliner, a chair for the individual conducting the biofeedback session, the biofeedback equipment, a personal computer, and lighting that can be dimmed. After space is established for the laboratory then the practitioner would begin searching for the type of equipment that would serve the goals of the practitioner. There are several nationwide companies that can be contacted to provide bids on biofeedback equipment. Some individuals prefer to buy individual biofeedback components for each response, often called "stand alone" modules. Another approach would be to purchase the preamplifier/amplifier components that various transducers and electrodes could be plugged into. In order to connect the biofeedback equipment to a computer a component called an analog-to-digital converter needs to be purchased.

C. Safety Considerations

There is a small chance of electrical safety problems when using biomedical instrumentation. In order to minimize risks Schwartz and associates in 1987 suggested that each power line piece of auxiliary equipment be evaluated periodically for electrical safety; all individuals should be kept out of arm's reach of all metal parts; and equipment should be properly grounded.

IV. TYPES OF BIOFEEDBACK

A. Electromyographic Biofeedback

Electromyographic (EMG) biofeedback is the most widely used biofeedback technique with both children and adults. EMG biofeedback provides information about the individual's striate muscle tension in the area where the electrodes are attached. As the muscle constricts it generates an electrical current between one motor neuron and the next. The EMG sensors pick up the intensity of that electrical current. Typically, there is one reference electrode that is used and two active electrodes. It is important to place the electrodes lengthwise over the muscle of interest so that the electrodes are picking up the electrical current as it moves from one motor neuron to the next within the same muscle. If the electrodes are placed on two different muscles, then the information obtained reflects the electrical difference between two different muscles. The muscles most commonly monitored are the frontalis, masseter and trapezius muscles. The frontalis is the forehead muscle that tenses when an individual is worried or under pressure. Some clinicians believe the tension in the frontalis area is one of the best indicators of overall body tension. The masseter muscle is connected to the jaw bone and contracts when an individual is tense or angry. The trapezius muscle contracts the shoulders when an individual is alarmed or chronically anxious. These muscles are often the focus in biofeedback training because they typically respond to stress and can be measured without much interference from other muscles. They can be a good starting point from which muscle relaxation training can be generalized.

B. Skin Temperature Biofeedback

Skin temperature feedback monitors fluctuations in surface body temperature. These are most often measured by monitoring finger, hand, or foot temperatures. A sensor is usually attached to the index finger of the hand. The sensor, a thermistor, is a heat-sensitive semiconductor in an epoxy bead.

Skin temperature monitoring is useful because skin temperature tends to become cooler as one experiences greater sympathetic nervous system (SNS) arousal and stress. Peripheral vasoconstriction and reduced blood flow to the tiny capillaries in the skin are what causes the skin temperature to decrease. During SNS arousal, changes in blood flow takes blood from the skin and sends it to the skeletal muscles, allowing large muscles to respond to the flight or fight challenge. This response in turn protects the peripheral parts of the body, by reducing blood flow to the hands or feet in order to reduce bleeding if these body parts were injured. Thus, it is suspected that when the person experiences greater parasympathetic nervous system arousal, changes in blood flow return the blood to the skin and smooth muscles. Increased blood flow to the skin causes increases in skin temperature, and this may reflect relaxation.

C. Galvanic Skin Response Biofeedback

A feedback dermograph measures the electrical conductance or electrical potential in the individual's skin. The galvanic skin response (GSR) biofeedback machine can monitor minute changes in the concentration of salt and water in sweat gland ducts. The natural metabolism of cells produces a slight voltage that varies as sweat gland activity changes. The lower the measurable voltage, in millivolts, the less there is of sweat gland activity. With skin conductance techniques an imperceptible electric current is passed through the skin. As the sweat glands become more active, the monitor registers the skin's increased ability to conduct electricity. The reverse of this procedure is called skin resistance.

The GSR has been used in lie detectors as a measure of emotional arousal. The sympathetic branch of the autonomic nervous system controls sweating. GSR biofeedback helps the individual gain control of the arousal produced by the autonomic nervous system. Two sensors or electrodes are usually placed on the ends of two fingers. Many clinicians prefer not to use GSR responses because they change rapidly and often respond to irrelevant stimuli.

D. Electroencephalographic Biofeedback

Electroencephalographic (EEG) biofeedback is another frequently used biofeedback training method with children and adults. EEG biofeedback gives information about the brain's electrical activity. Brain waves have been classified into four states: beta, which occurs when the individual is wide awake and thinking; alpha, which is associated with a state of calm relaxation; theta, which reflects a deep reverie or light sleep; and delta, which is associated with deep sleep.

In the typical procedure the subject is provided with feedback about the presence or absence of some specified amplitude and/or frequency of brain electrical activity. Often the goal of EEG biofeedback is to produce alpha waves because they are associated with relaxation.

E. Heart Rate, Blood Pressure, Pulse, and Volume Biofeedback

The heart rate monitor uses electrodes to measure the action of the heart muscle. Heart rate biofeedback usually involves measuring heart beats per minute. In general, greater SNS arousal is associated with a faster heart rate, and a relaxed state is associated with decreased heart rate. Blood pressure biofeedback monitors the diastolic and the systolic pressure of the cardiovascular system. Increases in blood pressure reflect greater SNS arousal; thus, in most cases the goal of blood pressure biofeedback is to reduce the pressure. Blood pressure is difficult to monitor as one has to use a blood pressure cuff that must be inflated and deflated to measure the changes in pressure. It is has been shown that the inflating and deflating of the cuff actually alters the blood pressure response. Newer technologies have been developed to overcome this problem; however, they are more expensive.

Blood pulse and volume are measured using a photoplethysmograph. A photoplethysmograph generates a small amount of infrared light that is monitored with a light sensor. As blood volume increases the density of the skin increases and less light passes through the skin and is reflected back and is registered by the light sensor. Blood volume feedback helps the individual constrict or dilate the blood vessels or artery being monitored. Blood pulse is also measured with a photoplethysmograph and is often used as an indirect measure of heart rate.

F. Sexual Response Biofeedback

Sexual arousal in males is usually measured by penile tumescence. A strain gauge is used and it measures the physical changes of the penis as arousal increases and decreases. Female sexual arousal is measured with a thermistor or photoplethysmograph that is placed near the clitoris. Sexual response biofeedback may be used in the treatment of sexual deviations as well as sexual dysfunctions.

G. Gastrointestinal Biofeedback

Measuring the activity of the gastrointestinal system can be accomplished by measuring the electrical activity on the surface of the skin where the stomach is. Muscular activity is screened out. Greater electrical activity is related to greater stomach motility. This type of biofeedback may be useful in treating stomach disorders that are affected by stress and anxiety.

V. CURRENT RESEARCH FINDINGS IN BIOFEEDBACK

A. Research on the Best Methods of Biofeedback

Studies indicate that initially feedback should be salient to the individual, continuous and given when small changes are made. As the individual begins learning to manipulate the response, then feedback can be contingent on greater change and may be given intermittently. The clinician can experiment with a variety of forms of feedback, many people prefer audio feedback as they can close their eyes while trying to relax.

It is important to include segments of "self-control" training in which the feedback is turned off and the individual is instructed to continue to manipulate the response without feedback. Research also indicates that home practice is necessary for lasting changes to occur. Practicing self-control of the physiological response for 10 to 20 minutes several times a week is recommended. It appears that it is best to have the patient plan out the practice schedule ahead of time and to practice earlier in the day. If the patient waits until right before they go to sleep they may fall asleep during the practice. As the patient gets better at controlling the response, he or she should be encouraged to do this while continuing normal activities.

Studies indicate that changes in symptoms come slowly with most changes occurring four to six weeks after biofeedback therapy has begun. It is important to explain to the patient that biofeedback does not work like most medication and that changes occur slowly and often accompany a real change in the person's behavior and attitude about the problem and how to cope with it. Also, biofeedback may not eliminate the symptoms but it may reduce the intensity, frequency, and/or medication usage.

B. Research Investigations on How Biofeedback Works

In the late 1970s and early 1980s research in biofeedback was focused on evaluating the different models of biofeedback discussed above. Many interesting findings were reported, but more questions were raised than were answered as to how biofeedback works. Much of the recent research on biofeedback has focused on evaluating the clinical efficacy of biofeedback, and little systematic work is now being done on discovering how it works. In order to address the question of how it works some researchers have attempted to design false feedback studies. Results of these studies have been mixed, with some studies reporting that even when false feedback is given subjects alter their response as instructed. Some researchers have compared biofeedback training with relaxation only and found that in both conditions, decreases in ANS arousal can be achieved. Other researchers are now examining the role of cognitions in the biofeedback process. The bottom line is that we are not sure how it works but studying this question allows for a fascinating journey into the mind-body research arena.

C. Research on Differences between Children's and Adults' Responses to Biofeedback

In general children are more open and responsive to biofeedback than adults. Children are usually fascinated with the equipment, and motivation and curiosity are high. Research on nonclinical populations response to biofeedback indicate that children between the ages of 8 and 12 are able to achieve greater changes in physiological responses using biofeedback than any other age group. For clinical groups biofeedback may be a good alternative to medication if the medical treatment has potentially negative short- and long-term consequences for the developing child. Research evaluating the effectiveness of biofeedback with children who have headaches indicates that more children improve and to a greater degree than do adults.

Besides play therapy, behavior modification, and some of the newly developed cognitive strategies, there are only a few individual therapy techniques to be used directly with children. Most interventions involve changing or teaching parenting skills, or manipulating the child's environment. Biofeedback offers the therapist a mode to teach the child concepts of self-control, stress management, and an opportunity to begin talking about feelings and stressors and how these may affect physical health. Most children have an external health locus of control in which powerful others have responsibility for their health. Biofeedback may help the child gain an internalized view that acknowledges one's own role in maintaining good health.

Although children may be more responsive in the therapy setting, they may have greater difficulty than adults in remembering to practice outside of the therapeutic settings and to record changes in their symptoms. Often a parent is recruited to gently remind the child to practice and record symptoms.

VI. CLINICAL USE OF BIOFEEDBACK

A. How and Why Biofeedback Is Used in Clinical Settings

A major use of biofeedback is to teach relaxation skills. A second use of biofeedback is to alter pathophysiological processes such as blood flow or SNS arousal for migraine headache patients, to decrease the flow of gastric juices for ulcer patients, to decrease muscle tension and increase proper posture for the chronic back-pain patient. Biofeedback should be considered as a therapeutic tool that can help introduce the client to therapy in a concrete and nonthreatening manner. It can be especially useful for the patient who focuses on physical problems or insists his problems are not physiological. Biofeedback can also be used to increase feelings of self-efficacy and self-control. The client learns quickly the connection between emotions, thoughts, and physiological responses.

Biofeedback may be used when there are no viable medical alternatives, or when the physician determines that medication should not be used. Sometimes patients do not want to take medication and biofeedback may be a treatment alternative. For example, a chronic back-pain patient may have to use pain medication to control the pain for the rest of her life because there are no other medical treatments to reduce the pain. The patient may choose to try biofeedback to help cope and reduce the pain instead of taking pain medication, which is addictive and may have undesirable side effects.

Biofeedback has also been used in modifying behavioral problems. Two examples are hyperactivity that is associated with attention deficit disorder and maladaptive behaviors that are associated with mental retardation. Motor responses may be monitored using biofeedback; the child is rewarded as the problem behavior decreases.

Biofeedback should be used clinically only after a competent medical diagnosis has been made and the examining physician has decided that biofeedback may be valuable. Patients coming directly to psychologists for biofeedback or other behavioral treatments of physical disorders should be referred first to a medical specialist for a thorough medical examination. The need for medical consultation in any biofeedback case is both an ethical and legal responsibility of the psychological practitioner.

B. Biofeedback, Relaxation Training, and *Stress Management*

The question has been raised as to the difference in effectiveness of outcome between biofeedback and relaxation training in reducing stress. This has been a controversial question as many clinicians and researchers argue that you can get the same benefits from relaxation strategies as from biofeedback for most problems. Furthermore, they point out that the relaxation strategies are not as costly nor do they require knowledge of complicated equipment. Only a few large-scale controlled outcome studies on the efficacy of biofeedback as compared to other behavioral techniques in the management of physiological disorders have been reported. Most of these do not find that biofeedback provides a distinct advantage over other behavioral procedures. The selectivity of physiological control often achieved by biofeedback methods would suggest that the methods would have a unique advantage in disorders in which the symptom is quite specific, for example, cardiac arrhythmias, seizure disorders, and various neuromuscular disorders. However, at the present time there is not enough research evidence to discount the idea that biofeedback may be better for some disorders, and that some people may respond better to biofeedback than relaxation therapy. As technology advances equipment is becoming less expensive and more user "friendly." Biofeedback may be particularly useful for children as cognitively they can understand concrete examples of what is happening in their bodies as compared to relaxation training that may be more abstract. In a culture that provides video games, robots, computers, and other high-tech games and toys for children, they are usually attracted and eager to participate in the biofeedback session.

C. Clinical Issues in Using Biofeedback

Biofeedback can be abused if it used outside of the context of therapy. It cannot be used in the same manner that one would administer medication. *Individual differences* must be noted and addressed using an individualized protocol before biofeedback can be successful. Also, the individual should be closely monitored and changes recommended if problems arise. Biofeedback may be successful in the clinic, but patients may not be able to modify their responses in the natural environment without biofeedback. Thus the development of self-control should be included in the protocol.

Sometimes a person's baseline physiological responses are normal, but the individual may experience exaggeration of SNS responses when stressed. Biofeedback should be focused on helping these individuals decrease SNS arousal during stressful situations. Thus, in biofeedback therapy it is important to teach biofeedback skills in a variety of situations and intensities of stimuli.

Biofeedback allows for discrete control of a response system. For example, one component of autonomic nervous system (ANS) activity can be modified without other ANS systems being called into play. Specific EEG patterns can be modified and discrete muscle groups as small as a single motor unit can be trained independently with the use of feedback. However, for the ANS it appears that increases in arousal-like activity are easier to obtain than decreases in arousal-like activity. Thus, researchers have more consistently demonstrated voluntary blood pressure and heart rate increases and skin temperature decreases than the opposite processes. This indicates that biofeedback may be more useful in lowering high levels of arousal such as those associated with clinical stress conditions or pathological states than normal or healthy states

The specific form and structure of the biofeedback training must depend largely on the individual characteristics of the patient, the physiological symptoms in question, the particular physiological system for which feedback is to be given, the nature of the disorder itself, and the goals of treatment. Through an accumulation of knowledge gained through basic and clinical research, including systematic case studies, certain generalizations may be possible. However, at this time generalization are made with caution. The biofeedback clinician must choose a specific procedure on the basis of all the facts in the case and his or her own understanding of the current technology and state of research knowledge. The astute clinician can proceed in a systematic manner through trial, error, and close observation of clinical outcomes as they occur for a given patient.

Compliance to the biofeedback practice may be difficult at times as positive effects usually do not always happen instantaneously. The patient must be prepared to expect that decreases in symptoms may not occur for several weeks. Patient motivation may be low because for some disorders there are no short-term aversive consequences such as in hypertension. Another motivation reducer is that the symptom itself may be reinforced in the natural environment. The patient may experience secondary gain. For example, a patient may use talking about her problem in social situations to gain attention. What will she do in social situations if she does not have a problem to discuss? The patient may also be a candidate for social skills training, so that as the symptom is reduced she will have acquired other skills to help her cope in social situations. Another possible area of motivational difficulty may arise from other behaviors strongly entrenched in the patient's repertoire that are in conflict with the aim of therapy. An example is a young man who has overextended himself in extracurricular activities and has poor time-management skills. This young man is quite able to learn the biofeedback skills but cannot find time to practice at home. This issue must be addressed by the therapist if treatment is to be successful.

If the patient is on medication that may effect the response that is being manipulated, consult with the patient's physician to determine if the medication can be kept at a constant level while biofeedback therapy is occurring. If during the biofeedback training the patient or physician wants to decrease or increase medication intake, ask that this be reported so that this information can be used to evaluate the success of the biofeedback therapy.

VII. OPPORTUNITIES IN AND FUTURE OF BIOFEEDBACK

A. Professional and Research Opportunities

Reports on studies of biofeedback have steadily declined over the past 10 years. This is unfortunate as there are still so many unanswered questions regarding how and why biofeedback works. The area of biofeedback research provides a wealth of opportunities, particularly as technology improves and instrumentation becomes more reliable and valid. There are now more training opportunities to learn biofeedback instrumentation and methodology. The Biofeedback Society of America encourages continued scientific investigations of biofeedback, and there are numerous high-quality scientific journals that publish biofeedback research, including *Psychophysiology; Biofeedback and Self-Regulation;* and *Biofeedback and Behavioral Medicine.*

On the professional level biofeedback techniques and therapy have become more widely accepted as a method of treatment for numerous mental and physical problems. Those interested in developing a profession in biofeedback can contact the two national societies, the Biofeedback Society of America and the American Association of Biofeedback Clinicians. There are also many state and regional biofeedback societies that provide training and scientific meetings.

B. Future Directions in Research, Clinical Practice, and Biofeedback Technology

Biofeedback is alive and well as there continues to be a steady output of high-quality research, greater acceptance of biofeedback as a clinical tool, and improvements in technology. Although biofeedback has been used to treat problems, it may have advantages in helping individuals develop self-regulation skills to prevent mental and physical health problems. For example, a study was reported in which children with no clinical problems were taught skin-temperature biofeedback. These children learned to relax and incorporated this in their daily schedule. They also demonstrated decreases in anxiety and depression scores, even though these scores were in the normal range. Biofeedback may have helped them achieve a greater degree of psychological health.

With the advent of greater access to personal computers people may be able to purchase inexpensive biofeedback devices that they can use at home to teach themselves self-regulation skills. Of course, as with all self-help approaches, misunderstanding of instructions, the problem, or proper follow-through may diminish the effectiveness of self-help biofeedback. However, combining home devices with some therapist assistance may be as effective as time-intensive, outpatient biofeedback training. These are just some of the future directions to be explored.

BIBLIOGRAPHY

Andrasik, F. (1994). Twenty-five years in progress: Twenty-five more? *Biofeedback and Self-Regulation, 19,* 311–324.

Miller, L. (1994). Biofeedback and behavioral medicine: treating the symptom, the syndrome, or the person? *Psychotherapy, 31,* 161–169.

Schwartz, M. S. (1987). *Biofeedback: A practitioner's guide.* New York: Guilford.

Shapiro, D. (1977). A monologue on biofeedback and psychophysiology. *Psychophysiology, 14,* 213–227.

Surwillo, W. W. (1990). *Psychophysiology for clinical psychologists.* Norwood, NJ: Ablex.

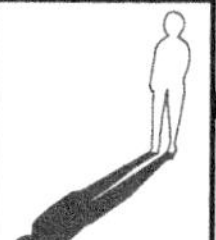

Brain Scanning/Neuroimaging

Richard J. Haier
University of California, Irvine

Co-Registration When one image is aligned, scaled and superimposed over another image so both fit the same space.
EEG Electroencephalogram
fMRI Functional Magnetic Resonance Imaging
MEG Magnetoencephalogram
MRI Magnetic Resonance Imaging
PET Position Emission Tomography
Pixel The smallest unit of an image; each pixel is quantified.
Radiotracer A radioactive substance that imaging devices measure to show where the tracer goes.
Region-of-Interest (ROI) Any brain area defined and located anatomically or mathematically.
SPECT Single-Photon Emission Computed Tomography
Stereotactic A method of defining brain area location using coordinates of a standard brain.
Tomography Process of making a mathematical picture.

A variety of MEDICAL IMAGING TECHNOLOGIES show the brain in ways not possible previously. Functional imaging is especially useful for identifying brain areas involved in specific cognitive tasks and states. Each imaging method has different strengths and weaknesses. There are several core issues concerning image analysis that must be considered by researchers and clinicians. The combination of advanced imaging technology with sophisticated psychological experiments is a powerful tool for helping understand the normal and abnormal brain.

I. BASIC CONCEPTS

A. Structural and Functional Imaging

Through the 1970s researchers had access to the living human brain mostly through the study of blood, urine, and spinal fluid. Only electroencephalograph (EEG) methods and occasional probing during brain surgery provided direct data on human brain functioning. Computed Axial Tomography (CAT) scans and early Magnetic Resonance Imaging (MRI) showed brain structures in considerable detail (see Fig. 1) but provided no functional information. That is to say, CAT and MRI scans may show tumors, strokes, and other forms of structural brain damage but they do not show brain activity during learning, memory, language processing, emotion, sleep, and other brain states. In fact, structural imaging may show the brain in fine anatomic detail but whether the patient is alive or dead is not apparent in the images. Functional brain imaging is designed to reveal regional brain activity while the person is engaged in a psychological task chosen to maintain the brain in a specific mode during the imaging procedure. Functional images, therefore, change in a person depending on the task performed or the state of

Copyright © 1998 by Academic Press.
All rights of reproduction in any form reserved.

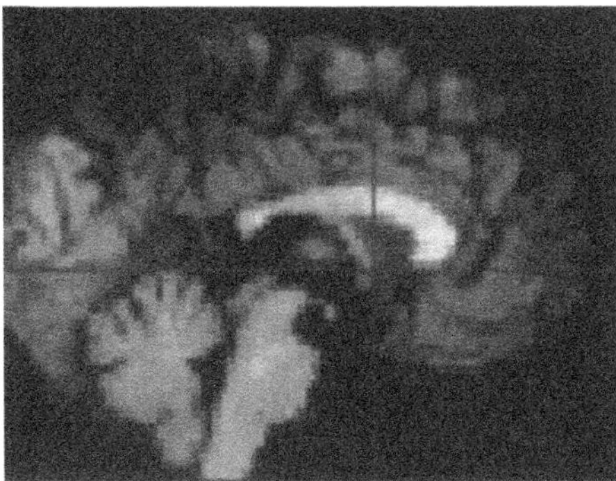

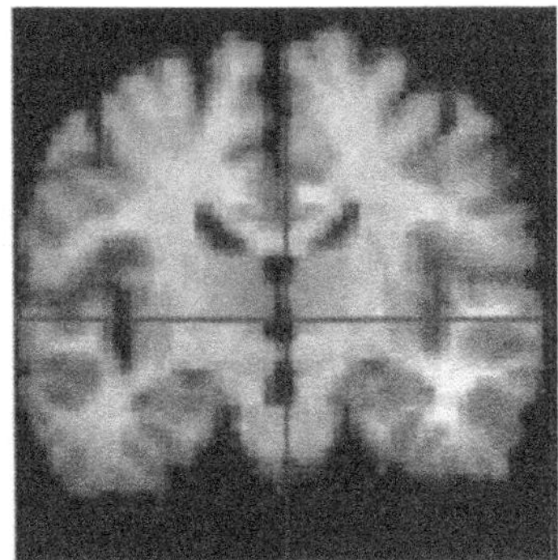

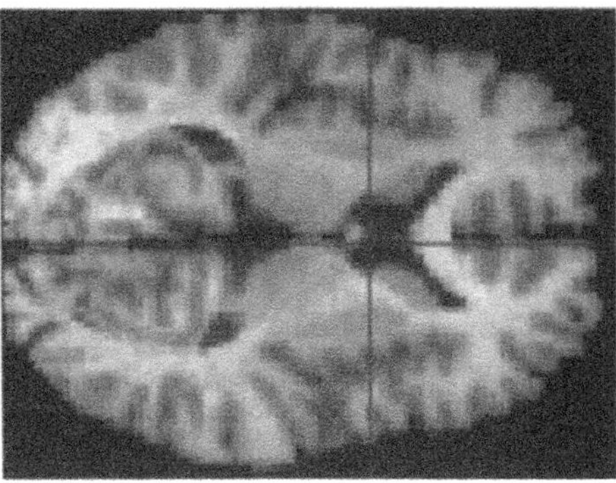

Figure 1 Image orientations. The upper left image shows an MRI slice in sagittal or side orientation; the front of the brain is on the right. The upper right image shows a coronal or cross section orientation looking through from the front of the brain. The bottom image shows an axial or top down view; the front of the brain is on the right.

the brain (awake, asleep, at rest, problem solving, etc.) whereas in structural imaging, the pictures look the same irrespective of the brain's work or state. For CAT scans and MRI, it does not matter if the person is performing a task of attention or memory, or whether the person is awake or asleep, or eyes open or closed. The structural image is the same and the tumor or stroke is revealed just as well. Structural imaging has been of great importance in making clinical evaluations regarding the extent and location of brain damage in individual patients. Researchers have also used structural imaging to compare anatomic measurements of brain size and volume among groups of interest. These data augment earlier autopsy studies and, in many instances, are more accurately assessed in the living brain undamaged by death and brain fixation procedures.

As dramatic as structural brain images can be, however, functional images have captured the imagination of many clinicians and researchers. These images show the brain responding to activation by cognitive tasks. Functional brain imaging techniques now available include Positron Emission Tomography (PET), Single Photon Emission Computed Tomography (SPECT), functional MRI (fMRI), topographic EEG, and Magnetoencephalogram (MEG, also known as Superconducting Quantum Interference Device or SQUID). The older methods of acquiring blood flow images with xenon gas are no longer used much in activation studies, although pioneering work was done with these techniques. Functional images show the brain at work and often reveal complex relationships between activation or deactivation in well-defined anatomic areas and specific cognitive processes. The interpretation of functional images depends on the psychological task or brain state engaged during the imaging and the sophistication of the task is a major factor to be considered.

B. Key Role of Psychological Tasks and Brain States

Functional imaging shows the brain "at work." The type and amount of work are specified in a task performed by the subject during the scanning procedure. Scans during two or more task conditions or states can be compared to show the brain areas that differ in activity between the conditions. Task condition is critical for functional imaging. During the early years of PET, many subjects were studied at rest with eyes closed and ears plugged; no task was used. These studies compared brain function during this "resting" state in one group of subjects to another group. The resting condition, however, is not particularly well controlled because subjects are free to engage in any cognitive activity to pass the time during the scan procedure. Moreover, even when a specific task condition is compared to a resting condition, the same problem remains. The choice of a control task, therefore, is often more complex than choosing a "resting" state. As cognitive psychologists and neuropsychologists have engaged in functional imaging experiments, the choice of tasks has become more sophisticated. Many tasks are chosen to maximize elemental cognitive processes and to minimize individual differences in performance and learning (habituation). These studies tend to focus on localizing brain areas involved in various aspects of cognition. Many a priori hypotheses from a cognitive neuropsychology perspective have been tested by comparing such tasks as generating words, listening to words, and speaking words. Other tasks are chosen to maximize performance differences among individuals to help identify relationships between brain activation and performance. These studies address questions concerning task difficulty, mental effort, and other parameters of performance. For example, one may use a test of reasoning to identify salient brain areas and then use easy and hard versions of the reasoning task to help identify relationships between mental effort and regional brain activation. The more complex the task, the more difficult it is to interpret the results in terms of elemental cognitive processes. Nonetheless, complex tasks can be used to examine performance differences and the functional relationships among brain areas. Because the manipulation of brain engagement and state are critical in functional imaging, these techniques are fundamentally psychological.

C. Standard Images and Types of Image Analyses

Empirical analyses of structural and functional neuroimaging data have evolved dramatically from 2D stereotactic based regions-of-interest to 3D anatomically precise localization. Much neuroimaging now uses structural MRI as the basis for individual or group data and superimposes (coregistration) functional data. MRI thus provides an accurate anatomical template for functional data. PET, SPECT, EEG, MEG and fMRI data all can be displayed on MRI images in 2 dimensions or 3 dimensions (see Fig. 2). A typical analysis begins by taking each image slice (from different brain levels) from each subject and averaging them into a group brain image. Individual brains vary enormously in size and shape, especially in cortex; internal features and regions-of-interest also vary considerably. This variation presents a problem for averaging individuals into a group image. Each person's image must be fit to a standard brain where shape and size are fixed. Each person's image is then pushed and pulled and stretched to fit the standard (see Fig. 3). There are many ways to define the standard and many ways to accomplish the fitting to it. For example, a standard brain outline can be derived from stereotactic atlases and internal areas can be located according to a grid system. Because the most popular atlases used for this purpose are based on only one person's brain, generalizations are limited. An alternative method is based on averaging a large number of brain images (e.g., MRI scans) and deriving an average outline, although there are a number of

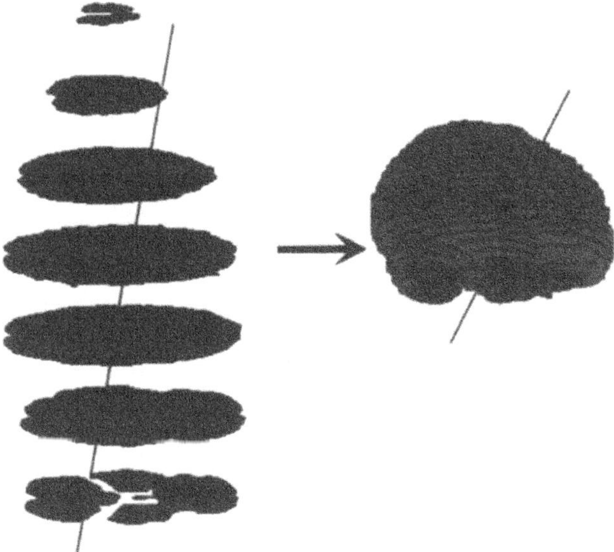

Figure 2 3-dimensional reconstruction. Shows how a series of axial slices from any imaging modality can be stacked to construct a 3-dimensional image.

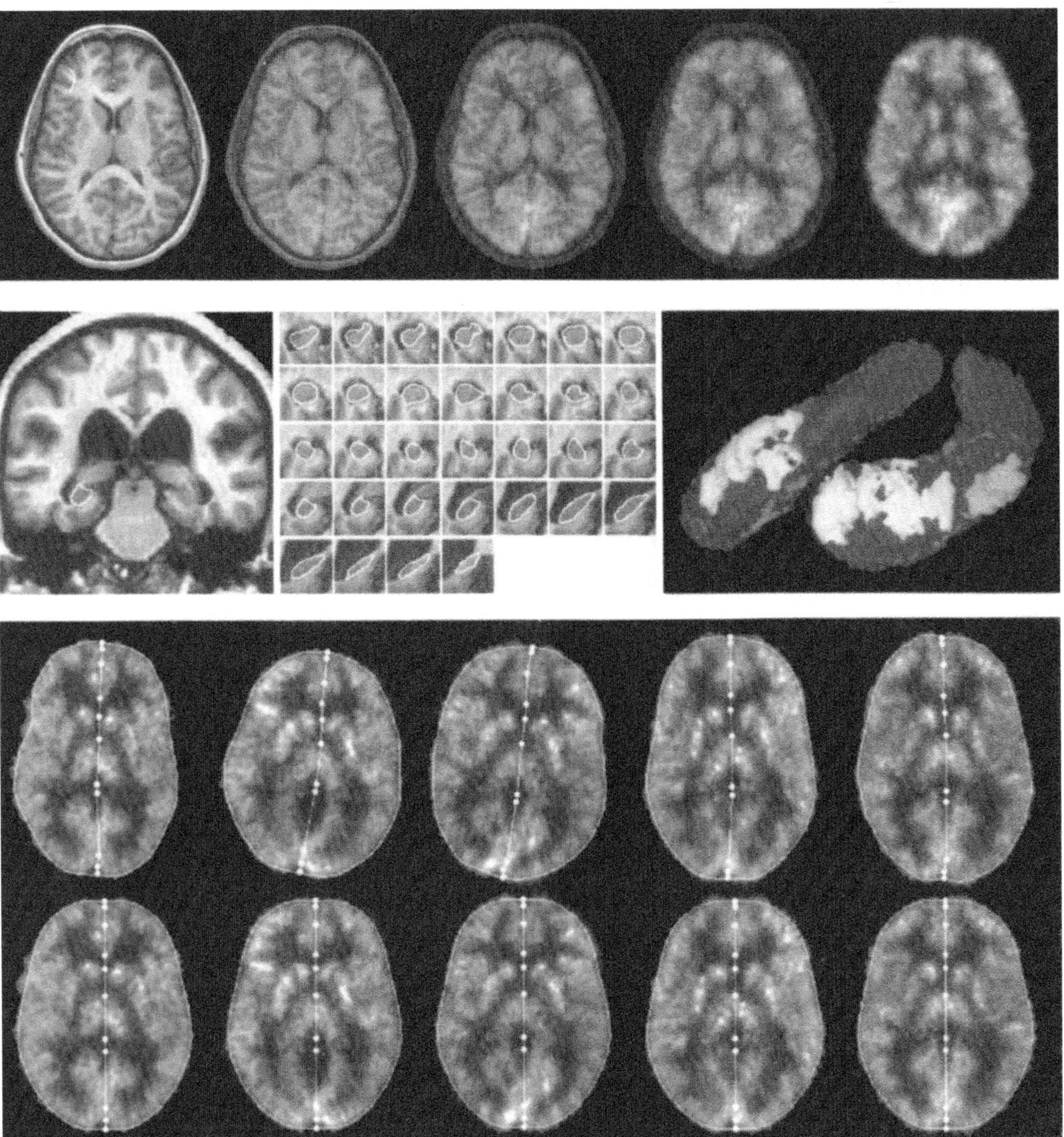

Figure 3 Top row: Gradient from structure to function. MRI (left) provides anatomical information about the brain showing the gray matter where cell bodies and dendritic connections are made, the white matter which is composed of the cell axons coursing between gray matter areas, and the cerebrospinal fluid filled spaces shown in black. PET (right) reveals the metabolic rate of glucose, the main energy source for brain activity. The images were formed by aligning the axial MRI and PET scans from the same person and then calculating images composed of pixel values drawn 100% from MRI, 75% MRI and 25% PET, 50% MRI and 50% PET, 25% MRI and 75% PET, and 100% PET. Subject is performing a memory task involving viewing words on a screen so visual cortex is activated (bottom of PET images on right). Middle row: Visualization of the hippocampus in 3 dimensions. Left: The hippocampus can be traced on MRI anatomical images cut in coronal sections. Middle: Each successive tracing of the 3D object is assembled. Right: 3D reconstruction of the successive surfaces for left and right hippocampus showing glucose metabolic activity (white) from aligned PET scan. Bottom row: Warping individual brains for comparison. Top shows the individual variation in size and shape among five normal subjects' PET scans (one slice each). Midline landmarks and brain edge identified on MRI scans matched to the PET are used to warp all images to the same configuration (bottom) so that individuals can be compared directly using statistical parametric mapping techniques. (Courtesy of Dr. Monte Buchsbaum.)

ways of doing this as well. Once the average outline is established, each person's image can be stretched, pulled, warped, or morphed to the standard using the brain outline or internal landmarks. Although there have been some attempts to standardize this process, no clear advantage of any method over others has been compelling to date.

Once standard images are created for a group of subjects, various statistical analyses are possible. A common analysis for functional data is based on a subtraction procedure. For example, each pixel value (e.g., glucose metabolism) in one group image is subtracted from the value of the corresponding pixel in a second group (see Fig. 4). Each of the thousands of resulting subtractions can be expressed statistically (e.g., as *t*-tests) and the value of each statistical comparison can be displayed pixel by pixel. Usually this is done for a significance level of probability so the resulting image shows at a glance, the brain areas where there is a statistically significant difference between the groups. Within a group, subtractions can be made between task conditions. This is one of the most frequently used analysis for group or condition analyses. Because of the very large number of tests, often thousands per slice, statistical corrections for multiple comparisons can be applied. A number of corrections have been proposed using multivariate methods, Monte Carlo simulations, resampling, and other techniques. All require assumptions that are more or less applicable to particular research circumstances and no single approach has been adopted as a standard. Because of high per-scan costs (due largely to hardware investment), most imaging studies report small sample sizes, further compounding the statistical problems. Replication of results, in combination with a priori hypotheses, is regarded by many researchers as the most effective way to overcome the statistical difficulties inherent in this kind of work.

In addition to subtraction of means, some data and research designs allow analyses based on individual differences. Correlations, for example, can be computed between task performance and functional data pixel-by-pixel or brain area-by-brain area. The subtraction analyses may identify a brain region activated by a task; whereas, the correlation analysis shows the correspondence between task performance and activation of specific areas. For instance, researchers can ask if brain activity increases more or less in a salient area in those people who have the best task performance. Correlations can also be computed among brain areas, even pixel-by-pixel, to reveal functional relationships throughout the brain. For example, the statistically significant correlations between one brain area, say the superior frontal lobe, with all other brain areas can be shown for a specific condition or in a specific group. The pattern of correlations can then be compared for other conditions or groups. Other statistical approaches like path analysis can be used to help identify functional neurocircuity.

It is also possible to display an individual brain im-

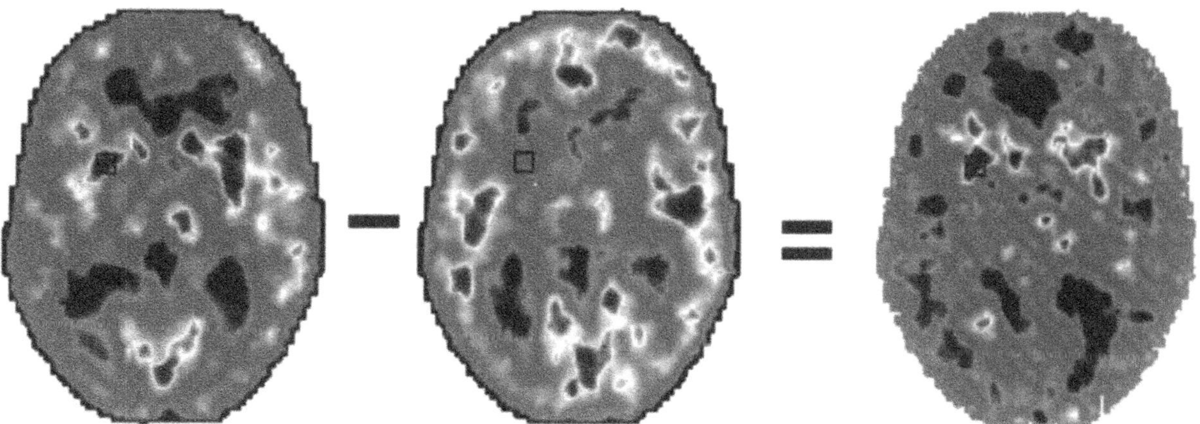

Figure 4 The image subtraction concept. After being warped to a standard, one image can be subtracted from another pixel by pixel. Here the middle image is subtracted from the left image and the resulting image is shown on the right. The box is 7 × 7 pixels and shows the subtraction in the left caudate area. The resulting image can be displayed as a significance probability map where the subtraction for each pixel is statistically summarized.

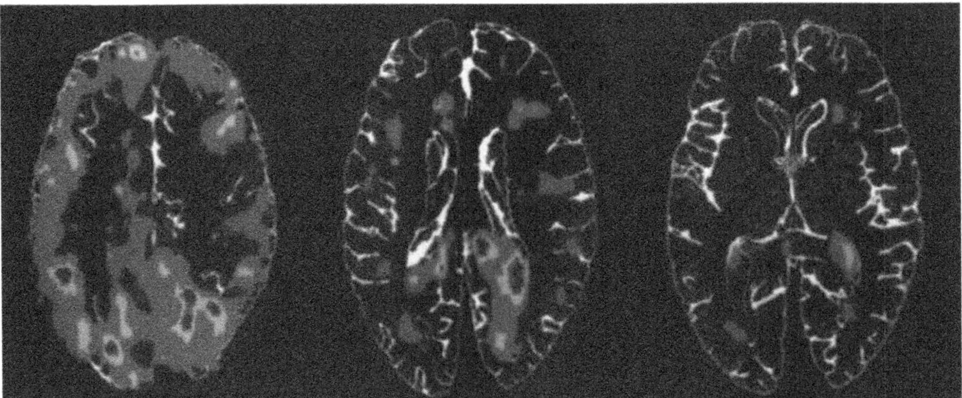

Figure 5 Standard score display. Shows three axial PET slices from a subject with Down Syndrome warped to a standard shape. Each pixel is displayed as a standard score for this subject based on the mean and standard deviation for each pixel measured in a control group. In these images, gray shows areas where the standard scores are greater than 2. (Courtesy of Dr. Richard Haier.)

age where each pixel is a standard score based on a group mean and standard deviation. For functional images, this allows a person's unique pattern of brain activity to be shown relative to a comparison group or task condition (see Fig. 5). Standard score images may be most useful for clinical applications including diagnostic classification and treatment strategies.

Specific examples of these analyses from several areas will be discussed after a review of the major brain/neuroimaging techniques.

II. POSITRON EMISSION TOMOGRAPHY (PET)

A. Methodology for Glucose Metabolic Rate (GMR)

PET is a functional imaging technique based on the use of positron emitting radiotracers. A number of positron emitters can be used for PET but the two most commonly used for brain imaging are fluorine (18) and oxygen (15). F18, for example, can be attached to an analog of glucose, 2-deoxyglucose, to form fluorodeoxyglucose (FDG). When FDG is injected into a person's blood stream, the deoxyglucose part enters the glucose pool and is used by neurons for energy. The more a neuron fires, the more deoxyglucose it uses and the more the neuron is labeled with F18. Thus, the harder a brain area works during a task, the more FDG it takes up. Following the injection of FDG, it takes about 32 minutes for the brain to use most of it. Therefore, whatever the brain is doing for the 32 minutes following the injection determines the pattern of glucose use. When FDG is used, the scanning begins only after the 32 minute labeling period. The person is not even in the scanner during this time. The person does perform a psychological task and the brain areas most active use the most FDG, resulting in regional patterns of GMR. At the end of the 32-minute task, the brain is labeled with F18; the more neuronal firing in any area, the more F18. As each positron decays spontaneously (as it strikes a free electron), two gamma rays are emitted at a 180° angle to each other. When the head is placed in the center of the scanner and surrounded by a ring of many detectors, a computer determines each time a pair of gamma rays 180° apart is detected. These coincident events are reconstructed mathematically showing the origin of each pair of gamma rays; the more positrons in an area, the more pairs of gamma rays are emitted. The resulting images show the pattern of accumulated brain activity over the 32-minute period—not the activity while the person lies in the scanner, because by this time there is no more FDG to be taken up by the brain. Even if the person suddenly died as the scanning begins, a colorful image can be made showing what the brain had been doing during the prior 32-minute labeling period. By contrast, if the person dies as the FDG is being injected, the subsequent scanning will show no image because the dead brain had no metabolism and took up none of the FDG. If a second task is to be studied in the same person, at least 10 hours (5 half-lives) must pass before a second injection of FDG can label the new activity. Most FDG studies use a between scan interval of 2 to 7 days, a logistical disadvantage compared to blood flow techniques. FDG studies have the advantage of quantification as glucose metabolic rate (GMR) following the method of Sokoloff and associates. Spatial resolution can range from about 3.5 mm in plane for the newest scanners to about 8mm for older models. Spatial resolution for PET is usually measured as Full Width Half Maximum (FWHM), a complex measure suggesting the smallest distance that can be resolved between two small points.

B. Methodology for Blood Flow

The use of O15 for PET requires a different procedure although positrons decaying into gamma rays detected by the same scanner are still the basis for the image. O15 is attached to water molecules. The radioactive water, emitting positrons, is injected or inhaled into the bloodstream and for the next 60 seconds, while a task is performed, the distribution of the water can be followed in blood flow. For this method, the person must be in the scanner during the 60-second uptake time of the O15 during which a task is performed. The images show blood flow patterns during the 60-second task performance; brain areas that are activated show increased blood flow. The half life of O15 is only about 2 minutes compared to about 2 hours for F18. Thus, for blood flow PET studies using O15, the person can be injected with a second dose after a 10 minute period (5 half-lives) and a different task can be studied. Often several tasks are studied in the same person over a session; each task is studied for 60 seconds and 10 minutes pass between tasks. This is advantageous for subtraction procedures. Spatial resolution for O15 images may not be as good as for F18 since the 32-minute uptake period produces more gamma ray detections than the 60-second period. While O15 PET studies have the advantage of providing several 60-second experiments in one session, 60 seconds is far too long a period for most psychological studies of cognitive processes best studied in milliseconds. For some psychological studies, FDG has the advantage of a relatively strong signal-to-noise ratio in a 32-minute experiment with hundreds of stimuli. Functional MRI, described below, also determines blood flow with a time resolution on the order of 2 seconds or better. Spatial resolution is also better and no radioactive injection is required. Therefore, most researchers using blood flow PET techniques are switching to fMRI (see below).

C. L-Dopa and Other Tracers

PET can also be used with other radiolabels so that receptor binding sites can be imaged. For example, F18 can be attached to L-dopa, a drug that binds to dopamine receptors. This fluorinated L-dopa can then be used to make images of dopamine system function. Such images have been used to study Parkinson's Disease, a disease of dopamine deficiency, and schizophrenia, a brain disorder treated with dopamine acting drugs. This kind of neuroimaging research has potential for predicting drug response of individual patients. For example, Buchsbaum and colleagues reported that schizophrenics with low GMR in some dopamine-rich brain areas (i.e., the basal ganglia) may show a good clinical response to a dopamine acting drug whereas a similar patient without low basal ganglia GMR will not respond to the same drug. In other studies, fluorinated cocaine has been used to image drug abusers to help understand the mechanism of addiction and, possibly, vulnerability to addiction. Many other positron-emitting receptor labels available for use in PET can image aspects of the serotonin, benzodiazapine, NMDA, and other neurotransmitter systems. This diversity for specific brain system imaging is an advantage over other imaging techniques, especially for the study of psychopathology.

D. SPECT (Single-Photon Emission Computed Tomography)

This is similar to PET in principle. However, the radioactive sources used to emit gamma rays do not produce pairs of gamma rays at 180° and they are not metabolically active so full quantification is not available. The sources are, however, very long lived so a local cyclotron is not necessary. Spatial resolution is not generally as good as PET but SPECT, because it is cheaper hardware and does not require short-lived isotopes, is more available than PET.

III. MAGNETIC RESONANCE IMAGING (MRI)

A. Methodology

MRI was first used as a structural imaging technique that had better spatial resolution than CAT scans for many organs without any radiation exposure. Originally called nuclear magnetic resonance (NMR), MRI uses a strong magnetic field to align spinning protons in hydrogen atoms throughout the body into a north/south orientation. The stronger the magnet, the greater number of protons are aligned. There is no subjective feeling of this alignment taking place while the person lies in the MRI scanner tube, surrounded by the powerful magnetic field. Radio frequencies are pulsed into the magnetic field very rapidly; each pulse briefly throws protons out of the magnetic north/south alignment but because the body is always in the magnetic field during the procedure, the protons realign immediately. As the protons lose and then regain alignment in the magnetic gradient, different radio frequencies that contain spatial information are produced. These frequencies are detected by antenna-like coils within the MRI scanner and provide the basic data for the mathematical reconstruction that produces the images. Because hydrogen is especially sensitive to the magnetic/radio frequency alternations, water is particularly well imaged so organs like the brain with high water content can be imaged in exquisite spatial detail, often about a millimeter or less (see Fig. 6).

By increasing the speed of acquiring enough information to make an image (under 50 milliseconds in some cases using the echoplanar technique), fast MRI now allows functional information to be collected as changes from one image to the next can be measured. These changes are related to blood flow and they can be imaged with fMRI (functional MRI). The hardware is basically the same as for structural MRI but advanced software and special magnetic coils allow the rapid scanning sequences that can show small changes in blood flow when the magnetic/radio frequency signals in one task condition are subtracted from another condition pixel-by-pixel, much like the routine subtraction procedures used in PET. These signal changes are then superimposed (coregistered) as colored areas on the person's structural MRI (see Fig. 7), typically acquired in the same session.

At this point in development, there is some controversy over whether the fMRI signal changes show actual blood flow or hemoglobin parameters related to oxygenation of the blood. The time resolution of fMRI is also difficult to determine because the images can be generated in much less than a second using very powerful magnets but it is not clear whether blood flow changes in response to a cognitive task occur in less than a second or two. These problems aside, fMRI is used for many cognitive studies. It has the appeal of wide availability because there are more than 5000 MRI units in the United State alone (PET is limited to about 50 centers) and it has no associated risks so that it can be used repeatedly in adults and in children.

IV. EEG AND MAGNETOENCEPHALOGRAM (MEG)

A. EEG

EEG recordings provide functional brain information. EEG was first used to make functional brain images of cortical electrical signals in the 1970s when computers allowed the integration of simultaneous EEG recordings from multiple electrode sites and interpolation among sites. Early EEG images displayed EEG parameters (e.g., alpha, beta, theta waves) interpolated across the surface of the cortex using from 8 to 16 electrode sites. The placement of the electrodes was standard, using head landmarks, and each person's data was fit to a standard brain outline, pioneering many of the techniques subsequently applied to PET and MRI. The pattern of EEG activity over the cortical surface could be displayed from task to task, millisecond by millisecond and, as computers became more powerful, these displays even could be shown in real time. Evoked potentials (EP), a special EEG technique that averages EEG to specific stimuli over many trials, also can be displayed as an image using the same interpolation methods. One of a number of early methods to display such images was Brain Electric Activity Mapping (BEAM). Spatial resolution for EEG and

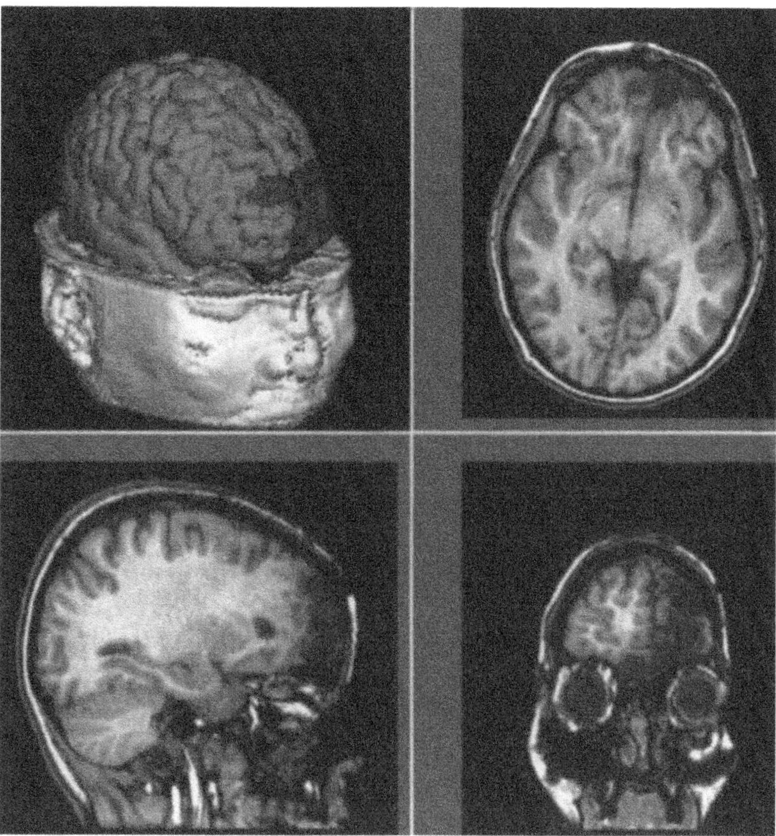

Figure 6 Structural MRI. Reconstructions are shown in one head injury patient with brain damage (dark areas) to the frontal lobe, especially in the right hemisphere. The upper left shows a 3-dimensional view, the upper right shows an axial view, the lower left shows a sagittal view and the lower right shows a coronal view. (Courtesy of Dr. Erin Bigler.)

EP images depend on the number of electrode sites. The more sites, the more accurate the interpolations among sites. Arrays of more than 100 electrodes currently provide the best spatial resolution. Time resolution is millisecond by millisecond, essentially real time, and far exceeds all other functional imaging techniques. EEG and EP also are relatively inexpensive and logistically easy to use. There is no restriction for repeated testing in adults or children. The spatial resolution with more than 100 electrode sites is similar to PET but only the cortical surface is shown most accurately. There are advances in computing the possible deep brain sources for cortical signals. Gevins and colleagues have pushed EEG and EP methods to their limits for describing complex temporal topographic patterns of electrical activity during sensory, motor, and cognitive tasks (see Fig. 8).

B. MEG

MEG uses supercooled detectors (SQUID—superconducing quantum interface device) to measure the extremely weak magnetic fields produced by the electrical activity in the brain that results from neurons firing. MEG can localize the source of these fields and provide functional images showing these sources as they change from one task or state to another. As an adjunct to EEG and EP mapping, MEG gets below the cortical surface and can map the entire brain, although best results come from cortical areas. Like fMRI, MEG results are typically coregistered on structural MRIs. Currently, MEG is limited to only a few centers worldwide; it is expensive and difficult to use. Hari and colleagues have published extensively on MEG and sensory activations.

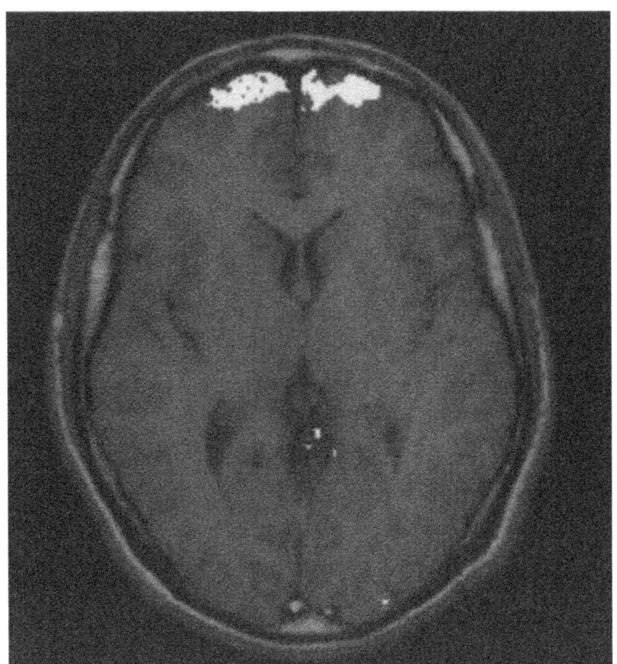

Figure 7 Functional MRI. The white areas show blood flow increases when this subject counted backward by 2s compared to resting. The functional information is superimposed on a structural MRI.

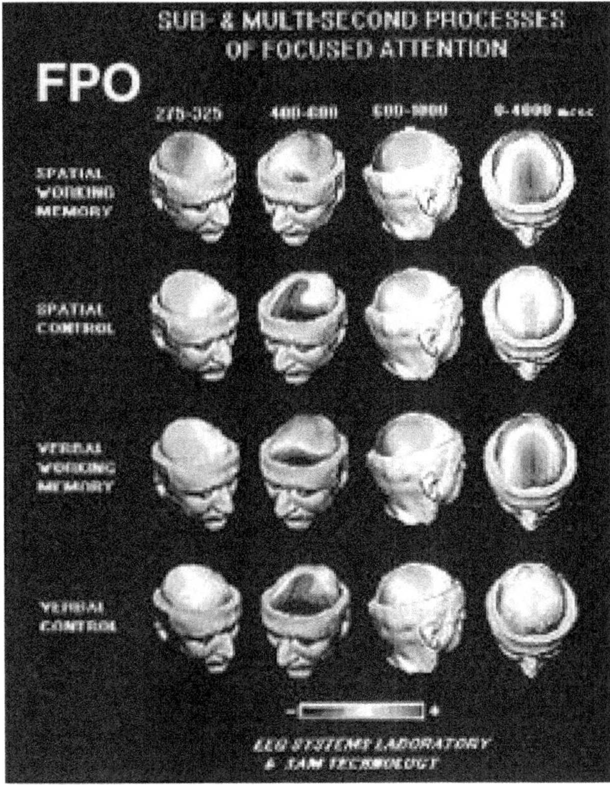

Figure 8 EEG measures from multiple electrode sites in four time ranges during four psychological tasks are displayed as cortical regional patterns of activity. This demonstrates the millisecond time resolution of this imaging technique. (Courtesy of Dr. Alan Gevins.)

V. NEUROIMAGING FINDINGS AND NORMAL BRAIN FUNCTION

Xenon blood flow, EEG, and CAT scan images have been used to characterize normal and abnormal brains for more than 30 years. PET research on normal brain function began about 1980 when controls were studied for comparisons to various brain disorders like schizophrenia and Alzheimer's Disease. For the last 10 years, many PET studies have studied only normal subjects performing a variety of tasks for the purpose of understanding normal cognition. Functional MRI has been used for this purpose only in the last few years but the use of fMRI is growing dramatically as more and more psychologists and neuroscientists gain access to study language processing, attention, reasoning, personality, emotion, learning and memory. Currently, many cognitive researchers and neuropsychologists favor fMRI or PET over topographic EEG, mostly because the latter is more limited to cortex assessment rather than whole brain, despite the temporal resolution superiority. MEG is the least available to researchers. Although the study of normal and abnormal cognition with neuroimaging complement each other, the focus of this review is on a relatively few recent findings in normals to give the flavor of how brain imaging is advancing our knowledge of cognition in key areas.

A. Language

One of the first cognitive areas studied with PET in normals was language processing. Researchers at Washington University, St. Louis, reported a number of subtraction comparisons between elemental language processing tasks and regional cerebral blood flow using the O15 method. In a classic study by Petersen and colleagues in 1989, normal subjects were imaged while viewing words, listening to words, speaking words, and generating words. Using the pixel-to-pixel subtraction technique, cerebral blood flow during each of these conditions was compared (e.g., listening minus viewing, speaking minus listening, generating minus speaking). Each task activated a distinct set of brain areas, demonstrating both that elemental cognitive tasks are somewhat localized and that the salient brain areas are organized into networks that underlie specific mental operations. One major goal of current research is to establish further the nature of these networks. Another goal is to understand disorders of language, especially in children. The radioactivity used in PET has limited functional imaging research in children but fMRI can be used without this concern.

B. Learning

Some PET studies in normal volunteers suggest that GMR decreases after learning a complex task, suggesting that the brain becomes more efficient, perhaps in learning what areas not to use for good performance. Other PET studies show a shift in the pattern of GMR use after learning, suggesting that different brain areas become involved. Some fMRI studies suggest that learning increases the size of the cortical brain area used during a task, suggesting that adjacent neurons are recruited to the effort. At this point, brain imaging studies of learning are preliminary and not completely consistent. Children with learning disabilities or attention deficit disorder have not been studied extensively, although a number of fMRI projects are underway. Even at this early stage of research, the results indicate the enormous potential for further work to help understand brain mechanisms of learning.

C. Memory

A large number of recent studies with PET and fMRI are providing evidence that, just as for language processing, memory involves localized areas organized into networks for specific functions. Imaging studies of normals show that some memory tasks activate the hippocampus, a part of the temporal lobe known to be important for various memory functions. PET studies of Alzheimer's Disease confirm lower activity in temporal lobe/hippocampal areas. In combination with genetic testing, functional imaging of these areas may have potential as an early screening for Alzheimer's Disease. Other memory studies address frontal lobe involvement. For example, Tulving and associates have advanced the idea that functional imaging results indicate that the left prefrontal cortex is more related to retrieval of semantic information and encoding novel aspects of it into episodic memory; the right prefrontal cortex is more related to retrieval of episodic memory. Other work by Cahill and colleagues published in 1996 has reported correlations between GMR in the amygdala while subjects watch an emotional video and recall of the emotional information three weeks later. Interestingly, in this study, there was no mean difference in amygdala GMR between the emotional and neutral conditions, but the correlation technique showed significant correlations between amygdala GMR and subsequent memory in only the emotional condition. In general, memory research, like language processing research, benefits from an extensive empirical literature that is the basis for sophisticated theories which support testing explicit hypotheses about the brain with neuroimaging. This allows relatively rapid progress on basic issues as well as generating new hypotheses.

D. Reasoning/Intelligence

Brain theories about the basis of high level reasoning and problem solving are not so advanced. Neuroimaging studies in this area are more exploratory. For example, in 1988 Haier and colleagues published a PET study of GMR in normal volunteers while they performed a difficult test of abstract reasoning, the Raven's Advanced Progressive Matrices (RAPM). The RAPM is a standard test that requires the subject to solve 36 problems, each one comprised of a series of nine symbols arranged in a pattern. One symbol, however, is always missing from the pattern. Once the subject understands the pattern, the missing symbol can be selected from eight possible choices. Scores on the RAPM are highly correlated with IQ. Surprisingly, this study found an inverse relationship between RAPM scores and brain GMR. The subjects with high RAPM scores (i.e., good performance) had lower GMR, especially in the temporal lobe. This was interpreted as evidence that the efficiency of brain energy use was more important for good cognitive performance on this complex task than the level of GMR. Whether brain efficiency involves task strategy, mental effort, characteristics of individual neurons, or other parameters has yet to be determined. Other PET research also reports inverse relationships between performance on complex tasks and brain function. A study of mild retardation and Down Syndrome reported by Haier and colleagues in 1995 showed higher brain GMR in both groups compared to matched controls. They speculated that a failure of normal developmental neural pruning could be the basis for a person having too many synaptic connections and redundant brain circuitry resulting in inefficient problem solving, low IQ, and high GMR. Standard score images for each retarded subject revealed considerable heterogeneity of GMR patterns. In the same study, MRI was used to measure brain volume. For the combined samples of mildly retarded, Down Syndrome, and controls, there was an inverse relationship between GMR and IQ and an inverse relationship between GMR and brain volume. There also was a positive relationship between brain size measured by MRI and IQ, consistent with many other studies. Clearly, the use of brain imaging to study complex reasoning in humans has potential for elucidating the biological basis of problem solving and individual differences in intelligence. At this stage, sophisticated theoretical formulations for hypothesis testing are awaiting the accumulation of additional empirical observations.

E. Sleep and Consciousness

Several PET studies have addressed patterns of GMR changes during REM and non-REM sleep. During dreaming, GMR is about the same as during the awake state but during deep non-REM sleep, whole brain GMR is down about 40% compared to the awake state. Other PET studies by Alkire and colleagues of anesthetic agents show even larger whole brain decreases during unconsciousness induced by propofol and by isoflurane. Moreover, the pattern of regional GMR decreases in propofol anesthesia suggests the biggest decreases are in brain areas rich in GABA receptors. This is an example of using neuroimaging to help discover possible mechanisms of action for specific drugs. Moreover, these data tentatively support a theory relating whole brain GMR reduction to loss of consciousness rather than a theory of a specific consciousness control center. Further imaging/anesthesia studies hold great promise for helping to establish the neural basis for consciousness and unconsciousness.

F. Aging

Chugani and colleagues have published several PET studies of children and young adults that show that GMR increases in most brain areas from birth to ages 3 to 5 years and then slowly decreases through about age 20. This pattern parallels the pattern of changes in synaptic density previously demonstrated in autopsy studies. Other imaging studies suggest continued small decreases in whole brain GMR with increasing age beyond 20 years but these data are not consistent among all studies. Grady and colleagues used PET blood flow imaging and reported in 1996 that normal aging appears associated with shifting or compensatory activation in various brain systems for some specific cognitive tasks. For example, during a face-matching task where young and old subjects performed the same, older subjects had more activation in frontal cortex and other areas than younger subjects. Whether this pattern is related to regional brain atrophy or other structural parameters is not yet known. Imaging studies with very large sample sizes are required to examine the various aspects of aging, cognition, and brain function.

G. Sex Differences

A number of brain structural differences have been noted between men and women in studies using structural imaging. Recent functional imaging with PET has yielded inconsistent results with some studies showing women having slightly higher brain metabolic rates than men but other studies showing no differences. Most of the studies addressing this issue were done in a resting condition. Task activation imaging studies published in 1995 show some intriguing male/female differences. For example, Shaywitz and colleagues studied language processing using fMRI. They found blood flow increases in specific frontal lobe areas during phonological processing in males; but in females, areas of increased activation were more diffuse. Haier and Benbow matched men and women for average or high mathematical reasoning ability in a PET study. Mean GMR did not differ much between any of the four groups but there were significant correlations between temporal lobe GMR bilaterally and mathematical reasoning scores in the men; there were no GMR/math score correlations in the women for any cortex area. More studies with large samples and a variety of tasks need to be done.

VI. CONCLUSIONS

A. Interpretation Issues

Even these brief descriptions of a few neuroimaging studies demonstrate the potential for new understandings of the brain. Brain images of structure and function are compelling glimpses into complex relationships. The most sophisticated neuroimaging techniques, however, are no more sophisticated than the research designs and methods that make use of them. High-resolution functional brain imaging is only as good as the psychological tasks used to probe or stimulate brain areas. A simple approach of finding brain areas activated by a simple task is a good start but is still simple. Tasks can also deactivate areas or circuits. Brain activation may also indicate excitatory or inhibitory activity. That is, when inhibitory cells are activated, GMR or blood flow will increase in that brain area although the effect of the increased inhibitory firing is decreased activity somewhere along the circuit. Moreover, the functional relationships among brain areas may be more important than specific areas alone. Even the range of activity within a brain area may be related to the range of task performance during which the activity was measured. This recognition of individual differences may produce additional surprising results when incorporated into research designs to augment standard group comparisons.

B. Future Advances

New neuroimaging studies can use increasingly sophisticated research designs incorporating levels of cognitive ability (e.g., bright and average subjects), task strategy alternatives (e.g., chunking or not chunking memorized items into categories), easy and hard versions of tasks (i.e., low and high mental effort), and a variety of tasks to probe specific brain areas and systems. The combination of neuroimaging techniques in the same subjects, even simultaneously, also promises to advance research. Structural MRI, for example, now is essentially necessary for exact anatomical localization irrespective of the functional technique used. Functional MRI and MEG results routinely are displayed on structural MRIs. In the future, neurosurgeons and researchers may use virtual brains created from a variety of imaging procedures to explore the relationships between structure and function as computer models of cognition generate responses to test stimuli. In the near future, human PET studies using different radiolabels and using drugs to manipulate brain state during task conditions will help discover which neurotransmitter systems are related to specific sensory, motor, and cognitive performance. Neuroimaging studies have already begun to bridge the gap between animal experiments and human studies because animal studies can provide specific hypotheses for human testing. Neuroimaging technology will likely advance our abilities to test hypotheses in ways beyond the scope of our current theories. These abilities will drive new theories of how the brain works normally and how it fails when it is broken.

BIBLIOGRAPHY

Alkire, M. T., Haier, R. J., Barker, S. J., Shah, N. K., Wu, J., & Kao, J. (1995). Cerebral metabolism during propofol anesthesia in humans studied with PET. *Anesthesiology, 82:* 393–403.

Bigler, E., Yeo, R., & Turkheimer, E. (Eds.). (1989). *Neuropsychological function and brain imaging.* New York: Plenum Press.

Buchsbaum, M. S. (1996). Neuroimaging: PET and the averaging of brain images. *American Journal of Psychiatry, 153*(4), 456.

Cahill, L., et al. (1996). Amygdala activity at encoding correlated with long-term, free recall of emotional information. *Proceedings of the National Academy of Sciences, vol. 93,* 8016–8021.

Gevins, A., Leong, H., Smith, M. E., Le, J., & Du, R. (1995). Mapping cognitive brain function with modern high-resolution electroencephalography. *Trends in Neurosciences, 18*(10), 427–461.

Haier, R. J. (1993) Cerebral glucose metabolism and intelligence. In P. A. Vernon (Ed.), *Biological approaches to the study of human intelligence.* Norwood, NJ: Ablex Publishing Co.

Haier, R. J., et al. (in press). Brain imaging and classification of mental retardation. In Soraci & McIlvane (Eds.), *Perspectives on fundamental processes in intellectual functioning.* Norwood, NJ: Ablex Publishing Co.

Petersen, S. E., Fox, P.T., Posner, M., Mintun, M., & Raichle, M. (1989). PET studies of the processing of single words. *Journal of Cognitive Neuroscience, 1*(2): 153–170.

Phelps, M. E., Mazziotta, J.C., & Schelbert, H. R. (1986). *Positron emission tomography and audoradiography.* New York: Raven Press.

Posner, M., & Raichle, M. (1994). *Images of mind.* Scientific American Library. New York: W. H. Freeman & Company.

Roland, P. E. (1993). *Brain activation.* New York: Wiley-Liss. John Wiley & Sons, Inc.

Shaywitz, B. A., et al. (1995). Sex differences in the functional organization of the brain for language. *Nature, 373,* 607–609.

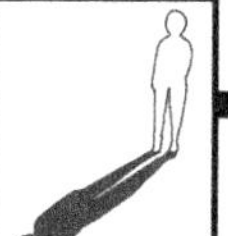

Child Sexual Abuse

Kathleen Coulborn Faller

University of Michigan School of Social Work

Analogue Studies Research studies, involving staged events (e.g., a visit to a stranger in a trailer) or naturally occurring events (e.g., a medical exam) in children's lives that have some characteristics in common with situations of sexual abuse. Researchers then question children in a variety of ways, some of which may involve attempts to manipulate children or to contaminate their responses, and draw parallels between their responses in these experiments and memory and suggestibility regarding allegations of sexual abuse.
Cognitive Distortions Rationalizations (in the case of sexual abuse) of sexual acts that are considered abusive; another term used for this phenomenon is "thinking errors."
Criminal Sexual Conduct Sexual acts that are crimes, with penalties of incarceration, probation, and parole. These acts either are nonconsensual or involve minors or others unable to give informed consent (developmentally disabled individuals; persons under the influence of alcohol or drugs). These acts are usually subcategorized in terms of degree, with first degree being the most serious.
Incest Sexual activity between two people related by blood.
Polygraph A lie detector test. It relies on measures of autonomic system arousal, usually heart rate, breathing rate, and galvanic skin response. Autonomic arousal is supposed to be associated with lying, but this has not been empirically demonstrated. The polygraph has high rates of false negatives and false positives and is inadmissible in most court proceedings.
Plethysmograph A means of measuring erectile response, using a strain gauge that encircles the penis. It is used in some sexual abuse treatment programs to measure changes in arousal to various sexual stimuli.
Prognosis Prospects for improvement. In the case of mental health treatment, it refers to appropriate response to therapy.
Sequelae Consequences or effects. In the case of sexual abuse, these are sexual and nonsexual behavioral and affective symptoms.
Statutory Rape Consensual sexual activity between a child who is below the age of consent (14 to 16, depending upon the state) and an adult. The activity usually involves sexual penetration.

CHILD SEXUAL ABUSE is an important mental health issue, and one characterized by significant advances in the last 20 years, with continuing developments and refinements. However, it is also a very controversial issue. In part, the controversy can be understood in light of the emotional dilemma sexual abuse creates. On the one hand, we assume that to sexually abuse a child is to engage in monstrous behavior with devastating consequences. On the other hand, we find it virtually impossible to believe that an adult would behave so reprehensibly toward a child. Thus, allegations of sexual abuse evoke the competing reactions of rage and denial. In some respects, these

Copyright © 1998 by Academic Press.
All rights of reproduction in any form reserved.

reactions are manifested in the quandary of whether to believe the child or believe the offender. Often this dilemma is heightened because the child is reticent in disclosure, and the offender is insistent and persuasive in denial.

The goal of this article is to enlighten this controversy and put the problem of sexual abuse in perspective, relying upon existing knowledge about sexual abuse. In fact, child sexual abuse is common, may have many manifestations—from horrendous acts to those that differ in degree from acceptable behavior, and results in a spectrum of *sequelae*—from pervasive to negligible.

In this article, sexual abuse will be defined, its prevalence and incidence addressed, its impact described, and professional interventions discussed. These interventions include child protection investigation, mental health assessment, treatment, and prevention.

I. DEFINITION OF CHILD SEXUAL ABUSE

For an event to meet the definition of child sexual abuse, there should be a victim, an offender, and a sexual act. Characteristics and subcategories of each component of the definition will be discussed in this section. In addition, the variability in definitions employed in both research and clinical practice will be noted. Finally, situations that are regarded as "gray areas" will receive attention.

A. Child Victim

Child victim status is defined primarily by age. However, there is some variability in what is considered the upper age limit. Research definitions, legal definitions, and treatment definitions of child victims may differ in their determination of when adult status or informed consent begins. Legal definitions of the upper age limit may differ by state and by statute (e.g. statutory rape, incest, criminal sexual conduct statutes). Also, some researchers have used a lower maximum age for boys than for girls. The maximum age used in research for girls is generally 16 or 18, but some researchers have used a maximum age of 12 for boys. Interesting assumptions about gender underlie this differential. This lower age seems to be based upon assumptions that boys are more capable of protecting themselves than girls and more desirous of sexual activity than girls. Hence boys' sexual experiences during adolescence that otherwise meet the definition of sexual victimization may not be considered abusive by researchers and others.

Research findings indicate that victims are fairly evenly distributed across the age span of childhood, that is preschoolers, latency-aged children, and adolescents. Diagnosis is more difficult for preschoolers because of their less well-developed communication skills and concerns about their suggestibility. Nevertheless, because of increased awareness of sexual abuse, allegations involving younger and younger children are coming to professional attention. Thus, there are cases involving the sexual abuse of infants.

For the relationship to be considered abusive, there usually is an age differential between the victim and the offender, the victim generally being at least 5 years younger than the offender, and 10 years younger when the victim is an adolescent. However, based upon her research of 930 women, Diana Russell pointed out that acts can be abusive without the age differential; for example, a brother may be only 3 years older than his sister, but still can impose his will for sexual activity upon her. A gray area is how to handle a situation of what appears to be consensual sexual activity between a teenager and a significantly older person, for example a 14-year-old girl and a 30-year-old man, or a 13-year-old boy and a 25-year-old woman.

More girls are reported than boys as victims, boys constituting one-fifth to one-third of cases, depending upon the source of the statistics. Although girl victims remain the majority, the proportion of girl victims is higher in intrafamilial cases than in extrafamilial ones. Thus, girls may be more vulnerable to family members, such as fathers, stepfathers, uncles, and grandfathers, and boys at relatively greater risk from persons in the community, such as coaches, boy scout leaders, and adolescents whom they admire.

Professionals who work with boy victims believe there is a greater failure to disclose sexual victimization by boy victims than by girls. This differential reporting is thought to be related to more support for girls, in the process of their socialization, to talk about their problems than for boys, and the fact that boys must overcome not only the taboo of sexual activity with an adult, but usually the taboo associated with homosexual activity, when they disclose.

B. Offender

A sex offender may be a male or female, although the vast majority are males, between 85 and 99% depending upon the study. As awareness of sexual abuse grows, so does the proportion of female offenders identified. Generally, offenders are adults or adolescents. A gray area in definition is how to classify latency-aged or even younger children who are sexual predators. Although many of these children are "abuse reactive," that is, maladaptively coping with their own sexual victimization by sexually accosting sexually naive or younger children, a substantial minority of child predators have not been sexually victimized. Some researchers and clinicians characterize them as "children with sexual behavior problems" to avoid stigmatizing them as sex offenders. Nevertheless, the acts they perpetrate may be quite serious.

There is some controversy about offender motivation, for example, some individuals asserting that the offender is motivated by a desire for dominance, not sexual gratification. Sexual abuse, like any sexual act, may fulfill a variety of needs, including the assertion of power, but what differentiates it for other exercises of power is its sexual content.

For some offenders (pedophiles), their preferred sexual object is a child, while other offenders experience and act upon sexual arousal to children because of a range of circumstantial factors. These factors include the availability of a child, the absence of an adult sexual partner, and an assault on the offender's self-esteem, such as a divorce or employment loss. Nevertheless, an initial act because of circumstances appears to enhance risk for subsequent sexual abuse to children. The proportion of sexual offenders who prefer children to those who do not is not known, but it is generally assumed that pedophiles are the minority. However, on average they have a greater number of victims.

C. Abusive Acts

Sexual abuse involves the full spectrum of sexual activity. These acts are designated and illustrated in Table I.

Table I Sexually Abusive Activities

Activities	Examples
1. Noncontact behavior	
A. Exposure	A. A coach wore his sweatpants low in front, with his penis hanging over the top, during girls' gym practice.
B. Voyeurism	B. A stepfather drilled a hole in the bathroom wall so he could observe his daughter toileting and bathing.
C. Lewd and lascivious talk	C. A mother told her son she wanted to suck his penis.
2. Fondling/sexual contact	2. A mother's boyfriend rubbed a 7-year-old girl's genital area on top of her panties while they watched *Pocahontas*.
	2. A 15-year-old brother grabbed his little sister's hand and placed it on his penis, saying "rub it."
3. Oral–genital contact	
A. Fellatio	A. A camp counselor cornered a 10-year-old boy in the shower and put his penis in the boy's mouth.
B. Cunnilingus	B. A grandfather bit his granddaughter's vagina.
C. Analingus	C. A 6-year-old boy described how it tickled when his friend's father "licked his butt."
4. Digital penetration of the vagina or anus	4. A 6-year-old girl said her brother's friend put a finger in her peepee and it hurt.
5. Penile penetration of the vagina or anus	5. A 4-year-old boy said, "Uncle Jimmy poked me in the butt and it stinged."
6. Sexual exploitation	
A. Child prostitution and	A. Sisters, aged 4 and 5, were fondled while naked, by men who were strangers and their pictures were taken. Their mother
B. Child pornography	B. Received money from the men.

This list of sexual acts progresses from the least intrusive and therefore possibly least traumatic to the most intrusive and possibly most traumatic. However, the judgment regarding trauma is from a professional perspective, not from a child's. Victims may have a different perception. Most clinicians and some researchers include noncontact behaviors—exposure, voyeurism, and lewd and lascivious remarks, in the definition of abusive acts. Activities that do not involve the adult in the sex acts directly, such as prostituting a child or using the child in pornography, are also subsumed under the definition.

II. THE EXTENT OF SEXUAL ABUSE

How widespread is the problem of child sexual abuse? We know about its extent from studies of prevalence and reported incidence. Both sources of information tell us sexual abuse is experienced by large numbers of children. How serious a problem is false allegations? Making this determination is more difficult, but there is some useful research. Prevalence, incidence, and the issue of false reports will be discussed in this section.

A. Prevalence of Child Sexual Abuse

The term, prevalence, is used to refer to the proportion of a designated population that has a particular problem or characteristic. In the case of sexual abuse, prevalence refers to the number of people who were sexually abused during childhood. Data about prevalence are gathered in retrospective studies of adults. This research may involve face to face interviews, self-administered questionnaires, or telephone surveys. Researchers may ask a single general question, such as "were you sexually abused as a child?" or multiple questions designed to approach the topic from several perspectives and gather information about a variety of relationships and experiences. Findings vary depending upon methodology, with studies using face-to-face interviews and multiple questions yielding higher rates of child sexual abuse. Taking into account the variability in findings, estimates are that, in the general population, between 1 in 3 or 4 women were sexually abused during childhood and between 1 in 6 to 10 men.

B. Incidence of Reported Sexual Abuse

Incidence refers to the number of reports of a particular phenomenon, usually occurring during a circumscribed time frame. In the United States, there are governmental and nongovernmental initiatives to gather incidence data on child sexual abuse.

Illustrative of governmental efforts is a provision in the Child Abuse Prevention and Treatment Act of 1974, which requires that the federal government collect annual statistics on reports of child maltreatment received by local Child Protection Agencies. These data include reports of child sexual abuse. Over the 20 years this information has been collected, there has been a steady increase in reports of child abuse and neglect, and a fairly steady increase in the proportion of sexual abuse cases among reports. According to the National Committee for the Prevention of Child Abuse (NCPCA), sexual abuse cases constitute about 11% of cases currently reported—in 1995 almost 350,000 cases. Currently, approximately one-third of reports are substantiated after investigation by Child Protective Services (CPS), or about 110,000 cases of child sexual abuse annually.

Although the number of cases from the CPS reports is considerable, a study of 1000 parents conducted by the Gallup Poll in 1995 yielded a projection 10 times larger, of one million children sexually abused during the previous year. Part of the reason that the Child Protective Services number is lower is that CPS only concerns itself with situations in which a caretaker is the abuser. Most extrafamilial sexual abuse cases are not handled by CPS, but by law enforcement. However, the higher number in the Gallup Poll projection likely also indicates a substantial number of cases do not come to professional attention. Moreover, even the Gallup Poll figure is probably a low estimate because parents would be unlikely to report themselves if they were sexually abusing their children, and they might even be reluctant to report relatives and friends.

C. False Allegations of Sexual Abuse

The modest substantiation rate noted in the discussion of NCPCA findings raises the question of false allegations. Why are so many more cases being reported than are being substantiated? Does this mean that two-thirds of the reports made are false? It does not. There are many reasons that a case may not be substantiated, other than that someone made a false claim of sexual abuse.

In studies conducted at the Kempe National Center on Child Abuse and Neglect, a very small proportion of unsubstantiated cases were determined to be false allegations, altogether about 5%. Another interesting finding is that adults are more likely to make false reports of sexual abuse to children than are children. The largest proportion of unsubstantiated cases involved "insufficient information." Illustrative would be situations in which the child protection caseworker could not locate the family, or the child refused to talk to the caseworker. The next largest proportion were "legitimate cause for concern, but no sexual abuse." In these cases, reporting was appropriate, but some more plausible alternative explanation for the source of concern about abuse was found. An example might be a case in which the source of the child's advanced sexual knowledge was observing adults engaging in sexual activity. This is not to say that false allegations are nonexistent. They do exist, but research to date indicates that true reports are very much more common.

III. EFFECTS OF CHILD SEXUAL ABUSE

The impact of sexual abuse depends upon many factors: the offender–victim relationship, the particular sexual act(s), the frequency and duration of the sexual abuse, the nature of inducements to participate and admonitions regarding disclosure, the response of nonabusive caretakers to disclosure, and the personality and personal history of the child. Research documents that the most important element in the child's recovery is having a caring and concerned, nonoffending parent. Thus, being believed and supported makes a great deal of difference in the long-term well-being of the victim.

Clinicians and researchers generally divide the effects of sexual abuse into sexual and nonsexual effects. These sexual and nonsexual emotional and behavioral impacts of sexual abuse also serve as indicators of its likelihood, when professionals are making a determination about whether a child has been sexually abused.

A. Sexual Sequelae

William Friedrich, a clinician and researcher at the Mayo Clinic, has played a leadership role in cataloging the sexual effects and researching differences in the rates of sexualized behaviors in children with and without a history of sexual abuse. Table II is drawn from version 3 of Friedrich's Child Sexual Behavior Inventory (CSBI).

Table II Items from the Child Sexual Behavior Inventory

1. Dresses like the opposite sex.
2. Stands too close to people.
3. Talks about wanting to be the opposite sex.
4. Touches sex (private) parts when in public places.
5. Masturbates with hand.
6. Draws sex parts when drawing pictures of people.
7. Touches or tries to touch mother's or other women's breasts.
8. Masturbates with toy or object (blanket, pillow, etc.).
9. Plays with a friend.
10. Touches another child's sex (private) parts.
11. Tries to have sexual intercourse with another child or adult.
12. Puts mouth on another child's/adult's sex parts.
13. Touches sex (private) parts when at home.
14. Touches an adult's sex (private) parts.
15. Touches animals' sex parts.
16. Makes sexual sounds (sighs, moans, heavy breathing, etc.)
17. Asks others to engage in sexual acts with him or her.
18. Rubs body against people or furniture.
19. Puts objects in vagina or rectum.
20. Tries to look at people when they are nude or undressing.
21. Pretends that dolls or stuffed animals are having sex.
22. Shows sex (private) parts to adults.
23. Tries to look at pictures of nude or partially dressed people.
24. Talks about sexual acts.
25. Kisses adults that they do not know well.
26. Gets upset when adults are kissing or hugging.
27. Overly friendly with men he/she does not know well.
28. Kisses other children he/she does not know well.
29. Talks flirtatiously.
30. Tries to undress other children against their will (opening pants, shirts, etc.).
31. Eats breakfast.
32. Wants to watch television or movies that show nudity or sex.
33. When kissing, he/she tries to put his/her tongue in other person's mouth.
34. Hugs adults that he/she does not know well.
35. Shows sex (private) parts to children.
36. Tries to undress adults against their will (opening pants, shirts, etc.).
37. Is very interested in the opposite sex.
38. Puts his/her mouth on mother's or other women's breasts.
39. Knows more about sex than other children their age.
40. Other sexual behaviors (please describe).

Sexualized behavior is the most common impact of sexual abuse, but according to Friedrich's research, it is present in only about 40% of children with a history of sexual abuse. Friedrich and his colleagues have assessed for the presence of sexualized behaviors separately for males and females and for children from ages 2 to 6 and 7 to 12 years. Preliminary data are available from research on version 3 of the CSBI. Children with a history of sexual abuse were compared to children from psychiatric and normal populations. Children with a history of sexual abuse rank higher than children in the other two groups on total score for sexualized behavior (sexually abused, 14.2; psychiatric population, 3.45; normal population, 3.5). In addition, 22 of the 40 items differentiate children with a history of sexual abuse from the other two groups, regardless of age and sex. These items are numbers 6, 8, 10–12, 17–19, 21, 23–28, 30, 32, 33, 35–37, and 39.

B. Nonsexual Symptoms of Sexual Abuse

Nonsexual symptoms are less definitively linked to sexual victimization because they are more likely than sexual symptoms to derive from other experiences and traumas. For example, while such behavioral and emotional symptoms can come from being sexually victimized, they can also be the result of physical abuse, neglect, divorce, auto accidents, or natural disasters. Nevertheless, Table III lists nonsexual symptoms and, where relevant, their possible relationship to subgroups of victims.

Table III Psychosocial Symptoms of Sexual Abuse: Nonsexual Behavioral and Emotional Indicators of Distress

1. **Sleep disturbances**
   - A. Night waking
   - B. Nightmares
   - C. Night terrors
   - D. Refusal to go to bed (in some cases, because it is the site of the sexual abuse)
   - E. Refusal to sleep alone
   - F. Inability to sleep
2. **Toileting disturbances**
   - A. Previously toilet trained (more common in young victims)
     - 1. Enuresis
     - 2. Encopresis
   - B. Refusal to go into the bathroom (in some cases, because it is the site of the sexual abuse)
   - C. Smearing feces (more common in very disturbed victims)
   - D. Hiding feces (more common in very disturbed victims)
3. **Eating disturbances**
   - A. Anorexia (characteristic of adolescent girl victims)
   - B. Bulimia (characteristic of adolescent girl victims)
4. **Avoidant reactions**
   - A. Fear of the alleged offender
   - B. Fear of persons of the same sex as the alleged offender
   - C. Refusal to be left alone
   - D. Fear of particular places that may be associated with abuse
5. **Somatic complaints**
   - A. Headaches (associated with nondisclosure)
   - B. Stomach aches (associated with nondisclosure)
   - C. Pelvic pain (may be related to affect or injury)
6. **Behavioral problems**
   - A. Firesetting (more characteristic of boy victims)
   - B. Cruelty to animals (more characteristic of boy victims)
   - C. Aggression toward more vulnerable individuals (younger, smaller, more naive, retarded individuals)
   - D. Delinquent behaviors (characteristic of older victims)
     - 1. Incorrigibility
     - 2. Running away (may be an adaptive response to avoid the offender)
     - 3. Criminal activity
   - E. Substance abuse
   - F. Self-destructive behaviors (characteristic of adolescent girl victims)
     - 1. Suicidal gestures, attempts, and successes
     - 2. Suicidal thoughts
     - 3. Self-mutilation
7. **School problems**
   - A. Inattention
   - B. Sudden decline in school performance
   - C. School truancy
8. **General disturbances of affect**
   - A. Low self esteem
   - B. Anxiety
   - C. Fear
   - D. Anger
   - E. Dissociation
   - F. Posttraumatic stress disorder

Caveat: A determination of sexual abuse cannot be made based upon the presence of these factors alone; however when noted in conjunction with sexual indicators and other positive findings, they increase the likelihood of sexual abuse.

The array of possible impacts is considerable. However, not every child is seriously affected. In fact in a 1993 survey of 45 comparative studies of the impact of sexual abuse, Kendall-Tackett, Williams, and Finkelhor found that about a third of the victims of child sexual abuse were reported to be asymptomatic. In addition, about two-thirds of children showed recovery during the first year to year-and-a-half after the abuse. Although children with a history of child sexual abuse had more symptoms than both clinical and nonclinical comparison groups—fear, PTSD, behavior problems, sexualized behaviors, and low self-esteem being the most frequently noted, no single symptom characterized the majority of children.

IV. INTERVENTION IN CHILD SEXUAL ABUSE

Awareness of the extent of sexual abuse and its effects on functioning have led to positive outcomes. First, the problem of child sexual abuse is being taken seriously. The time has passed when sexual abuse was regarded as a problem of insignificant proportions and an experience that was not very harmful. Second, the fact that there are mechanisms for reporting child maltreatment is illustrative of government and social policy commitment to address the problem of child sexual abuse, and child maltreatment more generally. Third, with reporting statutes has come greater professional and public awareness of child sexual abuse. Professionals are more likely to consider sexual abuse as a possible source of children's symptoms, and children's caretakers and others are more likely to notice symptoms. Moreover, media attention to sexual victimization has made the public more cognizant of the problem and may serve to decrease victims' sense of isolation.

In addition, there have been refinements in how governmental and mental health systems address child sexual abuse. In part, because of controversies about the truth of children's assertions about their sexual abuse, there have come advances in expertise in case investigation and assessment, the development of sexual abuse specific treatment programs, and efforts to prevent sexual abuse before it happens.

Crucial to long-term child well-being is sensitive and well-orchestrated intervention. If professionals can effectively investigate, evaluate, and ameliorate in situations of sexual abuse, children can survive their victimization and lead productive lives. The advances in assessment and treatment of child sexual abuse will be described in this section.

A. The Child Protection System (CPS)

Each state has a Child Protection System, whose responsibility includes investigation and intervention in all cases of child maltreatment involving children's caretakers. These investigations take place at the local, usually county level, and are conducted by child protection caseworkers. This response is structured to be immediate, and the involvement of CPS short term. Child protection caseworkers act as case managers and are supposed to refer children and families to ongoing therapy and other services. Not all of these caseworkers have mental health or competent, on the job training; their case loads are usually high; and the availability of treatment and other services may be limited. Consequently the promise of the Child Protection System is greater than the delivery.

B. Mental Health Assessment

In addition to CPS investigations, mental health professionals in a variety of contexts have become involved in the assessment of sexual abuse allegations. The goals of these mental health assessments are several: determining the likelihood of sexual abuse, making recommendations about child safety, proposing treatment plans, predicting *prognosis* for response to treatment, and assisting in legal intervention. With regard to the final goal, because sexual abuse is not only a mental health problem, but also a crime, mental health professionals may assist in litigation to protect children, to criminally prosecute alleged offenders, and to exact civil damages in cases involving sexual abuse.

There are a number of models for mental health assessment of possible sexual abuse. For example, models can involve the child alone, the child and other family members, and the offender alone. The appropriate model depends on the goals of the assessment, the nature of the child–alleged offender relationship, and the age and functioning of the child. Sensitive and careful assessments assist the child and others affected by the allegation in seeing the assessment process as health promoting rather than traumatic.

A somewhat unique characteristic of sexual abuse assessments for mental health professionals is the importance of determining whether an event (sexual abuse) occurred. Mental health skills need to be adapted and expanded to address this requirement. Mental health professionals must usually engage in direct inquiry about sexual abuse with the child and others, using nonleading questions. A variety of child interview questioning protocols have been developed to guide evaluators. One example is shown in Table IV.

Evaluators employing this protocol are urged to use open-ended questions (found at the top of the continuum) and only to resort to more close-ended questions when open-ended ones do not assist the child in communicating his/her experience. For example, if a child does not respond to a focused question, "Are there things you like about your grandpa?" the mental health evaluator might ask a multiple choice question, "Does he ever do special things with you, buy you things, or do any other nice things you can think of?" The more open-ended the question, the more confidence the mental health evaluator should have in the child's response and visa versa. However, both *analogue studies* and clinical research indicate most children require direct or focused questions to disclose sensitive material. If information is elicited using a close-ended question, the interviewer should follow this disclosure with a more open-ended question. Leading questions and coercion are inappropriate for use in an evaluation of a child for sexual abuse.

Table IV A Continuum of Questions for Assessment of Possible Sexual Abuse

Question type	Example
Open ended	More confidence
1. General question	1. Why did you come to see me?
2. Focused question	
A. People	A. What kind of a guy is your dad?
B. Body parts	B. Did you ever see a penis?
C. Circumstances of abuse	C. Tell me everything you remember about daycare?
D. Circumstances of prior disclosure	D. Did you tell your mom something happened?
3. Follow-up question	
A. Narrative cue	A. What happened next?
B. Repeat disclosure	B. You said he touched you?
C. Clarification	C. He touched you where?
D. Details of abuse	D. What did that touching feel like?
E. Details of context of abuse	E. Do you remember where this happened?
4. Multiple choice	4. Did it happen before or after Christmas or both?
5. Direct question	5. Did your daddy put his peepee inside?
6. Leading question	6. Your mom makes you suck her breast, doesn't she?
7. Coercion	7. You can't leave until you tell me what happened.
Close ended	Less confidence

Other special features of sexual abuse assessments include the following: Mental health professions should gather information on past and current history of the abuse allegation and of the people involved. Collaboration with other professionals, for example, examining physicians, child protection caseworkers, police officers, and lawyers, is integral to such assessments. The mental health professional must be able to clearly articulate criteria he/she uses in determining the likelihood of sexual abuse. In a review of such decision-making strategies in 1995, Faller found 12 sufficiently elaborated to be discussed. The criteria shown in Table V are found in these decision-making strategies.

An interesting and somewhat surprising finding from Faller's review was the number of mental health professionals who endorsed medical findings as an important factor. This is interesting because, of course, medical evidence is not gathered by mental health professionals. Furthermore, most cases of sexual abuse have no medical findings. The other items endorsed by the majority of mental health professionals were criteria derived from child interviews, specifically details about the sexual abuse and details about the context of the abuse.

C. Treatment

Mental health professionals assume that every sexually abused child deserves and needs treatment. And in fact, children who are victims of sexual abuse are more likely to receive treatment (from 44 to 73% of them receiving treatment, according to Finkelhor and Berliner) than are victims of other types of child maltreatment.

Table V Criteria Included in Guidelines for Decision Making about Sexual Abuse

1. **Child interview information**
   - A. **Sexual abuse description from the child**
     1. Detail about the sexual abuse
     2. Child's perspective evident in the description of abuse
     3. Advanced sexual knowledge for the child's developmental stage
   - B. **Offender behavior description, as described by the child**
     1. Use of inducements to participate in the sexual activity
     2. Admonitions not to tell about the sexual abuse
     3. Progression of abuse from less to more intrusive sexual acts
   - C. **Information about the context of the sexual abuse**
     1. Idiosyncratic event
     2. Where the abuse occurred
     3. When the abuse occurred
   - D. **Emotional reaction to the abuse by the child**
     1. Affect consistent with the abuse description
     2. Affect related to the offender
     3. Recall of affect during abuse
     4. Reluctance to disclosure
   - E. **Child functioning**
     1. Competency
        - a. Cognitive test results
        - b. Recall of past events
        - c. Ability to differentiate the truth from a lie
        - d. Ability to differentiate fact from fantasy
        - e. Child is not suggestible
     2. Child is motivated to tell the truth
     3. Consistency of the child's accounts
     4. Feasibility of the events the child describes
   - F. **Structural qualities of the child's account**

2. **Information from other sources**
   - A. **Child's behavior in other contexts**
     1. Statements to others about the abuse
     2. Nonsexual behavioral and emotional symptoms
     3. Sexualized behavior
     4. Evidence of advanced sexual knowledge
   - B. **Offender characteristics**
     1. Overall functioning
     2. Results of *polygraph*
     3. Results of *plethysmograph*
     4. Psychological test results
     5. Evidence of other victims
     6. Confession/admission
   - C. **Family**
     1. Information related to nonoffending parent
     2. Marital functioning and family functioning
     3. Family history of abuse
   - D. Other
     1. Medical findings
     2. Police evidence
     3. Witnesses

Treatment of child sexual abuse may only involve the child, the child and his/her family, or the offender and sometimes the offender's family. The relationship of the victim to the offender will usually have an impact on the structure of treatment. However, in intrafamilial sexual abuse, the offender's prognosis also affects whether his treatment will prepare him/her for some level of future contact with the child. Because of space limitations, the focus in this article will be on child victim treatment.

A variety of theoretical frameworks related to treatment and rehabilitation are being used in victim treatment, including psychodynamic, play therapy, cognitive behavioral, and eclectic, drawing upon psychodynamic, behavioral, and family systems frameworks. However, one thing they have in common is that they dictate a direct focus on the abuse in the course of treatment. For example, it is not recommended that the therapist merely focus on the child's self-esteem or avoidance of men without addressing the underlying cause of these problems, the experience of sexual abuse. [*See* BEHAVIOR THERAPY; COGNITIVE THERAPY; PSYCHOANALYSIS.]

A variety of treatment modalities are employed, the most common being individual, group, and family therapies. These may be employed concurrently or in progression, depending upon the structure of the treatment program, the functioning of the child, and the treatment issues being addressed. [*See* FAMILY THERAPY.]

Common treatment issues for victims are fears and phobias associated with the sexual abuse, the inability to trust adults, altered body image, guilt and responsibility associated with the abuse and its aftermath, anger because of the abuse, sexualized behavior, a need to understand aspects of the sexual abuse experience, and personal boundary and prevention issues.

A number of treatment manuals and descriptive writings have been developed that propose the structure of the treatment and even provide specific exercises to address treatment issues. These are geared to children at different developmental stages, and some have been especially developed for boys.

Illustrative of treatment manuals is one developed by Mandell and Damon for group treatment of 7- to 12-year-old sexually abused children. It includes guidelines for group membership selection and a rationale for group treatment. It also contains 10 modules and provides topics and exercises for each module. Issues covered in the curriculum are shown in Table VI.

Outcome studies of treatment efficacy for victims of sexual abuse are just beginning to be conducted. In 1995, Berliner and Finkelhor provided a summary of 29 treatment outcome studies. All of these treatments lasted less than a year and most were treatment of a few weeks. These studies demonstrated that children who receive treatment for sexual abuse improve, but only 5 studies demonstrated that it was the therapy, itself, rather than, for example, the passage of time, that led to the children's improvement.

In providing appropriate treatment, the mental health professional must consider the nature of the abuse, the child's age and functioning, the offender–victim relationship, and the impact and symptomology. The treatment approach and modality should take into account the child within his/her context and should be of sufficient length to address the child's treatment issues and symptoms. A systematic way of measuring the child's functioning before and after treatment is advisable. The child may need to return to treatment as subsequent developmental stages raise new concerns about past abuse and when new crises and traumas reactivate issues related to the sexual abuse.

Table VI Treatment Issues Developed by Mandell and Damon

1. Learning to trust others, beginning with other members of the group.
2. Identifying feelings (e.g., proud, special, jealous, worried, embarrassed, ashamed).
3. Telling the secret (i.e., disclosing the sexual abuse).
4. Feelings related to sexual abuse (e.g., betrayal, shame, guilt, responsibility, secrecy, protectiveness, helplessness).
5. The effect of sexual abuse on the victim, caretakers, and the family unit.
6. Recovery from sexual abuse.
7. Rebuilding and enhancing self esteem.
8. Protecting oneself in the future from sexual abuse and other harms.
9. Preparation for puberty.

V. PREVENTION OF SEXUAL ABUSE

Prevention of sexual abuse can be conceptualized as encompassing the following endeavors: (1) community and professional education; (2) prevention programs targeted at specific populations; and (3) prevention programs targeted at particular institutions.

A. Community and Professional Education

The Federal Statute that defines Child Protective Services (The Child Abuse Prevention and Treatment Act) restricts its federal grants for child abuse and neglect prevention and treatment services to states that provide education about child maltreatment (among other provisions). This provision is aimed at identifying maltreating families so that abuse can be stopped and its causes and effects ameliorated. However, because such education must define child maltreatment, it puts the community and professionals on notice about inappropriate forms of behavior toward children and, by doing this, can prevent some instances of child maltreatment, including sexual abuse.

Awareness of the unacceptability of child sexual abuse that derives from education also may serve as a deterrent for potential offenders. Some potential offenders may actually be ignorant about what sexual abuse is. In addition, it is fairly common for actual offenders to engage in "*cognitive distortions*" or rationalizations of their behavior. Examples might be telling themselves that because the behavior does not involve penile penetration, it is not abuse, or because the child is too young to understand, the abuse will not be harmful. It is possible, therefore, that potential offenders could be deterred and actual offenders could be led to cease sexual abuse by information that, for example "just touching" is abuse.

In addition, some potential offenders might be deterred by knowledge of the consequences of getting caught, information that could come from education. This might be professional education, community education, or information reported in the media. Although the media have provided some misinformation in their coverage of sexual abuse, they also have been the source of news stories that could have a deterrent effect, could lead to reporting of cases by victims or others, and could help victims feel less stigmatized and alone.

Another way education can be preventative is by causing earlier reporting of cases. That this is happening is suggested by changes in the types of cases that are being reported. In the 1950s and 1960s the clinical literature suggested that the modal case was one of an adolescent, who disclosed in the course of family conflict or after marital dissolution. Statistics from the most recent National Incidence Study, which gathers data on cases of child maltreatment coming to the attention of professionals, indicate that the children ages 3 through adolescence are at relatively equivalent risk for being identified as victims of sexual abuse.

B. Prevention Programs Targeted at Specific Populations

The dominant approach to prevention of child sexual abuse has been to rely on victims to avoid potentially abusive situations, to resist attempts to victimize them, and to report attempted and successful sexual abuse. This approach has been summarized as "say no, yell, and tell." Sexual abuse prevention programs have been developed for and delivered to children from preschool age through adolescence. Most are delivered in school settings. Some programs involve classroom teachers and parents. There were initial concerns by program designers about program content because of the sensitivity of the topic and anticipated parental resistance. Because of this, many programs focused on "stranger danger" and avoided addressing the possibility that the offender could be, and in fact was much more likely to be, someone known to the child. Presently, many programs are imbedded in broader "personal safety" programs that address a variety of risks children may encounter. These include safety when crossing the street and riding a bike, physical abuse, bullying, and kidnapping.

These prevention programs have been the targets of considerable criticism. First, and justifiably, they have been criticized for making the child responsible for prevention. This especially is an issue with preschoolers. There have been concerns that the victims will not be successful at saying no, resisting, and yelling help and then will blame themselves if they are unable to protect themselves. Critics have queried, "Why not target the offenders rather than the potential victims?" Better still, programs in high school aimed at potential parents and potential perpetrators might be more efficacious.

Prevention supporters counter these arguments as follows: If children receive this training as children, they will not victimize children when they become adolescents and adults. Further, supporters state that the fact children receive this kind of training may inhibit offenders from trying to abuse them. Offenders will fear children are on guard.

Second, prevention programs have been criticized because of their impact on the recipients. Specifically, there are worries that the programs may engender fear and cause trauma. Moreover, they may create a gulf between children and important adults in their lives because these programs put children on notice that adults, even those closest them, may not be trustworthy. In addition, prevention programs have been criticized as the source of some false allegations of sexual abuse. However, outcome studies indicate that only a very small minority of children experience an elevation in anxiety because of participation in prevention programs. No empirical support has been found for the assertions that prevention programs result in fears of caretakers or generate false allegations of sexual abuse.

Third, prevention programs have been challenged for their lack of effectiveness. For example, children may not understand all of the concepts they are being taught; may not be able to use the concepts to defend themselves; and may soon forget what they have learned. These criticisms have especially been leveled at preschool programs. Prevention program supporters reply that critics are expecting too much of the programs. These programs should be one of several approaches to preventing sexual abuse. Moreover, it is unrealistic to expect a program of an hour or even of several hours over time, to have a lasting or lifetime effect. Regular, periodic doses of prevention that occur at least on a yearly basis are what is needed.

Although prevention programs are far from a panacea, they can be beneficial. Finkelhor and colleagues recently conducted a national telephone survey of youth and their parents related to these programs. This study was funded by the Boy Scouts of America and intended to address some of the above noted criticisms. Using a representative sample of 2000 young people, ages 10 to 16, these researchers found that about 70% had participated in a prevention program, 36% in the past year. Younger children were more likely to have participated in the previous year. The vast majority of both the youth and their parents rated the programs positively and 26% of youth reported using some of the skills they had learned. Girls, African American children, and children from lower socioeconomic status families rated programs more positively.

C. Prevention Programs Targeting Particular Institutions

With the growing awareness of the problem of child sexual abuse has come an appreciation that certain institutions are vulnerable. That is, they may attract adults with a sexual interest in children. These persons are drawn to these institutions, sometimes because they naively find children's company preferable, without any awareness of their sexual attraction to children, but other times with the clear knowledge they are looking for prey. Both types of adults choose vocations and avocations that afford them ready access to children. These include jobs in day care centers, positions as boy scout and cub scout leaders, volunteer assignments as big brothers and big sisters, work as camp counselors, employment in recreational programs for youth, religious vocations such as the priesthood or the ministry, work in group homes for trouble youth and in residential treatment programs, and positions as foster parents.

Compared to prevention programs that target children, those in vulnerable institutions have been slow to develop. Generally they have been inspired by the surfacing of scandalous cases. As a rule, these prevention programs include five components: (1) screening for potential pedophiles; (2) prevention material that is delivered to children in these institutions; (3) educational material provided to adults in the institutions; (4) rules that reduce risk; and (5) procedures for investigating complaints.

Since these institutions either rely on volunteers or pay staff modestly, their reluctance to take on the issue of sexual abuse and develop prevention programs is understandable. Nevertheless, the importance of prevention in these contexts cannot be overstated. The majority of youth affected in these institutions are males, and boy victims are more likely than girls to respond to the trauma of sexual abuse by victimizing others. Therefore, preventive interventions in these institutions can have far-reaching impacts, because of the number of children they can save and the number of perpetrators they can stop.

VI. CONCLUSION

Although child sexual abuse is a common and serious mental health problem, it is not unmanageable nor unspeakable. Prevention programs and early identification can decrease the extent of sexual abuse and ameliorate its impact. Impressive progress has been achieved in the last 20 years. Despite present challenges to children describing sexual victimization, adults recalling abuse during childhood, and mental health professionals who attempt to assist child victims and adult survivors, the prospects for further progress in preventing and treating child sexual abuse are good.

BIBLIOGRAPHY

Executive summary of the third National Incidence Study (NIS-3). Washington, DC: USDHHS, National Center on Child Abuse and Neglect.

Faller, K. C. (1996). *Evaluating children suspected of having been sexually abused: APSAC Study Guide.* Newbury Park, CA: Sage Publications.

Finkelhor, D., & Berliner, L. (1994). Research on the treatment of sexually abused children. *Journal of Child and Adolescent Psychiatry, 34(11),* 1408–1422.

Finkelhor, D., & Dziuba-Leatherman, J. (1995). Victimization prevention programs: A national survey of children's exposure and reactions. *Child Abuse and Neglect: The International Journal, 19(2),* 129–141.

Friedrich, W. (1993). Sexual victimization and sexual behavior in children. *Child Abuse and Neglect: The International Journal, 17(1),* 59–66.

Gil, E., & Johnson, T. C. (1993). *Sexualized children.* Rockville, MD: Launch Press.

Jones, D., & McGraw, M. (1987). Reliable and fictitious accounts of sexual abuse to children. *Journal of Interpersonal Violence, 2,* 27–45.

Kendall-Tackett, K., Williams, L. M., & Finkelhor, D. (1993). Impact of sexual abuse on children: A review and synthesis of recent empirical studies. *Psychological Bulletin, 113(1)*, 164–180.

Mandell, J., & Damon, L. (1989). *Group treatment for sexually abused children*. New York: Guilford Press.

Saunders, B., & Williams, L. (Eds.). (1996). Special section: Treatment outcome research. *Child Maltreatment 1(4)*, 293–352.

Wurtele, S., & Miller-Perrin, C. (1992). *Preventing child sexual abuse: Sharing the responsibility*. Lincoln, NE: University of Nebraska Press.

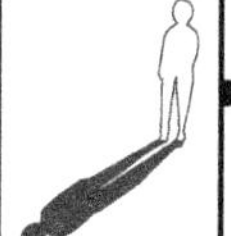

Classifying Mental Disorders: Nontraditional Approaches

Theodore R. Sarbin
University of California, Santa Cruz

Ernest Keen
Bucknell University

Contextualism A worldview that requires taking into account the entire context in which actors' behavior takes place. For human beings, the context is largely symbolic and languaged so that one must consider the meanings that persons assign to aspects of their worlds.
Discourse Analysis Analysis of the verbal and nonverbal communication contexts within which meanings of the world and its events and objects are constructed.
Historical Act The root metaphor of contextualism, the basic concept for interpreting conduct as addressing the world in its narrative flow, thus assuming a past and anticipating a future.
Internality A characteristic of traditional diagnostic language that locates the crucial context for understanding the causes of conduct as internal to the actor, tending to neglect other contexts.
Mechanistic A worldview for understanding conduct in terms of the properties of machines, such as the transmission of energy.
Narrative The story, implicit or explicit, that contextualizes and gives meaning to human conduct; the story may be idiosyncratic but most often is borrowed from the stock of stories that comprise a culture.
Nosology A classification system of diseases assumed to be discrete entities, such as tuberculosis or measles.
Root Metaphor The basic concept, often implicit, of a particular worldview that facilitates some interpretations of the world and forecloses others. The machine and the historical act are root metaphors for, respectively, the mechanistic worldview and the contextualist worldview.
Strategic Actions Intentional acts performed by a person directed toward solving identity and existential problems.

Classifying for purposes of research or intervention is a feature of the scientific method. Traditional methods for CLASSIFYING MENTAL DISORDERS emerged from 19th century advances in the biological sciences basic to the science and practice of medicine. Underlying such advances was the explicit adoption of the world view of mechanism, the root metaphor of which was the transmittal of forces. In this context, physicians constructed systems for classifying organic disease. These systems provided the model for traditional psychiatric diagnostic and classification systems.

Nontraditional classification systems flow from an alternate worldview—contextualism, the root meta-

Copyright © 1998 by Academic Press.
All rights of reproduction in any form reserved.

phor of which is the historical act in all its complexities. Instead of relying on the medically inspired concept of psychopathology, nontraditional practitioners speak of "unwanted conduct." This practice explicitly recognizes that a moral judgment is being made on the strategic actions that people employ to solve their problems in living. In the nontraditional method described in this article, classification is not of disease processes but of interactional strategies and the conditions that influence the success or failure of such strategies.

I. INTRODUCTION

As a preamble to an article on alternate ways of classifying mental disorders, we point to a built-in source of ambiguity. The use of the construction, "mental disorders," together with the phrase "mental health" in the title of the encyclopedia, reflects an implicit acceptance of a particular worldview from which the traditional approaches to classification are generated. The use of the word "mental" implies an assured and nonproblematic ontological status for the concept of mind, notwithstanding the many critiques of the concept, and by the claim that "mind" is an exemplar of the human tendency to transfigure a metaphor to a literal entity. Lost in the history of lexicography is the recognition that at one time mind was a verb, useful for talking about silent and unseen actions, such as thinking, imagining, and so on.

For the most part, the traditional approach treats "mind" as a literal entity, often as a quasi-organ parallel to the brain, or as an epiphenomenon arising from the workings of the brain. In actual practice, mental health professionals do not deal with "minds," but with persons whose actions fail to meet a particular society's standards of propriety or fail to meet self-imposed standards. It is an illusion that therapists aid in reconstructing "minds," although they may be instrumental in modifying beliefs and values, in reinforcing strategies for managing interpersonal relations, in changing habits, and in acquiring self-knowledge.

"Disorders" is also an unsettled concept. The term implies a departure or deviation from "ordered" conduct. It is important to note that the supraordinate concepts "ordered" and "disordered" (staples of mental health and mental illness doctrines) are derived from a particular worldview, probably unrecognized by the vast majority of mental health workers. The worldview is that of the machine, the root metaphor of which is the transmission of forces. Being "in order" or "out of order" (disordered), although apt constructions for describing the condition of a clock, a motor, or a computer, are misleading when applied to the acts of human beings. As a descriptor for unacceptable conduct, "disorders" is derived from traditional practices for classifying absurd or unwanted conduct—such practices being consistent with the mechanistic worldview that the "mind" operates like other machines—as a vehicle for the transformation of forces.

Related to the mechanistic conception of order is another implicit meaning of "disorder." The concept of "social order" grew out of the belief in an orderly universe. Thus, "disorder" is applied to violations of the normative expectations for human conduct in everyday life. Shared constructions of the social order supply the context within which conduct may be classified as mentally disordered, deviant, nonconforming, abnormal, inept, or improper. Further, the shared constructions provide the background for legitimating interventions such as hospitalization, incarceration, or other systematic effort to restore order to the social group the equilibrium of which has been disrupted by the conduct of the "disorderly" or "disordered" person.

II. THE PURPOSES OF CLASSIFICATION

Behind any classification system is one purpose or more that provides the basis for distinguishing and defining categories. In Western culture, classifications of "mental disorders" have been designed to serve the purposes of the science and practice of medicine: (1) to select and guide treatment and (2) to facilitate research. In medical science, classifications are employed as a means of identifying diseases. For historically documented reasons, the classification of unwanted conduct has followed the patterns laid down by medical science for classifying organic disease. In regard to treatment, there are marked differences in the goals of treatment of measles and treatment for unwanted conduct (such as phobias). For measles, the ministrations of the doctor are in the service of providing a *cure*. For the person seeking help to control unwanted conduct, "cure" may be a less apt term than one that describes helping an individual to achieve his or her purposes in ways that are less objectionable to relevant others or more acceptable to oneself.

Medical research also explores the causes and treatments of diseases. Knowledge of treatment efficacy depends on research. However, in order to conduct research, particular instances must be located in classes in order to process data from a collection of similar cases. The literature of psychiatry and clinical psychology is replete with research reports that are indeterminate because traditional classification by "disorders," which, like diseases, are categories based on "symptoms," has not been sufficiently reliable nor valid.

If we add to treatment another purpose of classification, prevention, then examining the contexts that influence persons to engage in unacceptable conduct will influence the choice of categories for distinguishing among kinds of unwanted behavior. Such a move in the purpose of classification would require abrogating pretensions to being "objective" and value-free. The problem with the value commitments that attend the notion of "disease" is not that they are value commitments, for example, that the patient is not responsible for behavior "caused" by some internal happening. Any intervention into the life of another person engages a value commitment. The problem rather is that practices based on the notion of "disease" or "disorder" follow from the profession's commitment to a counterproductive set of values that positions the person as without agency.

III. THE TRADITIONAL APPROACH TO CLASSIFICATION

To write about nontraditional ways of classifying persons whose conduct fails to meet contemporary standards of propriety requires that we first lay out the boundaries of traditional classification systems the better to show contrasting features. We take as the prime exemplar of traditional classification systems the *Diagnostic and Statistical Manual of Mental Disorders,* Fourth Edition, published by the American Psychiatric Association, with the most recent edition (hereinafter referred to as *DSM-IV*) published in 1994. *DSM-IV* provides a detailed nosology, a critical analysis of which opens the door to an understanding of the underlying worldview that guides the practice of classifying deviant conduct. The claimed purpose of the nosology is to provide a means of establishing reliable diagnoses. [*See* DSM-IV.]

A. The Mechanistic Conception of Unwanted Conduct

The history of science makes clear that the mid-nineteenth century witnessed tremendous progress in the science of biology. This progress was directly related to the mechanization of biology. All biological phenomena were to be explained in terms of the mechanistic transmission of physical and chemical forces. Scientific explorations sought principles that were invariant. During this period medical doctors took on the task of explaining abnormal behavior by extrapolating from the findings of the rapidly developing field of neuropathology. The context for this development was the surface resemblance of symptoms of neuropathology to unwanted conduct for which no neuropathology could be found. During this period Emil Kraepelin formulated his initial classification of psychiatric diseases, a classification that assumed all abnormal behavior to be related to organic causes, even in the absence of organic signs and symptoms. "Organic" and "functional" were the terms of convenience to identify whether or not neuropathology was demonstrable. The remote influence of the ideology that influenced Kraepelin's formulations can be deduced from the explicit claim in *DSM-IV* that "nonorganic" mental disorders have a biological basis.

The mechanistic framework inherited from Kraepelin creates serious problems for professionals engaged in the therapeutic enterprise. First, *DSM-IV* continues to manifest only marginal reliability, in spite of Herculean efforts by its creators. Second, the validity of the categories all too often fails traditional scientific tests and settles for negotiation and consensus among professionals. And third, the tendency to expand both the number of diagnoses, as well as the number of criteria, yields a continuing expansion of the category "mental disorder" into what might, from a less mechanistic point of view, be seen as the necessary travails and tragedies of everyday life. (The first *Manual,* published in 1952, listed 106 categories. *DSM-IV* lists 357 diagnostic categories.)

Beginning with the question of reliability, it has

been convincingly demonstrated that the accumulation of more categories and more criteria adds only marginally to the reliability of diagnostic practice. The self-advertised theoretically neutral "descriptive" character of diagnostic language may minimize unproved explanatory hypotheses, but it can yield no more agreement among practitioners than the language it uses to describe persons or behavior. For example, the stipulation that something must have been present for "at least 6 months" offers precision in a fairly trivial way compared to the difficulties of reliably assessing whether a set of actions is "disabling" or "not disabling." No behavior exists as simply disabling or not disabling, independent of the social and psychological context, most of which is beyond the specifiable stipulations of diagnostic manuals.

Marginal reliabilities compromise research by including in samples persons whose conduct is heterogeneous but who are lumped together into diagnostic categories. More serious is the questionable validity of diagnostic categories in the course of selecting treatment programs. Traditional classification manuals fail to deal with the question of whether a "mental disorder" exists apart from a culturally specific context—whether, in other words, the label for a disorder names a part of nature that is independent of the social constructions of clinicians and the authors of diagnostic manuals. The controversy of a quarter century ago, whether homosexuality is a "disorder," is not an exception in its clear dependency on normative judgments and negotiations that occur in a historical and cultural context. Most unacceptable conduct, even if reliably identified, is "disordered" only in terms of a culturally relative standard. Cross-cultural research has shown no consistency across cultures in the use of traditional diagnostic categories, for example, "schizophrenia." It is unclear whether this lack of consistency indicates different social constructions by clinicians or different causal antecedents. Professionals are not justified in construing that the meaning of a set of behaviors in one culture is the same in another culture, in the same way that diabetes in one culture is the same in other cultures.

Finally, in addition to the expansive and fluid character of the catalogue of disorder through its five editions, the *Manuals*' tendency to medicalize all human discomfort inspires even more questionable logic. The latest such version is the creation of "shadow syndromes," which are formulated to legitimate treatment for persons whose conduct fulfills only some of the *Manual*'s criteria for a disorder. Extrapolating from the proliferation of diagnostic entities over the various editions of the *Manual,* one might predict that through the typical negotiation process of the experts, some of these syndromes will come out of the shadows and enter the next version of the *Manual* as certified "disorders."

IV. THE CONTEXTUALIST CONSTRUCTION OF DEVIANT CONDUCT

But there are practitioners and scholars who operate from a different worldview, namely, contextualism—a worldview the root metaphor of which is the historical act in all its complexity. Novelty and change are features of this alternative worldview that provides the foundation for a nontraditional approach to the classification of intentional actions. Historical acts are engaged in by people. Further, historical acts are narrated, told as accounts, anecdotes, and stories in which men and women make choices to resolve their everyday problems of living. Because contextualists construct the world in terms of historical actions, they look for *reasons* for such actions, unlike the mechanistically inclined clinician who would look for *causes*.

The contextualist worldview directs us to see human beings not only as biological specimens, but as agents, as doers, as performers and problem solvers. In so doing, we are perforce obliged to develop understandings of how human beings employ narrative structure to shape their life histories.

A. Happenings and Doings

Completely overlooked in the constructions of traditional psychiatric classification is a simple distinction, that of *happenings* and *doings*. Examples of happenings are ruptured spinal discs, toothaches, brain tumors, and carcinoma. Such happenings are attributable to causes, empirically established or hypothesized. As exemplified in *DSM-IV,* abnormal actions are caused by happenings—the transmission of forces in the brain or in the metaphorical mind. Neurotransmitters, phrenological bulges, chemical anomalies have been sought as the causes of abnormal behavior. The diagnostic drama guided by traditional classification has no room for the client as agent, as doer, as capable of intentional action.

On the other hand, doings are the agential, intentional, purposeful actions of persons attempting to participate in a drama based on their self-defining narratives. Slapping a child, seeking a mystical experience, declaring that one is host to multiple personalities, avoiding a confrontation, are examples of doings, of actions.

The distinction between happenings and doings is helpful in understanding how the traditional diagnostic system and its vocabulary of symptoms has contributed to the medicalization of distress. In the absence of a strong competitor, the language of the medical model was embraced by neighboring professions to describe unwanted conduct. To refer to an action as a "symptom" is to adopt a special linguistic system. The use of "symptom" carries the implication "symptom of something." The "something" is a happening that is the presumed *cause* of the symptom—in traditional medicine, a microbe, a tumor, a morphological anomaly, a toxin, a chemical imbalance, and so on.

The application of the mechanistic worldview with its emphasis on causal happenings has worked well in organic medicine. A perusal of *DSM-IV* makes clear that the model was adopted in its entirety by modern biological psychiatry. The *Manual* is explicit in proclaiming that the diagnosis and treatment of "mental disorders" belong to the domain of medical practice.

Classifications of any kind must follow from some articulated theory. Although the authors of *DSM-IV* claim to being atheoretical, it is apparent that the claim is a veiled cover for a weakly defined theoretical system that is reminiscent of Kraepelin's mechanistic framework, that is, that all deviant conduct is caused by anomalies in organic systems. On this framework, *DSM-IV* fails because of the large proportion of cases for which no biochemical or other organic substrate can be found.

B. Unwanted Conduct

We employ "unwanted conduct" rather than "psychopathology" to emphasize the moral judgmental component of diagnosis. Every society creates procedures and practices for marginalizing persons whose public actions fail to meet propriety norms. Beginning in the mid-nineteenth century, the responsibility for controlling such marginalized persons was assigned to physicians practicing in institutions variously named mad houses, lunatic asylums, and mental hospitals. The criteria for detention included atypical imaginings ("hallucinations"), nonconforming beliefs ("delusions"), and incomprehensible or absurd gestural or speech behavior. Behind these criteria were implicit premises about maintaining public order. Authority figures (parents, police, magistrates, and doctors) made the initial judgment whether any particular item of conduct was to be classified as unwanted. Those whose nonconforming behavior was under scrutiny were labeled as mad, insane, lunatic, crazy, and more recently, mentally ill.

In the twentieth century, the scope of psychiatric practice included diagnosing and treating men and women who were self-referred. Not regarded as mad or insane, such self-referred patients sought help from medical doctors on the belief that they were suffering from ill-defined but nonetheless genuine "nervous" ailments. Hysteria was the diagnostic label employed to denote a wide variety of such "nervous" conditions. In due course, clinicians sorted the presenting complaints into a number of classes identified by labels derived from Greek or Latin roots, such as neurasthenia, psychasthenia, anxiety, hypochondriasis, and depression. These terms sometimes reflected unwanted "feelings." Persons seeking help for dealing with unwanted "feelings" would verbalize their complaints with vague and ambiguous expressions, such as "I am anxious," "I am depressed," "I can't concentrate," "I'm sitting on a volcano." Taken together, these complaints are subsumed under the general medical term "dysphoria."

Clinicians who subscribe to the medical model regard dysphoric complaints as symptomatic of a bodily dysfunction. It has become common practice among physicians to prescribe medications to reduce the extent of the dysphoria by altering the body chemistry. A radically different approach would be taken by contextualist clinicians who are sensitive to the notion that distress follows from the failure of strategic actions to solve problems of living. The self-reports of distress that are expressed in the language of "feelings" are construed as the patient's sense-making of proprioceptive and interoceptive changes associated with failed strategies to solve existential or identity problems. Contextualist clinicians direct their attention to the *reasons* for the unresolved strains-in-knowing rather than to reports of "feelings" that are adjuncts to personal problem solving. Their focus is on understanding the antecedents of the unsatisfactory attempts at problem solving, or expanding the library of plots for interpreting distress, and on the exploration of alternative strategies for maintaining an acceptable self-narrative.

V. ASSUMPTIONS AND ALTERNATIVES

The difficulties with traditional methods of diagnosis can be specified in terms of four assumptions routinely built into diagnostic manuals (1) internality; (2) physicality; (3) individuality; and (4) the value judgments accompanying the concept of disease. For each of the assumptions undergirding traditional modes of classification, we propose an alternative assumption that is consistent with the contextualist perspective.

A. Internality

The current system envisions each abnormal psychological condition to be a malfunction generated from within the person. In a given situation, one person may behave in accordance with common sense expectations while another may not. The latter will be labeled abnormal, deviant, disordered, disturbed, and so on. The difference between the two cases does not come from the social context that traditional diagnosticians assume to be the same for both. What is taken to produce acceptable conduct from one and unwanted conduct from the other are processes internal to the person.

The most elemental of diagnostic decisions, for example, that of orientation to time, place, and person, depends on this diagnostic procedure borrowed from the standard neurological examination. Like that examination, what is being assessed is assumed to be inside the person. More elaborate diagnostic judgments, such as deciding between "depression" identified as a disease, and "mourning a death in the family," which is not so identified, depend, for example, on sadness in the absence of mourning. Such a judgment influences the traditional clinician to locate the cause of the phenomenon inside the body rather than externally, in human relationships.

It is clear that most human behavior is oriented to concrete immediate situations. Human behavior is jointly produced not only by a person and a situation, but each of these factors also responds to the other over time to create a dialectical whole, such as a relationship. When a relationship contextualizes a behavior, as is always true even in diagnosis, the meanings of any behavior must take into account the dialectical determinants. The complex of avoidant actions identified by the label "agoraphobia," for example, does not exist inside the person. The actions are ways of coping with situations that have developed over time. Nontraditional approaches that depart from the disease model begin with the individual's history of trying various ways to cope with his or her environment. Traditional diagnosis underplays the agential character of human behavior because "diseases" are ordinarily understood to be happenings that take place inside the person.

B. Physicality

The traditional diagnostic system construes a person as a complex biological machine the controlling mechanisms of which are the neurochemical patterns of the brain. Information processing is seen as the central function of the brain, a conception that extends from neural transmissions to perceptions of the environment. This information is selected for its relevance to a given stimulus situation. Such selection is not always without error. The result of acting on mistaken perceptions is conduct that may violate social norms, leading to a psychiatric diagnosis.

Observing a person confounding imaginings, rememberings, and current perceptions, a clinician would invoke the diagnostic label "hallucinating schizophrenic." Or, observing a person confounding irrelevant sad feelings with nonpresent situations, the clinician might entertain the diagnosis "depression." In these instances, information appears to be scrambled, and there is a strong presumption that the brain, as the organ of information processing, is malfunctioning and the unwanted behaviors are thus believed to be caused by chemical imbalances in the brain.

Information, however, is not merely physical. To be sure, information can be reduced to a "signal" that can be described in the vocabulary of physics, but the signal never embodies meaning. In this sense, meaning is not physical but is constructed—the achievement of human beings who have acquired linguistic and epistemic skills. To sustain the premise that abnormal behavior is the product of exclusively physical processes would be like saying that the science of acoustics can reveal to us the meanings carried by human speech. The concepts and theory of sound waves and temporal patterns can tell us about human speech in their own terms, and that is hardly trivial. But scientists who do such work make no claims that their instruments can tell us anything about the meanings of words and sentences, the logic of theory, or the motives of actors who try to communicate with one another. To extend physical science into realms of meanings and motives is to claim too much. It is to persevere in a metaphysical belief that the only reality is the reality of the physical world, a belief that ignores the arguments and demonstrations that realities are social constructions.

C. Individuality

The current system envisions abnormal psychiatric conditions as affecting encapsulated individuals. While cultural differences in the incidence of unwanted conduct are well known, and some patterns of behavior are culturally specific, as anorexia is to modern industrially advanced cultures, the goals of treatment, as well as the interpretation of the problem, rarely extend beyond the distressed individual. Although the stresses of poverty, for example, may increase the incidence of many abnormal conditions, current practice assumes that abnormal behavior happens to individuals independent of social contexts. To take more seriously conditions such as poverty, and to make them medically relevant, one can of course add a note to the diagnostic statement, codified as the marginally salient Axis IV in *DSM-IV.* An impartial examination of demographic data of persons diagnosed as psychopathological would suggest that the mental health professions should advocate as therapeutically relevant such conditions as full employment, adequate welfare safety nets, and a livable minimum wage. But this practice is marginal exactly because taking it seriously would require economic, political, and governmental intervention rather than psychiatric or psychological attention. The entry of the treatment professions into politics would undermine the value-free pretenses of the diagnostic system. Such political involvement, especially since it pretends to be scientific rather than political, runs many risks already revealed to us in the awkwardness of courts of law where psychiatric (diagnostic) testimony becomes a part of society's decision to blame wrongdoers—or to excuse them. The risks already incurred by our diagnostic pretenses to scientific accuracy could stretch wildly the current legitimacy of the treatment professions. There is, of course, no simple solution to these problems, but it is clear they are made much worse by the notion of discrete diseases, some of which traditionally supply an excuse, others of which do not.

Empirically demonstrable is the fact that such socioeconomic variables as poverty can be relevant to diagnosis, a fact that cannot be acknowledged so long as mental illness is seen as an individualistic phenomenon. Behavior that has traditionally been labeled mental illness is hardly a private matter analogous to such patently medical conditions as diabetes or cancer where internality and physicality are demonstrable.

D. Value Judgments Accompanying the Concept of Disease

The current system envisions mental illnesses, like other illnesses, as conditions to be eliminated. Diseases, in our current understanding, rarely have value and meaning beyond that of deserving the most concerted efforts to eliminate them. The more internal, physical, and individual the diagnostic concepts and procedures, the less are abnormal actions perceived as addressing some aspect of a person's effort to position himself or herself in the world of social norms and moral expectations. An individual's complaints of depression and anxiety are not valued for their indexing a struggle with a personal decision or with a moral dilemma. They are merely "symptoms" that, when sufficiently aggregated, indicate a disease, and a disease is to be cured.

Just as the elimination of pain by analgesic drugs may mask a bodily ailment, so may the elimination of anxious or depressed behaviors mask a moral crisis. Furthermore, the individual diagnosed may, on the authority of the mechanistically oriented professional, misinterpret his or her own life narrative as internal happenings. Beyond that, the profession might address the possibilities for preventive measures. It can of course be argued that such a "public health" approach in psychiatry may have to pretend to know with some precision the societal and family conditions that engender contranormative behavior. The parameters of the ideal family or neighborhood or school have yet to be spelled out. The prevailing practice of dealing with instances of human distress as "diseases" removes from the profession any pressure to allocate research resources to filling gaps in knowledge necessary for implementing prevention programs.

VI. DIAGNOSING WITHIN A CONTEXTUALIST FRAMEWORK

A. Early Efforts to Construct a Contextualist Framework

The diagnostic procedures based on Kraepelinian doctrine have been the subject of earlier critical works. During the first four decades of the twentieth century, the Swiss-American psychiatrist, Adolf Meyer, promoted a contextualist view of unwanted conduct. He rejected the idea that the causes of deviant conduct would be discovered with advanced anatomical and histological technology. Instead, he urged his colleagues and students to attend to the whole person in his or her social and cultural milieu. His focus was not on purported biological happenings but on the person's ineptitude in adjusting to his or her life circumstances.

The history of the first half of the twentieth century credits Meyer's contextual approach with having a widespread impact on the direction of American psychiatry. A number of well-known texts promoted Meyer's contextualist views. These texts made use of formulations drawn from the social sciences and the humanities, among them discourse analysis, role-taking, socialization, learning theory, pseudocommunity, overinclusion, and so on.

Meyer's approach had a positive impact on the development of American psychiatry, but his contextualism faded into obscurity when the psychiatric profession enthusiastically adopted psychoanalysis as its quasi-official theory. The displacement of Meyer's contextualist framework by psychoanalytic doctrine may be attributed to the fact that the hydraulic model advanced by Freud was consistent with the mechanistic perspective that was already entrenched in the medical sciences. In addition, Meyer, unlike Freud, had no self-proclaimed disciples, no professional institutes to promote his contextualist formulations, and no organized corpus of writings.

More recent challenges to the validity of the Kraepelinian-inspired *DSM-IV* have been made in critical works by scholars working from contextualist behaviorism and from social psychological orientations.

B. The Narrative Framework

The contextualist model sensitizes the clinician to focus on the master question: "what is the client or patient *trying to do?*" Answers to this question will inevitably be in the form of a narrative that includes the parts played by other actors in the client's drama. The constructed narrative provides clues for a diagnosis in terms of the class of strategic actions employed. The clinician's answer to the master question satisfies the original purpose of diagnosis—namely, to guide the therapist and the client in developing a treatment plan.

Classification for purposes of scientific research should consider the narrative context within which a distressed person is trying to do something. Also relevant to scientific classification is the issue of how the client's narrative fits or fails to fit into the narratives of the client's family, social group, or subculture. Sorting cases into categories to explore differences and similarities requires attention to crucial attributes, including meanings, of the behavior itself. Science cannot ignore these narrative meanings and contexts in deciding whether cases are similar or different.

Unwanted behavior, then, is performed by agents whose purposes are crucial, even if such purposes may not be clear to relevant others or to the agents themselves. The talk, actions, and expressions of feelings that are the results of failed strategies to fulfill the requirements of an ongoing self-narrative are the raw data from which the clinician formulates a diagnosis. This alternative approach assumes that the narrative context must be understood if the puzzling behavior is to be understood. The narrative that guides a particular failed effort must be specified, as well as the fit or lack of fit, between such a narrative and the larger narratives of the social context. Usually, there is a lack of fit, which appears as a violation of norms and values held by social groups and codified in cultural traditions.

The narratives that fit these traditions may be referred to as "conventional," and those that do not, as "unconventional." Those people whose behavior issues from a life-narrative that is incomprehensible or grossly nonconforming become candidates for psychiatric diagnosis. These are not people without self-narratives; they are people with unconventional narratives, and/or an unwillingness to disclose them. For example, it is not comprehensible to most of us how someone might seriously suspect a man's unconventional narrative in which he identifies himself as Jesus Christ. In the case of such a client who is apparently convinced of the authenticity of his claims, diagnosticians have no way to understand this conviction and this narrative except to construct the inference: "the man is psychotic." The logic of that inference is consistent with *DSM-IV* criteria that qualifies the client's claim as a delusion and as sufficiently "bizarre" to assign the diagnosis of schizophrenia (if the belief had been held for 6 months or more).

While this diagnostic term ought scientifically be seen as a *description* of the patient's conviction, it is usually taken as an *explanation*. This elision of description to explanation is one of the outcomes of employing the disease model. It renders unnecessary any understanding of the narrative as a context for unwanted conduct, or understanding the social or moral circumstances that provided the context for the particular narrative. The illicit shift from description to explanation is in great measure responsible for the standard professional practice of ignoring the patient's life story.

However, it is important to note that not all behavior that is subject to professional diagnosis is merely an unconventional narrative. In a case of homicide, a truck driver strangled his wife in the heat of an argument in which she declared she had been unfaithful and was about to leave him for her lover. This threat not only confirmed his prior suspicions, it enraged the client. "I couldn't control myself, I was so mad. The anger inside me had to come out. I exploded." While this case is not one of clinical diagnosis for purposes of treatment, it is one of legal diagnosis for purposes of adjudication. To call him "insane" at the time of the murder would be to say that his behavior was caused by stimuli the provocative power of which controlled his behavior. He himself was helpless, the argument would go (and has gone); his being an agent of his actions would not be considered a factor.

At the same time, we recognize that the man was following a well-known and not unpopular narrative plot of "punishing an unfaithful wife." The narrative does not excuse his behavior, but it makes it intelligible. It collects those circumstantial factors together in a way that, in fact, is how we understand his behavior. It bears on why he did it, when we understand the "why" as searching for reasons, rather than causes.

This kind of contextual understanding does not resolve the question of whether or to what degree the man should be excused for his actions. It certainly avoids the possibility that the extreme behavior was caused by a diagnosable disease. And yet such contextual understanding is absolutely essential in order to understand the action, which, given the circumstances and the stock of cultural narratives about unfaithful wives and angry husbands, is quite easy to understand. This understanding addresses the question of what this man was trying to do. It opens up a psychological investigation of his strategic actions, given a particularly vivid set of circumstances.

This case, like most behaviors that come to professional attention, deals with a struggle in which both social and moral questions abound—questions about what one is to do, who one is to be. Except for behavior that is casual or genuinely accidental, human beings behave in such a way as to work toward achieving their goals, one of which is to be a certain kind of person. Was the truck driver to perceive himself as a cuckold? Was he to perceive himself as a failure in not controlling his wife? He not only wanted to punish her, but also likely wanted to persuade her, and he certainly did not want his manhood challenged.

These themes are congruent with common narratives in certain pockets of society, and they are not without influence. Grasping such meanings is what clinicians must do in order to have any intelligent grasp of clients' conduct. Such interpretive psychological work certainly does not suggest that a disease was the proximate cause of a death, as traditional diagnostic thought could imply. Finding a basis for such interpretive work is the point of the alternative model to which we now turn.

C. Strategic Actions

As an alternative construction to the implicit theory underlying *DSM-IV*—that unwanted conduct is caused by anomalous happenings in the biological machinery—the contextual construction takes its point of departure from the premise that people are agents. They are performers, actors, doers, discourse partners. This premise turns attention to a person's actions, not to postulated happenings in the brain or in the metaphorical mind. The actions of interest are in the service of resolving strain-in-knowing, particularly those actions that give rise to self-judgments or to other-declarations that such actions are unwanted. Strain-in-knowing is a response to conditions that interfere with the continuity of the person's self narrative. These are the conditions that are ordinarily subsumed under the heading of emotional life.

Strain-in-knowing occurs when there is a discrepancy between the demands of emotional life and the actor's current constructions (beliefs and values). An alternate way of formulating strain-in-knowing is the expenditure of effort to locate or position oneself in relation to the world of occurrences. Sometimes identified as anxiety, disequilibrium, threat, or unassimilated input, the center of the concept is "I have a problem."

The implicit and explicit behaviors intended to resolve strain-in-knowing may be called "strategic action." Often intelligible to the actor, strategic actions are not necessarily intelligible to others, for only the actor is the potential beneficiary. In cases we call abnormal, such strategic actions may become habitual and automatic, a condition that makes it difficult for actors to explain their conduct in ways that are intelligible to others. Strategic actions to resolve strain-in-knowing may appear to others as obscure or meaningless, or as potentially dangerous or embarrassing.

It is important to add a disclaimer that strain-in-knowing is not a passive phenomenon taking place in the metaphorical mind. The multifarious behaviors that are traditionally regarded as abnormal or incomprehensible may be parsimoniously classified as phases in the construction of a self-narrative. Whether successful or not, strategic actions in the service of resolving strain-in-knowing become a part of the lived narrative.

We present herewith a brief sketch of a model that derives from various contextualist frameworks. The model returns personal agency to the matrix of constructions that are employed to understand human action. The central feature of the model is a list of "strategic actions" that can serve as the scaffolding for a contextualist classification system. Strategic actions may be classified as follows:

- instrumental acts (including rituals);
- tranquilizing and tension-releasing acts;
- attention deployment acts;
- acts to change beliefs and values;
- nonaction.

These classes of strategic actions are connected to antecedent events and subsequent effects, the latter having a feedback function. Strategic actions are employed to neutralize strain-in-knowing. Any particular strategic act has two potential effects: the first, if successful in satisfying the intentions of the actor, would eliminate or modify the perceived source of strain, the second would provide a relevant audience with opportunities to give warrants of social validation or invalidation for the particular strategic action. In this model, the persons and institutions that enforce values are part of the external world of occurrences. The moral judgments of others are inputs that must be instantiated, matched against the beliefs and values that make up the person's self-narrative.

The antecedent events to strain-in-knowing require no detailed analysis—the cognitive psychology of the 1960s and 1970s has given us a template. The world of occurrences may be sorted into discrete domains or ecologies: the self-maintenance domain, the time–space domain, the social domain, the moral domain, and the transcendental domain. Sensory inputs are also generated within the body, the proximal world of occurrences. Human beings (and other sentient organisms) try to match sensory inputs with their systems of knowledge. In problematic situations, the actor directs his or her efforts to the world of occurrences to gain confirming or disconfirming inputs. During the interval when no match is made, the condition of strain-in-knowing prevails. In short, the actor strives to match the inputs against a construction—a self-narrative—derived from his or her prior experience. Of special interest is the observation that efforts to find a match are not always successful.

The prototype for sense-making is the ethological concept of vigilance. When an animal, human or other, registers inputs through vision, hearing, olfaction, and so on, it tries to match the sensory inputs against its available constructions. In the primeval world, the construction might be represented by the question: Is the stimulus event to be instantiated as benign or hostile? The choice of subsequent actions follows from the type of instantiation.

The problems in living that are the starting places for both traditional and nontraditional professionals are in the social, moral, and transcendental domains.

Positioning oneself in these domains or ecologies involves mapping input against existing constructions, that is, against the beliefs and values that have become part of the actors' ongoing self-narratives. Any particular self-narrative is built up from answers to the social identity question: Who am I? to the moral identity question: What am I in relation to moral standards? and to the transcendental identity question: What am I in relation to such abstractions as God, the universe, departed ancestors, and so on. When inputs from the social, moral, or transcendental domains produce incompatible or conflicting answers to the identity question, the person experiences strain-in-knowing, a condition that involves *effort* to match inputs with existing constructions and/or to seek confirming or disconfirming inputs for putative matches. This is a proactive process. Effort involves physiological participation that produces interoceptive and proprioceptive inputs. These inputs feed back into the proximal world of occurrences, thus, the actor's task includes attending to the additional sensory inputs generated in efforts at sense-making.

The use of strategic actions is not exclusive to people in distress who are the clients and patients of mental health professionals. We are all strategists in order to deal with our everyday strains-in-knowing, in our need to make sense of the welter of inputs from the various domains. It is only when the strategies fail to resolve the strain and/or are not given warrants of validation by significant figures—parents, spouses, teachers, employers, doctors—that the person becomes a candidate for diagnosis and treatment.

Each class of actions has a target: *instrumental acts* are directed to the external world, to change the relations between the person and some aspect of the world of occurrences. Inputs from the social domain, for example, that cannot be matched to one's self-narrative lead to an unvoiced interpretation: my identity is at risk. The person may choose between the traditional fight-or-flight instrumentalities in their many attenuated forms. A particular instrumental act may reduce strain-in-knowing and simultaneously be validated (or invalidated) by persons who have the power to pass moral judgment. The alleged Oklahoma City bombers are said to have constructed a belief that "the government" was evil. They equated a federal building with "the government" and destroyed it. Other citizens engage in less extreme forms of instrumental action: they write letters to their senators or change the relation to the distal domains by withdrawing from social relations, or becoming a hermit. *Ritual behavior* is included in the strategy of instrumental acts because it is mediated by the belief that, like direct action, rituals and ceremonials can influence the world of occurrences.

The *tranquilizing and releasing* strategy is directed toward changing bodily sensations that may be indirect effects of sense making efforts. Alcohol, drugs, sex, hot baths, cold showers, vigorous exercise, and the excitement of gambling are examples of the choices of actions that modify inputs from the internal ecology. The use of the strategy by itself does not certify that one is a candidate for a clinic or a sanitarium. The moral judgment of relevant others on the particular tranquilizing or releasing strategy is the act that identifies the strategy as acceptable or as not acceptable.

Examples of the strategy of *attention deployment* are the acts that are subsumed under such traditional labels as hypochondriasis, conversion reactions, and participation in imaginary worlds. The person's attentional resources focus on inputs other than those from the social and moral domains that are the usual antecedents to strain-in-knowing among humans. A common deployment is to attend to bodily sensations, thus avoiding critical inputs from the social world. A variant of the strategy of attention deployment is involved participation in an invented set of self-narratives, as in classic multiple personality.

Changing one's beliefs and values is a strategy directed to influencing the structure of knowledge. It is the strategy of choice for clinicians who work in the tradition of cognitive psychology. For example, a suicidal client holds the belief that suicide (an instrumental act) will solve his or her problems. The clinician takes on the task of modifying that belief. For example, a sample of women who held suicidal beliefs repudiated such belief following individual and group therapy, skills training, and other interventions. As with other strategies, change in beliefs may neutralize strain. When the person acts on the beliefs, or makes them public, the possibility exists for others to declare the beliefs good or bad. Persons who claim to have been abducted by extraterrestrial aliens, for example, are likely not to receive warrants of validation from most professionals.

The fifth category is labeled *nonaction*. The person may have tried the available strategies and they have not worked, either in the direct reduction of strain or in gaining social validation. Under these conditions, strain-in-knowing increases. Not succeeding in neutralizing strain, the person may strive to reduce involvement in the world, lest any actions may lead to inputs that would increase the strain. Traditional diagnosticians would scan the *DSM* categories for one of the 10 mood disorders, a procedure that would locate the individual's suffering as a happening.

In this connection, an alternative approach to "depressive disorders" should be mentioned. The nonaction of the so-called depressed person is interpretable as a subtle form of strategic action, the goal of which is to convince others that one is a helpless, hopeless, or worthless figure in a self-narrative. Specific kinds of "depressed" actions influence others to respond in specific ways. The "helpless" person, for example, calls out responses from others that are qualitatively different from the responses called out by persons who claim to be "hopeless."

This briefly sketched model is radically different from the medical model in that moral judgment is an acknowledged component. The appellation "unwanted conduct" and similar terms are moral judgments rendered either by relevant others or by self. This component is ordinarily omitted from psychiatric discourses that focus on hypothesized internal mechanisms only after the initial moral judgment has been rendered by relevant others or by self.

VII. CODA

The dominance of *DSM-IV* has clouded the fact that a variety of alternative approaches have been, from time to time, put forth for diagnosing psychological problems. These approaches have been eclipsed by the attempt to standardize procedures—an effort driven more by bureaucratic and insurance pressures than by scientific goals. In a historical and critical analysis of *DSM* some of these motivations have been laid bare. At century's end, the economic goals of the therapeutic professions continue to favor quick categorization of patients. A convincing argument has been made that the *DSM*s have evolved into instruments that serve bureaucratic and financial functions more fully than they do scientific ones. When critically examined the *DSM*'s claim to theoretical neutrality cannot be sustained. In fact, the *DSM* authors take pains not to conceal a strong biological bias. Critics have argued that the current dominance of *DSM* prematurely closes off scientific analysis. More specifically, the authors of *DSM* have failed to examine their underlying assumptions, particularly those embedded in their unarticulated theoretical structure and in their choice of root metaphors. Given the state of knowledge, it is premature to posit a theoretical structure that would support the notion of clearly delineated diseaselike entities. The root metaphor of mechanistic causal forces defines not only the clinical reality but human behavior in general, and it does so in a way that transforms historical actions of persons in identifiable sociocultural contexts into physicalistic happenings like infections and mechanical breakdowns that occur independent of human intentionality.

The narrowness of this perspective is obvious. It not only neglects most of the considerable advances made in social psychology and social anthropology in recent decades, it negates common sense views like those of Adolf Meyer half a century ago to be examined to construct systems for organizing the actions of people.

"Problems in living" are neither "mental" in any simple distinction from somatic, nor are they "disorders" in any obvious contrast to an order we can identify as natural. The intellectual resources available to the task of classifying people's problems in living are rich, varied, and often very much more precise and elaborate than the *DSM*s, but they have been neglected for reasons other than their scientific relevance to the task.

*DSM*s of the traditional kind are bound to become increasingly unworkable as the number of diagnoses approaches 500 and as the number of criteria approaches 2000. This development, together with the promulgation of critical inquiries that continue to illuminate the flaws in *DSM* systems, will direct professionals to entertain nontraditional theoretical premises. It is our belief that *DSM* systems will be replaced with systems based on the premise that human beings are agents that engage in intentional strategic actions to maintain their self-narratives. It is likely that scientists of the next century will look back at traditional *DSM*s with somewhat the same puzzlement that is now expressed about the claims of phrenology in the nineteenth century and the claims of lobotomists in the twentieth century.

ACKNOWLEDGMENT

We acknowledge with thanks critical readings of an earlier draft by Ralph M. Carney, James C. Mancuso, and Karl E. Scheibe.

BIBLIOGRAPHY

Berger, P. L., & Luckman, T. (1967). *The social construction of reality: A treatise on the sociology of knowledge.* Garden City, NY: Doubleday.

Borges, E. (1995). A social critique of biological psychiatry. In C. Ross & A. Pam, *Psychology, 64,* 1117–1119.

Follette, W. C., & Houts, A. C. (1996). Models of scientific progress and the role of theory in taxonomy development: A case study of the DSM. *Journal of Consulting and Clinical Psychology, 64,* 1120–1132.

Goffman, E. (1959). *The presentation of self in everyday life.* Garden City, NY: Doubleday.

Kirk, S. A., & Kutchins, H. (1992). *The selling of DSM: The rhetoric of science in psychiatry.* Hawthorne, NY: Walter deGruyter.

Kleinman, A. (1988). *Rethinking psychiatry: From cultural categories to personal experience.* New York: Free Press.

Lief, A. (Ed.). (1948). *The commonsense psychiatry of Adolf Meyer.* New York: McGraw-Hill.

Mirowski, J., & Ross, C. E. (1989). *The social causes of psychological distress.* New York: Aldine de Gruyter.

Sarbin, T. R. (1997). On the futility of psychiatric diagnostic manuals (DSMs) and the return of personal agency. *Applied and Preventive Psychology, 6,* 568–570.

Sarbin, T. R. (1977). Contextualism: A world view for modern psychology. In Landfield, A. (Ed.), *1976 Nebraska symposium on motivation.* Lincoln, NE: University of Nebraska Press.

Sarbin, T. R., & Keen, E. (1997). Sanity and Madness: Conventional and Unconventional Narratives of Emotional Life. In W. Flack & J. Laird (Eds.), *Emotions and psychopathology: Theory and research,* pp. 130–142. New York: Oxford University Press.

Wiener, M. (1989). Psychosocial transactional analysis of psychopathology: Depression as an exemplar. *Clinical Psychology Review, 9,* 295–321.

Clinical Assessment

Eileen Gambrill
University of California, Berkeley

Antecedents Events that immediately precede behavior and influence its frequency.

Behavior Any measurable or observable act or response. Behavior is defined broadly in some perspectives to include cognitions, feelings, and physiological reactions which, although they are not directly observable, are defined so that they can be measured.

Behavioral Approaches to understanding behavior in which learning histories and current environmental contingencies of reinforcement are emphasized. Behavioral approaches differ in the relative degree of attention devoted to thoughts and images.

Clinical Inference Assumptions about the causes of a problem.

Cognition Internal events such as thoughts (beliefs, self-statements, attributions) and images.

Consequences Events that follow behavior and influence its frequency.

Contingency The relationship between a behavior and the events that follow (consequences) and precede (antecedents) the behavior.

Diagnosis A label given to a client with particular characteristics that is assumed to reflect etiology and to have intervention implications.

DSM-IV Official classification system of mental disorders published by the American Psychiatric Association.

Psychodynamic Approaches to understanding behavior, in which unconscious mental and emotional processes (e.g., motives and conflicts) stemming from early childhood experiences are emphasized. Approaches differ in attention given to interpersonal processes, biological factors, and the cultural context.

Validity The extent to which a measure measures what it was designed to assess. There are many different kinds of validity (e.g., predictive, content, concurrent, construct).

CLINICAL ASSESSMENT involves the clarification of presenting problems and related factors including identification of outcomes that will be focused on. It should offer guidelines for selection of intervention methods.

Goals of assessment include describing clients, their problems and desired outcomes as well as their life situations, understanding why problems occur (inferring causes), deciding on what methods are most likely to achieve desired outcomes, and obtaining a base from which to evaluate progress. Assessment requires the search for and integration of data that are useful in deciding how to remove complaints. It involves (1) detecting client characteristics and environmental factors related to problems; (2) integrating and interpreting data collected; and (3) selecting outcomes to focus on. It should indicate what situational, biological, or psychological factors influence options, create demands, or cause discomfort. Decisions must be made about

Copyright © 1998 by Academic Press.
All rights of reproduction in any form reserved.

what data to collect, *how* to gather this, and *how* to organize it. Assessment should indicate the specific outcomes related to complaints, what would have to be done to achieve these outcomes, how these could most effectively be pursued, and the potential of attaining them.

The assessment methods that are used differ because of differences in theoretical perspectives which influence the kind of data collected as well as the uses and functions of these data. Clinical inferences vary in how closely they are tied to concrete evidence. Carrying out an assessment is like unraveling a puzzle or locating the pieces of the puzzle. Certain pieces of the puzzle are sought rather than others depending on the clinician's theoretical orientation and knowledge, and puzzle completion may be declared at diverse points. Issues of practicality also arise. The aim of all methods is to yield data that are useful, reliable, and valid. Specialized knowledge may be required and critical thinking skills are needed to weigh the value of evidence and examine the soundness of assumptions. Although decisions must typically be made on the basis of incomplete data, without a sound assessment framework, opportunities to gather useful data may be lost and ineffective or harmful plans may be suggested. Data should be gathered that are of value in helping clients. Collecting irrelevant data wastes time and money and increases the likelihood of incorrect decisions. Assessment should offer clients more helpful views of problems and a more helpful vocabulary for describing problems and options.

There is general agreement that an individualized assessment should be conducted which considers cultural differences. This does not mean that this is indeed done and practice perspectives differ in what is focused on. Individualized assessment avoids the patient uniformity myth in which clients (or families, or groups) are mistakenly assumed to be similar. Behavior consists of different response systems, which may or may not be related depending on the unique history of each individual: (1) overt behavior (for example, avoidance of crowds) and verbal reports (verbal descriptions of anxiety); (2) cognitions (thoughts about crowds); (3) physiological reactions (for example, increased heart rate when in crowds). Each person may have a different pattern of responses in a situation. Only through an individualized assessment can these unique patterns and related situations be discovered. Suicidal potential should be assessed as relevant. Recognizing the signs of pathology is important anytime this would be helpful in understanding what can be accomplished and how it can be accomplished. A clear agreement between clinicians and clients about the focus of helping efforts increases the likelihood that intervention will focus on outcomes that are of concern to clients.

I. THE GUIDING ROLE OF PRACTICE THEORIES

How problems are structured is a key part of clinical decision-making. Assessment frameworks differ in what is focused on, the kinds of assessment methods used, and how closely assessment is tied to selection of intervention methods. Preferred practice theories influence what clinicians look for and what they notice as well as how they process and organize data collected. Practice theories favored influence beliefs about what can be and is known about behavior and how knowledge can be developed. Dimensions along which theories differ include the following:

- Unit of concern (individual, family, community)
- Goals pursued (e.g., explanation and interpretation alone or understanding based on prediction and influence)
- Clarity of goals pursued
- Criteria used to evaluate the accuracy of explanations (e.g., consensus, authority, scientific)
- Range of problems addressed with success
- Causal importance attributed to feelings, thoughts, and/or environmental factors
- Range of environmental characteristics considered (family, community, society)
- Causal importance attributed to biochemical causes
- Attention devoted to past experiences
- Degree of optimism about how much change is possible
- Degree to which a perspective lends itself to and encourages empirical inquiry (finding out whether it is accurate)
- Degree of empirical support (evidence for and against a theory)
- Attention given to documenting degree of progress
- Ease with which practice guidelines can be developed
- Degree of parsimony

Practice frameworks differ in the value given to observation of interactions in real-life settings, in whether significant others are involved in assessment, and how directive clinicians are. They differ in degree of attention paid to cognitions (thoughts), feelings, environmental characteristics (such as reactions of significant others), genetic causes, and/or physiological causes. Different frameworks are based on different beliefs about the causes of behavior. Beliefs about behavior, thoughts, and feelings, and how they are maintained and can be changed influence what data are gathered and how data are weighted and organized. History shows that beliefs can be misleading. For example, trying to assess people by examining the bumps on their head was not very fruitful. However, for decades many people believed that this method was useful.

Problems can be viewed from a perspective of psychological deficiencies or from a broad view in which both personal and environmental factors are attended to. For example, a key point of feminist counseling is helping clients to understand the effects of the political on the personal, both past and present. Frameworks that focus on psychological characteristics are based on the view that behavior is controlled mainly by characteristics of the individual. In interactional perspectives, attention is given not only to the individual but to people with whom he or she interacts. The unit of analysis is the relationship between environmental events and psychological factors. It is assumed that both personal and environmental factors influence behavior. Interactional views differ in how reciprocal the relationship between the individual and the environment is believed to be and in the range of environmental events considered. In contextual, ecological perspectives, individual, family, community, and societal characteristics are considered as they may relate to problems and possible resolutions. A contextual framework decreases the likelihood of focusing on individual pathology (blaming the victim), and neglecting environmental causes and resources. Practice perspectives that focus on individual causes of personal problems may result in "psychologizing" rather than helping clients. Assessment frameworks differ in the extent to which they take advantage of what is known about behavior, factors related to certain kinds of problems, and the accuracy of different sources of data.

Forming a new conceptualization of presenting problems, one that is shared by both the clinician and the client that will be helpful in resolving problems is an integral aspect of assessment. The kind of conceptualization suggested will depend on the theoretical orientation of the clinician. It is important to arrive at a common view of the problem, as well as agreement as to what will be done to change it. This common view is a motivating factor in that, if clients accept it and if it makes sense to clients, there will be a greater willingness to try out procedures that flow from this account. Mutually agreed-on views are fostered in a variety of ways, including questions asked, assessment procedures used, and rationales offered. Focused summaries help to pull material together within a new framework. Identifying similar themes among seemingly disparate events can be used to suggest alternative views.

II. SIGN AND SAMPLE APPROACHES

Traditional assessment is based on a sign approach in which observed behaviors are viewed as indicators of more important underlying (and unobserved) personality dispositions (typically of a pathological nature) or traits. Traits can be defined as a general and personally determined tendency to react in consistent and stable ways. Examples are "aggression" and "extraversion." Inherent in sign approaches such as psychoanalytic approaches is the assumption that observable behavioral problems are only the outward signs of some underlying process, which must be altered to bring about any lasting change. A focus of change efforts on the behavior itself, according to this model, would not succeed, because no change has supposedly been brought about in underlying causative factors. A clinician may conclude that a child who has difficulty concentrating on his school work and sitting in his seat is hyperactive. The observed behaviors are viewed as a sign of an underlying disorder. The underlying hypothetical constructs are viewed as of major importance in understanding and predicting behavior. Dispositional attributions shift attention away from observing what people *do* in specific situations to speculating about what they *have*. Inconsistencies in behavior across situations are not unexpected within this approach because it is assumed that underlying motives, conflicts, wishes may be behaviorally manifested in many different ways.

The interactions between wishes, the threats anticipated if wishes are expressed, and the processes used to cope with or defend against conflictual situations are of interest in psychodynamic frameworks. Important elements in such processes are believed to be beyond conscious recognition of the individual experiencing them even when they may be recognized or inferred by others. The concepts of "positions" (developmental stages) and "mechanisms" (psychological processes such as defense mechanisms) are central concepts. Defensive aims, processes, and outcomes are of interest. Defense mechanisms include suppression, undoing, repression, role reversal, projection, and regression. The defenses are believed to be heightened under conditions of high emotion, stress, and conflict. Motives include the wish to avoid unpleasant, overwhelming, or out-of-control states. Some unconscious processes anticipate such outcomes. Classification of phenomena is in terms of deflections from volitional consciousness and rationally intended actions: as intrusions and omissions. For example, recurrent dysfunctional alterations in self-esteem and interpersonal behavior (such as those seen in the personality disorders) are viewed as involving both intrusive, inappropriate schemas and omissions of realistic learning of new schemas. It is assumed that the "dynamic unconscious" constantly undergoes symbolic changes which in turn affect feelings and behavior. Other aspects of psychoanalytic approaches include an emphasis on verbal reports concerning early histories and efforts to alter inner processes by verbal means. Compared to behavioral assessment, less attention is devoted to environmental variables that may influence behavior because of the assumed core relevance and stability of underlying dispositions.

There are many different kinds of psychodynamic assessment frameworks. For example, there are variants of object relations theory, each of which may have a somewhat different approach to assessment. The nature of a client's past interactions with their parents is viewed as central. However, there are differences in what is focused on by clinicians of different psychodynamic persuasions. In object relations theory, the concepts of mirroring and self objects are key ones. Attention is given to internal mental representations of the self and significant others. It is assumed that how we feel about ourselves and act toward others is a reflection of internal relationships based on experience. The term "object relations" refers to the interplay between the images of self and others. This interplay results in wishes, impulses, thoughts, and feelings of power (or its lack). Ego psychology emphasizes identification and support of strengths and working within the "defenses" rather than breaking them down. Proponents consider resistance to change natural and work with and support adaptive strengths. Defense mechanisms, such as rationalization of actions and projection of feelings onto others are identified but not necessarily discussed.

Behavioral assessment involves a sample approach. In a sample approach, direct observation of behavior in real life settings (or, if this is not possible, in situations that resemble these) is valued. A behavioral approach is based on an interactional view in which it is assumed that behavior is a function of both organismic variables (genetic history and physiological states) and the environment. Labels are used as summarizing categories rather than as terms indicating some underlying characteristic (usually a disorder). Unlike in sign approaches where the cause of behavior is assumed to be underlying dispositions, the cause of behavior is assumed to lie largely in environmental differences. Behavioral frameworks differ in the relative amount of attention devoted to thoughts and environmental contingencies. Differences in focus are so marked that they have resulted to the formation of different journals and societies. Differences in emphasis are related to the role attributed to thoughts in influencing behavior. This role varies from a causal to a mediating role. In the former, reflected in cognitive–behavioral frameworks, thoughts are presumed to cause changes in feelings and behavior. In the latter, reflected in applied behavior analysis, thoughts are assumed to influence feelings and behavior in a mediating (not causal) manner. It is assumed that one must look to past and present environmental contingencies to account for both thoughts and feelings.

In cognitive–behavioral methods, attention is devoted to thoughts as well as behaviors. Thoughts of interest include attributions for behavior, feelings, and outcomes, negative and positive self-statements, expectations, and cognitive distortions. Attention is devoted to identifying the particular kinds of thoughts that occur in problem related situations. Cognitive–behavioral approaches differ in their assumptions about the kinds of thoughts that underlie behavior. However, all share certain assumptions such as the belief that individuals respond to cognitive representations of environmental events rather than to the events per se. It is assumed that learning is cognitively mediated and that cognition mediates emotional and behavioral dysfunction. [*See* BEHAVIOR THERAPY; COGNITIVE THERAPY.]

In applied behavior analysis, environmental contingencies are focused on. A contingency analysis requires identification of the environmental events that occasion and maintain behavior. There is an interest in describing the relationships between behavior and what happens right before and after as well as "metacontingencies"—the relationships between cultural practices and the outcomes of these practices. There is an emphasis on *current* contingencies. Attention is directed toward the change of "deviant" environments rather than the change of "deviant" client behaviors. There is an interest in identifying functional relationships. A behavioral analysis includes a description of behaviors of concern as well as evidence that specific antecedents and consequences influence these behaviors; it requires a functional as well as a descriptive analysis.

Although there are differences, all behavioral approaches share many characteristics that distinguish them from sign approaches. Assessment is an ongoing process in behavioral assessment. This contrasts with some traditional assessment approaches in which assessment is used to "diagnose" a client in order to decide on treatment methods. What a person *does* is of interest in behavioral approaches rather than what she *has*. Behavior is of great interest, especially the behaviors of individuals in real-life contexts. Identifying variables that influence the frequency of behaviors of interest is a key assessment goal. Behavior is assumed to vary in different contexts because of different learning histories and different current contingencies as well as different levels of deprivation and fatigue. There is an emphasis on clear description of assessment methods as well as clear description of problems and outcomes. It is assumed that only if complaints are clearly described can they be translated into specific changes that would result in their removal. The emphasis on behavior and the influence of environmental contingencies call for the translation of problems into observable behaviors and the discovery of ways in which the environment can be rearranged. Clients are encouraged to recognize and alter the role they play in maintaining problems. For example, teachers and parents often reinforce behaviors they complain about. Assessment is individualized; each person, group, family, organization or community is viewed as unique. Data about group differences do not offer precise information about what an individual does in specific situations and what cues and consequences influence their behavior.

The focus on behavior has a number of implications for assessment. One is the importance of observing people in real-life contexts whenever feasible, ethical, and necessary to acquire helpful data. A range of assessment methods is used including observation in real-life settings as well as role plays. Multiple assessment methods are also called for because of the lack of synchrony in overt behavior, physiological reactions, cognitions (thoughts), and feelings. Assessment and treatment are closely related in a behavioral model. It is assumed that assessment should have treatment utility. There is an emphasis on the use of validated assessment methods. The principles of behavior are relied on to guide assessment and intervention. There is a preference for limited inference and a focus on constructing repertoires (on helping clients to acquire additional knowledge and skills that will increase opportunities for reinforcement). Clients are viewed in terms of their assets rather than their deficiencies. The preference for enhancement of knowledge and skills requires a focus on behaviors that are effective in real-life contexts. In a task analysis, the specific behaviors that are required to achieve an outcome are identified. For each step, performance is clearly described as well as the conditions in which it is expected to occur.

A. Some Important Distinctions

The form of a behavior (its topography) does not necessarily indicate its function (why the behavior occurs). Identical forms of behavior may be maintained by very different contingencies. Just as the same behavior may have different functions, different behaviors may have identical functions. The distinction between motivational and behavioral deficits is also important. If a desired behavior does not occur, this may indicate either that the behavior exists but is not reinforced on an effective schedule or is punished (a motivational deficit) or that the behavior is not present in the client's repertoire (a behavior deficit). Motivational deficits are often mistaken for behavioral deficits. Motivational and behavioral deficits can be distinguished by arranging conditions for performance of a behavior. For example, clients could be requested to role play behaviors and asked whether similar or identical behaviors occur in other situations. Behavior surfeits are often related to behavior deficits. For example, aggression on the part of a child may be related to a lack of friendship skills. It is also important to distinguish response inhibitions from behavior deficits. Emotional reactions such as anxiety may interfere with desired behavior.

B. Past History

Although the past is viewed as important in influencing current behavior in just about all perspectives, assessment frameworks differ in how much attention is devoted to the past and what is focused on. Past experiences are a major focus in psychodynamic assessment frameworks. Knowledge about past circumstances may be of value when it is difficult to identify current maintaining factors and may be helpful in preventing future problems. Information about a person's past may provide valuable information about unusual social histories related to problems. An understanding of how problems began can be useful in clarifying the origins of what seem to be puzzling reactions. New ways of viewing past events may be helpful to clients. Information about the past can be useful in encouraging clients to alter present behaviors and may help clients understand the source of current reactions. Demographic indicators about a client's past behavior in certain contexts may be better predictors of future behavior than personality tests or clinical judgments.

Information about the past offers a view of current events in a more comprehensive context. Major areas include medical history, educational and work history, significant relationships, family history and developmental history. Helpful coping skills may be discovered by finding out what clients have tried in the past to resolve problems. Research concerning autobiographical memory suggests that memories change over time, making it difficult to know whether reports are accurate. From a psychodynamic perspective, accuracy would not be an issue. Rather, the client's memories of events, whether accurate or not, are the substance of import. It is assumed in fact that memories may be distorted by unconscious motives/conflicts and so on. Excessive attention to past troubles may create pessimism about the future and encourage rationalizations and excuses that interfere with change, especially if this is not fruitful in selecting effective plans.

C. What about Psychiatric Labels?

Labels are used in assessment in two main ways. One is as a shorthand term to refer to specific behaviors. The term hyperactive may refer to the fact that a student often gets out of his seat and talks out of turn in class. A counselor may use "hyperactive" as a summary term to refer to these behaviors. Labels are also used as a diagnostic category which is supposed to offer guidelines for knowing what to do about a problem. Here, a label connotes more than a cluster of behaviors. It involves additional assumptions about the person labeled which should be of "diagnostic" value. The *Diagnostic and Statistical Manual of Mental Disorders* (*DSM-IV*) of the American Psychiatric Association describes hundreds of terms used to describe various disorders. [*See* DSM-IV.]

Methodological and conceptual problems connected with the use of diagnostic categories include lack of agreement about what label to assign clients and lack of association between a diagnosis and indications of what intervention will be effective. Psychiatric labels have been criticized for being imprecise (saying too little about positive attributes, potential for change, and change that does occur, and too much about presumed negative characteristics and limits to change). Both traits and diagnostic labels offer little detail about what people do in specific situations and what specific circumstances influence behavior. There is no evidence that traits have dispositional properties. Little cross-situational consistency has been found in relation to "personality traits." Some behaviors may appear "trait-like" in that they are similar over time and situations because of similar contingencies of reinforcement. Degree of consistency should be empirically explored for particular classes of clients and behavior rather than assumed. Acceptance of a label may prematurely close off consideration of promising options. The tendency to use a binary classification system (people are labeled as either having or not having something, for example, as being an alcoholic or not), may obscure the varied individual patterns that may be referred to by a term. Critics of the *DSM* highlight the consensual nature of what is included (reliance on agreement rather than empirical criteria) and the role of economic considerations in its creation. Some argue that psychiatric classification systems encourage blaming victims for their plights rather than altering the social circumstances responsible for problems.

Labels that are instrumental (they point to effective interventions) are helpful. For example, the understanding of anxiety disorders has advanced requiring the differential diagnosis among different categories (simple phobia, generalized anxiety, panic attacks and agoraphobia). Failure to use labels that are indeed informative may prevent clients from receiving appropriate intervention. Labels can normalize client concerns. Parents who have been struggling to understand why their child is developmentally slow may view themselves as failures. Recognition that their child has a specific kind of developmental disability that accounts for this can be a relief.

III. SOURCES OF INFLUENCE

Influences on behavior include other people's actions, the physical environment, tasks and materials, physiological changes, thoughts, genetic differences, and developmental factors. Material and community resources and related political, economic, and social conditions influence options. It is important to obtain an overview of the client's current life as this may relate to problems, including relationships with significant others, employment, physical health, recreational activities, and community and material resources available. Antecedents of behavior, like consequences, have a variety of sources. In addition to proximal antecedents (those that occur right before a behavior), distal antecedents may influence current behavior. Past or future events may be made current by thinking about these. These thoughts may then influence what we do, feel, and think. *Setting events* are antecedents that are closely associated with a behavior but are not in the situation in which behaviors of concern occur. For example, an unpleasant exchange with a teacher may influence how a child responds to his parents at home. The earlier event alters the likelihood of given reactions in subsequent situations. Preferred practice theories influence the attention given to various sources. Problems vary in the complexity of related factors. Problems may be complex because significant others lack needed skills, have interfering beliefs, or are threatened by proposed changes. Distinguishing between problems and efforts to resolve these will avoid confusion between the results of attempted solutions and effects of the original concern. Expected role behavior in a certain culture may limit change. Ongoing discrimination against a group may limit opportunities. Clients may lack needed information or skills. A *behavior deficit* may exist (the client may not know how to perform a given behavior).

A. Other People/The Nature of the Client's Social Relationship

With any presenting problem, the possible influence of significant others in the maintenance of a problem should be explored. Behavior occurs in a context. How significant others respond makes up an important part of our environment. Significant others are those who interact with clients and influence their behavior. Examples include family members and staff in residential settings. Significant others are often involved in assessment. For example, in family therapy, family members participate in assessment. Understanding relationships among family members is a key part of assessment in family therapy. Interactions between couples is closely examined in relationship counseling. Clients may lack social support such as opportunities for intimacy, companionship, and validation or the opportunity to provide support to others. Social interactions may be a source of stress rather than a source of pleasure and joy. It is important to assess the nature and quality of the client's social network and social support system.

B. The Physical Environment

The influence of the physical environment should be examined. Physical arrangements in residential and day care settings influence behavior. Unwanted behaviors may be encouraged by available materials. For example, toys that are visible to children may distract them from educational tasks. Temperature changes affect behavior as do degree of crowding and noise level. Characteristics of the community in which clients live that may influence complaints and possible intervention options should be assessed. Neighborhood quality influences well-being. For example, children who live in lower quality environments (e.g., there is little play space, housing is in industrial neighborhoods, upkeep of streets is poor) are less satisfied with their lives, experience more negative emotions, and have more restricted and less positive friendship patterns. There is a relationship between number of nonaccidental injuries to children and the physical conditions of the home which is related to socioeconomic status.

C. Tasks and Activities

The kind of task confronting an individual may influence the rate of problem behavior. Particular tasks or activities may be high-risk situations for unwanted behavior. Many studies have found a relationship between the kind of task and deviant behavior such as self-injury. Problems may occur because a task is too tedious or difficult or because an individual is uncomfortable or bored, or is told to do something in an unpleasant manner. In these instances, altering antecedents may correct the problem.

D. Biophysiological Factors

Presenting problems may be related to neurological or biochemical factors. Such factors may place boundaries on how much change is possible. Malnutrition, hypoglycemia, and allergic reactions have been associated with hyperactivity, learning disabilities, and mental retardation. Biochemical abnormalities are found in some children with serious behavior disturbances such as those labeled autistic. However, this only establishes that abnormalities in biochemistry are present, not that they cause a certain disorder (e.g., cause certain behaviors). Biochemical changes may be a result of stress related to social conditions such as limited opportunities due to discrimination. Drugs, whether prescribed or not, may influence how clients appear and behave. Certain kinds of illness are associated with particular kinds of psychological changes.

Drugs, alcohol, environmental pollutants, and nutritional deficiencies may influence health and behavior. Accidents may result in neurological changes which result in concomitant psychological changes. Even when brain damage can be shown to exist, this does not show that it causes any particular behavior. Premature acceptance of biophysical explanations will interfere with discovering alternative explanations that yield intervention knowledge. Behavior changes may be due to brain tumors. Hormonal changes associated with menopause may result in mood changes which may be misattributed to psychological causes. On the other hand psychological changes may be misattributed to hormonal changes. There are gender differences in return of diffuse physiological arousal (DPA) to baseline levels; men take longer to return to baseline levels. These gender differences have implications for understanding and altering aggression among family members. Whenever physiological factors may be related to a problem as, for example, with seizures, depression, fatigue, or headaches, a physical examination should be required. Overlooking physical causes including nutritional deficiencies and coffee, alcohol, or drug intake may result in incorrect inferences.

E. Cognitive–Intellectual Characteristics

People differ in their intellectual abilities which may influence problems and outcomes. Genetic differences have been found in intelligence as well as in shyness, temperament, and conditioning susceptibility. The importance of assessing what people say to themselves in relevant situations is emphasized in many assessment frameworks. For example, in cognitive–behavioral approaches, clients' internal dialogues (what they say to themselves) and the way this relates to complaints and desired outcomes is explored and altered as necessary. Certain thoughts may occur too much, too seldom, or at the wrong time. A depressed client may have a high frequency of negative self-statements and a low frequency of positive self-statements. In a radical behavioral perspective, thoughts are viewed as covert behaviors to be explained, not as explanations for other behaviors, although it is assumed they can serve a mediating function and influence both feelings and behaviors. The thoughts and feelings in a situation are assumed to be a function of the contingencies experienced in this situation or in situations that are similar or associated in some way. A causal role may be misattributed to thoughts because the histories related to the development of thoughts is overlooked. The role of thoughts can be examined by varying certain ones and determining the effects on behavior.

F. Feelings

When feelings are presented as a problem or are related to a problem, associated personal and environmental factors must be identified. Assessment frameworks differ in the role attributed to feelings and in factors sought to account for feelings. Some emphasize the role of thoughts in creating feelings. Others emphasize the role of unconscious conflicts and motives related to early childhood experiences. Other frameworks focus on the role of environmental contingencies in influencing emotional reactions. For example, in a radical behavioral approach, feelings are viewed as by-products of the relationships between behavior and environmental events. Feelings can be used as clues to contingencies (relationships between behavior and environmental events). Changing feelings will not make up for a lack of required skills, or rearrange contingencies required to attain desired outcomes.

G. Cultural Differences

Cultural differences may affect both the problems that clients experience as well as the communication styles and assessment and intervention methods that will be successful. An individualized assessment requires attention to cultural differences that may be related to problems and potential resolutions. Culturally sensitive practice requires knowledge of the values of different groups and their historical experience in the United States, and how these differences may influence the client's behavior, motivation and view of the helping process.

Different groups may prefer different problem-solving styles and have different beliefs about the causes of problems. The norms for behavior vary in different groups. It is important to be knowledgeable about cultural differences that may be mistakenly viewed as pathology. The degree of acculturation (the process of adaptation to a new or different culture) is important to assess. This influences drop-out rate, level of stress, attitude toward clinicians, and the process and goals that are appropriate. Knowledge of problems faced and preferred communication styles of people in different generations will be useful. Bicultural individuals are members of two or more ethnic or racial groups.

H. Developmental Considerations

Assessment requires knowledge about developmental tasks, norms, and challenges. Information about required behaviors at different ages and life transitions can be helpful in assessment. Knowledge of what is typical behavior at different times (developmental norms) can be useful in "normalizing" behavior—helping clients to realize that reactions they view as unusual or "abnormal" are in fact common. Knowledge about typical changes in different phases of the life cycle (e.g., adolescence, parenthood, retirement) allows preventative planning. The following kinds of information will be helpful: (1) norms for behavior in specific contexts; (2) tasks associated with certain life-situations such as parenthood and retirement; (3) the hierarchical nature of some developmental tasks (some behaviors must be learned before others can be acquired). Different kinds of norms may be used in the selection of outcomes. Criterion referenced norms rely on what has been found to be required to attain a certain outcome through empirical analysis. Another kind of norm is what is usual in a situation. However, what is usual may not be what is desirable. For example, although it may be typical for teachers to offer low rates of positive feedback to students in their classroom, it is not optimal. The similarities of contingencies for many people at a given age in a society may lead one to assume incorrectly that biological development is responsible. The role of similar contingencies may be overlooked. Acceptance of a stage theory of development may get in the way of identifying environmental factors that can be rearranged.

I. Reviewing Resources and Obstacles

Assessment involves identification of personal assets and environmental resources that can be used to help clients attain desired outcomes, as well as personal and environmental obstacles. Personal resources and/or obstacles include cognitive–intellectual abilities and deficiencies, physical abilities and handicaps, social skills and social-skill deficits, vocational and recreational skills, financial assets, and social support systems. Clients differ in their "reinforcer profile" and in degree of motivation to alter problematic circumstances. Environments differ in opportunities for certain kinds of experiences (see discussion of physical environment). Resources such as money, housing, vocational training programs, medical care, or recreational facilities may be unavailable. Limited community resources (such as day care programs, vocational training programs, recreational centers, high-quality educational programs, parent training programs) and limited influence over environmental circumstances may pose an obstacle. Child maltreatment is related to poverty. Unemployment is related to substance abuse and spouse violence. Agency policies and practices influence options. Lack of coordination of services may limit access to resources. Clients may receive fragmentary, overlapping, or incompatible services.

IV. SOURCES OF INFORMATION

Sources of data include interviews, responses to written or pictorial measures, data gathered by clients and significant others (self-monitoring), observation in the interview as well as in role play or in real-life settings, and physiological indicators. A variety of electromechanical aids are available for collecting data such as wrist counters, timers, biofeedback devices, and audio- and videotape recorders. Familiarity with and knowledge about different methods, as well as personal and theoretical preferences and questions of feasibility influence selection. Preferred practice theories strongly influence selection of assessment methods. For example, in individually focused psychodynamic approaches, self-report and transference effects within the interview may be the main source of data used.

In behavioral approaches, self-report is supplemented whenever possible by other sources of data such as observation in real-life settings, role play, and/or self-monitoring. (Clients keep track of some behaviors, thoughts, or feelings and surrounding circumstances in real-life). Some sources, such as self-report in the interview, are easy to use and are flexible in the range of content provided. However, accuracy varies considerably. The question is: what methods will offer a fairly accurate description of reactions or conditions of concern and related events? Individual differences will influence a client's willingness to participate in a given manner. Accuracy of decisions can be improved by using multiple methods, drawing especially on those most likely to offer accurate relevant data.

Self-report is the most widely used source of information. There are many different types of self-report including verbal reports during interviews and answers on written inventories. Interviews also provide an opportunity to observe clients. Advantages of self-report include ease of collecting material and flexibility in the range of material that may be gathered. Structured interviews have been developed for both children and adults in a number of areas. These may be completed by the clinician, the client, or significant others. The accuracy of self-reports depends on a number of factors including the situation in which data are collected and the kinds and sequence of questions asked. Helpful questions in assessing the accuracy of self-reports include the following: (1) Does the situation encourage an honest answer? (2) Does the client have access to the information? (3) Can the client comprehend the question? (4) Does the client have the verbal skills required to answer questions? Special knowledge and skills may be required when interviewing children. Play materials and storytelling may be used to gather data about children's feelings and experiences.

Measures that have uniform procedures for administration and scoring and that are accompanied by certain kinds of information are referred to as *standardized measures*. Thousands of standardized questionnaires have been developed related to hundreds of different personal and/or environmental characteristics. Standardized measures are used for a variety of purposes including: (1) describing populations or clients, (2) screening clients (for example, making a decision about the need for further assessment or finding out if a client is eligible for or likely to require a service), (3) assessing clients (a more detailed review resulting in decisions about diagnosis or assignment to intervention methods), (4) monitoring (evaluating progress), and (5) making predictions about the likely futures of clients (for example in relation to use of a particular intervention method). As always, a key concern is validity. Does a measure assess what it is presumed to assess? Reliability must also be considered. How stable are responses on a measure given a lack of real change? Unstable measures are not likely to be valid. How sensitive will a measure be to change?

Personality tests may be used to collect assessment data. *Objective tests* include specific questions, statements, or concepts. Clients respond with direct answers, choices, or ratings. *Projective tests* such as the Thematic Apperception Test, incomplete sentences test, and the Rorschach Inkblot Test are purposefully vague and ambiguous. It is assumed that each person will impose on this unstructured stimulus presentation unique meanings that reflect his or her perceptions of the world and responses to it. Psychoanalytic concepts underlie use of most projective tests. These tests focus on assessing general personality characteristics and uncovering unconscious processes. Tests are used not as samples of the content domain (as in behavioral approaches), but as signs of important underlying constructs. Whereas content validity is of great concern in a behavioral perspective, this is not so within a traditional approach. In fact, items may be made deliberately obscure and vague.

Valuable information can be obtained from data clients collect (self-monitoring). As with any other source of data, not all clients will be able or willing to participate. Observation of relevant interactions in real-life settings offers a valuable source of information. This is routinely used in applied behavior analysis. If observation in real-life settings is not possible, observation in role plays may provide a useful alternative. Physiological measures have been used with a broad array of presenting problems including illness such as diabetes and dermatitis and problems such as smoking, anxiety, sexual dysfunction, and rape. Measures include heart rate, blood pressure, respiration rate, skin conductance, muscle tension, and urine analysis. Physiological measures are useful when verbal reports may be inaccurate. Certain kinds of desynchronies between verbal reports of fear and physiological measures may provide useful assessment data. Whenever presenting problems may be related to physical causes, a physical examination should be obtained. Failure to do so may result in overlooking physical causes.

V. ASSESSING THE VALUE OF DATA

Assessment methods differ in their accuracy. For example, self-report of clients or significant others may not accurately reflect what occurs in real life. Observers may be biased and offer inaccurate data. Measurement inevitably involves error. One cause of systematic error is social desirability; people present themselves in a good light. Criteria that are important to consider in judging the value of assessment data include: (1) reliability, (2) validity, (3) sensitivity, (4) utility, (5) feasibility, and (6) relevance. *Reliability* refers to the consistency of results (in the absence of real change) provided by the same person at different times (time-based reliability), by two different raters of the same events (individual-based reliability) as in inter-rater reliability, or by parallel forms of split-halfs of a measure (item-bound reliability). Reliability places an upward boundary on validity. For example, if responses on a questionnaire vary from time to time (in the absence of real change), it will not be possible to use results of a measure to predict what a person will do in the future.

Validity concerns the question: Does the measure reflect the characteristic it is supposed to measure? For example, does behavior in a role play correspond to what a client does in similar real-life situations? Assessment is more likely to be informative if valid methods are used—methods that have been found to offer accurate information. *Direct* (e.g., observing teacher–student interaction) in contrast to *indirect* measures (e.g., asking a student to complete a questionnaire assumed to offer information about classroom behavior) are typically more valid. Validity (accuracy) is a concern in all assessment frameworks; however, the nature of the concern is different in sign and sample approaches. In a sign approach, behavior is used as a sign of some entity (such as a personality trait) that is at a different level. The concern is with *vertical* validity. Is the sign an accurate indicator of the underlying trait? *Horizontal* validity is of concern in a sample approach. Different levels (e.g., behavior and personality dispositions) are not involved. Examples include: (1) Does self-report provide an accurate account of behavior and related circumstances? (2) Does behavior in role play reflect what occurs in real life? Different responses (overt, cognitive, and physiological) may or may not be related to an event. For example, clients may report anxiety but show no physiological signs of anxiety. This does not mean that their reports are not accurate. For those individuals, the experience of anxiety may be cognitive rather than physical.

The *sensitivity* of measures is important to consider; will a measure reflect changes that occur? The *utility* of a measure is determined by its cost (time, effort, expense) balanced against information provided. *Feasibility* is related to utility. Some measures will not be feasible to gather. Utility may be compromised by the absence of empirically derived norms for a measure. *Norms* offer information about the typical (or average) performance of a group of individuals and allow comparison of data obtained from a client with similar clients. The more representative the sample is to the client, the greater the utility of a measure in relation to a client. *Relevance* should also be considered. Is a measure relevant to presenting problems and related outcomes? Do clients and significant others perceive it as relevant?

VI. THE SOCIAL CONTEXT OF ASSESSMENT

Assessment takes place in the context of a helper–client relationship. The nature of this relationship is considered important in all practice frameworks. Influence of the clinician on the client has been found even in very nondirective approaches. The role of the relationship is viewed differently in different practice perspectives. Great attention is given to the diagnostic value of transference and countertransference effects in psychodynamic therapies and the relationship itself is viewed as the primary vehicle of change. Traditionally, transference has been viewed as a reenactment between the client and the counselor of the client's relationship with significant others in the past, especially parents. Countertransference effects refer to feelings on the part of helpers toward their clients. Transferences are distinguished from therapeutic or working alliances within psychodynamic perspectives. Understanding and analyzing how the client relates to the clinician are of major importance. The way the client relates to the clinician is considered to be indicative of the client's past relationships with significant figures in the past and is thus viewed as a key source of information about the client. Within other perspectives such as cognitive–behavioral approaches, the relationship is viewed as the context within which helping occurs. The interpersonal skills of the clinician are viewed as essential for facilitating a collaborative working relationship, validating and supporting the client, and encouraging clients to acquire valued behaviors.

There is a continuing need throughout assessment to explain the roles and requirements of the client and the counselor, the process that will occur, and the rationale for this. Introductory explanations include an overview of mutual responsibilities and of the framework that will be employed. Because different client behaviors may be required during different phases of assessment and intervention, this "socialization" of the client is an ongoing task. Behavioral clinicians tend to be more directive than psychoanalytically oriented clinicians. They more frequently give instructions, provide information, influence the conversation, and talk more. Clinicians may err by being too directive or too nondirective. Overly directive clinicians may not recognize the need to help clients to explore and to understand their behavior. In contrast, nondirective counselors may err by assuming that self-understanding is sufficient to achieve desired outcomes (when it is not).

VII. COMMON ASSESSMENT ERRORS AND THEIR SOURCES

Errors may occur in any of the three steps involved in assessment: (1) detection of characteristics of the client and his or her life situation that are related to problems and desired outcomes; (2) integration and interpretation of data gathered; and (3) selection of outcomes to pursue in order to remove complaints. Errors made in the first two steps will result in errors in the third step. Examples of common errors are noted below. They result in incomplete or misleading assessment. Some errors involve or result in inappropriate speculation—assuming that what is, can be discovered simply by thinking about the topic.

- Hasty assumptions about causes (failure to search for alternative accounts)
- Speculating when data collection is called for
- Confusing the form and function of behavior
- Using misleading and/or uninformative labels
- Confusing motivational and behavior deficits
- Focusing on pathology and overlooking assets
- Collecting irrelevant material
- Relying on inaccurate sources (e.g., anecdotal experience)
- Being unduly influenced by first impressions
- Being misled by superficial resemblances of a client to other clients in the past or to a stereotype

Errors in detection include inadequate selection of modalities (e.g., confining attention to thoughts), inadequate selection of data collection methods (e.g., reliance on the interview alone), and errors in the data collection method itself (e.g., observer bias). Inaccurate or incomplete accounts of problems and related factors may occur because attention is too narrowly focused on one source (for example on thoughts or feelings). The fundamental attribution error is made when behavior is attributed to internal dispositions of the individual, overlooking the role of environmental causes. Sources of error in integrating and interpreting data include focusing on consistency rather than informativeness of data, hasty generalization based on limited samples, and inadequate conceptualization of problems due to theoretical biases (e.g., focus only on environmental factors) or superficial knowledge of practice frameworks. Another source of error at this stage is use of vague language that is not informative (e.g., psychological jargon). Errors in selection of outcomes to focus on may occur due to error in the first two phases.

Studies on clinical decision-making indicate that decisions are made on the basis of quite limited data. Even though a great deal of data are gathered, only a small subset is used. Clinicians tend to gather more data than are needed and, as the amount of data gathered increases, so does confidence in its usefulness, even though accuracy may not increase. Clinicians have a tendency to confuse consistency of data with informative value. Irrelevant as well as relevant data may be influential. Clinicians, like other individuals, are affected by limited information-processing capacities and motivational factors. As a consequence, they do not see all there is to see. Because of preconceptions and biases, things that are not actually present may be reported and events that do occur may be overlooked. There is a behavior confirmation tendency. Data are sought that are consistent with preferred theories and preconceptions, and contradictory data tend to be disregarded.

It is easy to recall bizarre behavior and pay excessive attention to this, ignoring less vivid appropriate behavior. The frequency of data that are available is overestimated. Many factors that are not correlated with the true frequency of an event influence estimates of its frequency and how important it seems (such as how visible it is, how vivid it is, and how easily it can be imagined—that is, how available it is). Chance availability may affect clinical decisions—that is, certain events may just happen to be available when thinking about a problem, and these have an impact on what is attended to. Clinicians in given settings are exposed to particular kinds of clients, which may predispose them to make certain assumptions. For example, a psychologist who sees many severely depressed individuals may be primed to attend to signs of depression. Base rate data that are abstract tend to be ignored, which increases the probability of inaccurate inferences. A lack of concern for sample size and sample bias can lead to incorrect judgments. General predictions about a person that are based on tiny samples of behavior in one context are not likely to be accurate, especially when behaviors of interest occur in quite different situations. Not distinguishing between description and inference may result in incorrect assumptions. Use of multiple methods in a contextual practice framework provides the greatest opportunity for sound assessment.

VIII. ETHICAL ISSUES AND FUTURE DIRECTIONS

Lack of assessment competencies may result in the selection of ineffective and/or harmful intervention methods. It is thus incumbent on clinicians to use valid methods that are useful in selecting effective intervention plans. This may require training. There are great stakes in how problems are framed and considerable resources are devoted to influencing how people think about problems. Many problems once viewed as sins were then seen as crimes and more recently are considered to be mental disorders. Explanations influence how people are viewed. In past years, pathology was often attributed to housewives who wanted to work. Incorrect explanations of problems often harm clients. Knowledge about social, political, and economic factors that influence the very definition of personal and social problems will help clinicians to consider problems in their social context and decrease the likelihood of pathologizing clients.

A discussion of clinical assessment would not be complete without noting the increased attention given to evolutionary influences. It is easy to lose sight of the fact that humans are the result of a long evolutionary process and that we carry anatomical, physiological, and psychological characteristics related to this history. An evolutionary perspective adds a valuable dimension to understanding aggression and caregiving in society, whether directed toward family members or strangers, as well as defeat states such as depression and the experiences that may be responsible. Computers will play an increasing role in helping clinicians to handle the many different kinds of data that must often be integrated. There has been considerable interest in the integration of different approaches to clinical practice. Some have explored the possible integration of behavioral and psychoanalytic approaches. Others have investigated the relationship between classical psychodynamics and object relations perspectives. Discussions here concern the nature of inferred conflict and how mental phenomena of interest are formed. Accurate descriptions of assessment perspectives will increase the likelihood that points of convergence and differences are correctly identified. Continuing research efforts are needed to identify valid assessment methods and indicate assessment frameworks that are most likely to help clients. Increased interest in clinical reasoning bodes well for enhancement of assessment competencies.

This article has been reprinted from the *Encyclopedia of Human Behavior, Volume 1.*

BIBLIOGRAPHY

Bellack, A. S., & Hersen, M. (Eds.) (1988). "Behavioral Assessment," 3rd ed. Pergamon, New York.

Bergen, J. R., & Kratchowill, T. R. (1990). "Behavioral Consultation and Therapy." Plenum, New York.

Ciminero, A. R., Calhoun, K. S., & Adams, H. E. (1986). "Handbook of Behavioral Assessment," 2nd ed. Wiley, New York.

Gambrill, E. (1990). "Critical Thinking in Clinical Practice." Jossey-Bass, San Francisco, CA.

Gilbert, P. (1989). "Human Nature and Suffering." Erlbaum, Hillsdale, NJ.

Goldstein, M., & Hersen, M. (Eds.) (1990). "Handbook of Psychological Assessment." Pergamon, New York.

Horowitz, M. J. (1987). "States of Mind: Configurational Analysis of Individual Psychology," 2nd ed. Plenum, New York.

Kirk, S., & Kutchins, H. (1992). "The Selling of DSM: The Rhetoric of Science in Psychiatry." Aldine de Gruyter, Hawthorne, NY.

Nay, W. R. (1979). "Multimethod Clinical Assessment." Gardner, New York.

Wetzler, S., & Katz, M. M. (1989). "Contemporary Approaches to Psychological Assessment." Brunner/Mazel, New York.

Cognitive Therapy

Marjorie E. Weishaar
Brown University School of Medicine

Automatic Thoughts Thoughts that are involuntary and difficult to inhibit.
Cognitions Thoughts and images.
Cognitive Distortions Habitual errors in logic.
Cognitive Organization A model of cognitions arranged hierarchically which reflects the accessibility and stability of various types of thoughts, beliefs, and assumptions.
Cognitive Shift The change from flexible thinking, which allows reappraisal and reevaluation, to more rigid thinking characteristic of psychological distress.
Cognitive Specificity Thoughts and images that are specific to diagnostic categories. For example, the cognitive themes of anxiety are danger and threat.
Continuity Hypothesis Hypothesis that psychological syndromes are exaggerated and persistent forms of normal emotional responses.
Schemas Cognitive structures that hold core beliefs and, when triggered, generate affect-laden thoughts and images.

COGNITIVE THERAPY is a form of psychotherapy that posits that how an individual perceives and interprets events strongly influences how that person responds emotionally and behaviorally. It combines cognitive and behavioral techniques to teach patients to challenge biased perceptions and the underlying assumptions that may cause them to distort current situations. It is best known as an effective treatment for unipolar depression. Since its establishment 30 years ago, it has been applied to a wide range of psychological problems and clinical populations. Outcome studies have demonstrated its usefulness in the treatment of depression and have suggested that cognitive therapy has some preventive effects against future depressive episodes. Current research is investigating whether cognitive therapy can prevent a first episode of depression among those at risk. In addition, cognitive therapy techniques are being used in schools to promote cooperation and self-esteem. Thus, this form of therapy can be used to promote mental health at the individual and community levels.

I. COGNITIVE THERAPY AND MENTAL HEALTH

Cognitive therapy is a system of psychotherapy that emphasizes the role of information processing in human behavior and psychological distress. It posits that how people perceive, interpret, and assign meanings to events strongly influences their emotional and behavioral reactions. It also maintains that significant

Copyright © 1998 by Academic Press.
All rights of reproduction in any form reserved.

life experiences shape core beliefs about the self and the world. These core beliefs, in turn, affect how new information is incorporated. Cognitive therapy is thus concerned with both the idiosyncratic meanings of events for people and the ways in which these meanings are generated and maintained. Although the content of cognitions (i.e., thoughts and images) may be highly personal, the mechanisms of cognitive processing are believed to be universal.

Cognitive therapy was developed in the 1960s by psychiatrist Aaron T. Beck. It is derived from empirical findings from studies of depressed patients. Beck found that depressed patients' thinking is saturated with themes of deprivation, defeat, and loss. Moreover, their judgments are absolute and rigid. Usually, information processing proceeds in a fairly flexible manner, so that initial impressions or primary appraisals may be checked and verified or adjusted. Beck observed that during depression this flexibility is lost, making it extremely difficult for depressed persons to generate alternative interpretations of events, solutions to problems, or new ways of behaving. Cognitive deficits, such as impaired perception, recall, and long-term memory, interfere with reasoning. Errors in logic, or *cognitive distortions,* become more apparent and create a negative bias to thinking.

Cognitive distortions are present in the thinking of nondepressed persons as well, for no one has perfect understanding. However, in the case of depression, anxiety, or other syndromes, these distortions are rigidly applied and initial impressions are not reevaluated. Self-correction is limited. In addition, in psychological distress, errors in thinking are combined with maladaptive assumptions, leading the patient in a negative spiral. Cognitive distortions include overgeneralization, dichotomous thinking, arbitrary inference, selective abstraction, personalization, and maximization and minimization. The goals of cognitive therapy are to return the person to more flexible thinking and to modify maladaptive beliefs and assumptions which may be risks for further depression. Cognitive therapy teaches people to identify and correct the distortions in their thinking to regain flexibility. It also teaches them to assess the utility of their beliefs and assumptions and to modify them if necessary. Beliefs are modified by examining them logically and considering alternative interpretations and through behavioral experiments designed to challenge specific assumptions.

The cognitive model of depression has found support for descriptive aspects of its theory and for its treatment efficacy. Cognitive therapy has also been applied to a number of other psychological disorders, including anxiety, personality disorders, substance abuse, eating disorders, stress, and marital conflict. More recently, it has been applied to nonclinical problems, such as management problems in business and conflict resolution in schools.

An important finding of treatment outcome studies in depression has been the apparent benefit of cognitive therapy in relapse prevention. This finding has generated studies of depression prevention with populations at risk. Thus, cognitive therapy may be helpful in preventing depression, not just in treating people once they have become depressed. Additionally, school intervention programs that teach cognitive skills such as problem solving, disputing negative self-talk, and improving self-esteem promote positive adjustment at a community level. In this sense, cognitive interventions may contribute to public health.

In theory and in practice, cognitive therapy addresses a spectrum of mental health, from treating psychiatric diagnoses to enhancing the functioning of those at risk for depression or poor social adjustment. This article reviews the cognitive model of psychopathology, describes characteristics of healthy cognitive functioning and presents information on how cognitive therapy may be used to promote mental health.

II. PRINCIPLES OF COGNITIVE THEORY

A. Cognitive Organization

Cognitive therapy envisions a cognitive organization that is hierarchically structured and cognitive mechanisms that selectively take in or screen out relevant information. The most accessible cognitions in this hierarchy are voluntary thoughts which appear in stream-of-consciousness reports. Less accessible, but more stable, are automatic thoughts, which arise without awareness and are difficult to inhibit, especially at times of emotional arousal. At the next level are beliefs and assumptions, including values. At the deepest level, out of the person's awareness, are core beliefs embedded in cognitive structures called *schemas.* The cognitive model proposes that these schemas are latent until triggered by a personally relevant life event. In depression, for example, a life event might trigger a schema of loss, deprivation, or defeat. This would be the mechanism that sets in motion the negative cognitive shift. As a consequence of the cognitive shift, much positive information is filtered out by cognitive distortions, and negative self-relevant information is accepted. The person is thus flooded by negative automatic thoughts.

Automatic thoughts are important in cognitive therapy because they are accessible and reflect core beliefs. They are also full of cognitive distortions. Cognitive therapy works directly on correcting biased thinking by challenging the validity of automatic thoughts. It also works at a structural level to modify maladaptive beliefs and assumptions contained in schemas. It is presumed that these schema-level beliefs are a cognitive vulnerability to various psychological disorders and, if not addressed, pose a risk of recurrence for that disorder.

B. Cognitive Specificity

Although individuals have idiosyncratic thoughts, themes appear within diagnostic categories. Studies comparing the cognitive content of depression and anxiety have found that the cognitions of depressed patients reflect themes of loss, defeat, worthlessness, and deprivation, and anxious patients express themes of danger and threat.

C. Continuity Hypothesis

The cognitive model of psychopathology emphasizes well-being on a continuum. Various psychopathological syndromes are viewed as exaggerated and persistent forms of normal emotional responses. Thus, there is "continuity" between the content of normal reactions and the excessive responses seen in psychological disorders. This hypothesis fits an evolutionary perspective, for it suggests that disorders are extreme manifestations of adaptive strategies. In addition, the notion of continuity makes psychological syndromes more understandable, because people in general can identify with the less severe forms of the behaviors. Indeed, extrapolating from observations of psychopathology gives information about the more subtle biases common in everyday reactions. For example, the intense fear of negative evaluation in social phobia is an exaggeration of the normal social vulnerability and self-consciousness felt in many social interactions. Positive bias and positive illusion, noted in many nondepressed individuals, have an extreme expression in the expansiveness and self-aggrandisement of mania.

Cognitive therapy research has identified cognitive risk factors for various disorders. As a psychotherapy, it is biased in its attention to deficits and limited in its generalizability from clinical samples. Thus, conceptualizations of mental health must be tempered with evidence from social, developmental, and cognitive psychology, which investigate normal populations but are often biased in the direction of generalizing from contrived, laboratory situations. Cognitive models of several disorders are presented here to elucidate cognitive risk factors to mental health. These risk factors are considered in the design of interventions to treat and prevent psychological distress. In addition, contributions from other branches of psychology are presented to consider how healthy cognitive functioning can be promoted.

III. COGNITIVE MODEL OF DEPRESSION

The cognitive model posits that in nonendogenous, unipolar depression, life events activate highly charged negative schemas which override more adaptive schemas and set negatively biased cognitive processing in motion. The activation of schemas is the mechanism by which depression occurs, not its cause. Depression may be caused by any combination of genetic, biological, stress, or personality factors. Regardless of its cause, the same cognitive changes occur in depression. Cognitive distortions bias perceptions and interpretations, judgments and problem-solving skills become limited, and thinking reflects the cognitive triad: a negative view of the self as a failure, a negative view of one's personal world as harsh and unyielding, and a negative view of the future as hopeless. As a consequence of pessimism, hopelessness, or apathy, the depressed person becomes less active, avoids social contact, and takes fewer risks. Reduced performance is then taken as a sign of failure or worthlessness, reinforcing the negative view of the self.

Although the cognitive model is not explicitly causal, it does propose that schemas containing negative beliefs about the self and the world are a cognitive vulnerability to depression. Examples of depressogenic schemas are, "I am unlovable" and "I can never get what I want." Schemas are believed to be established by early learning experiences which are reinforced over time. As they are used to explain further events, schemas become anchored and are both self-perpetuating and difficult to change.

Cognitive therapy also considers the interaction of personality and stressful life events in the onset of depression. Two broad personality types have been identified among depressed patients: autonomous and sociotropic. Autonomous individuals are most likely to become depressed when thwarted from achieving their goals or when confronted with failure. Sociotropic types are most sensitive to personal rejection or to loss of a relationship. Although these are pure types at opposite ends of a continuum of personality styles, they allow investigation of the relationship between life events and various cognitive vulnerabilities. Current research supports the association between sociotropy and depressive symptoms.

Beck's original formulation of depression describes nonendogenous, unipolar depression. He later refined his theory to include six separable but overlapping models: cross-sectional, structural, stressor–vulnerability, reciprocal interaction, psychobiological, and evolutionary. This reformulation was made to describe comprehensively the onset and maintenance of various types of depression. It was articulated in response to such developments in psychology as the growing interest in Bowlby's attachment theory, the emergence of evolutionary psychology, and findings on marital interaction and depression. For example, the original cognitive model exemplifies the stressor–vulnerability model. The maintenance of depression seen in marital discord demonstrates the reciprocal interaction model.

A further clarification of the cognitive theory of depression addressed the misconception that cognitive therapy states that only the thinking of depressed persons is inaccurate or distorted. Research from the field of social cognition demonstrates that the thinking of nondepressed persons tends to be distorted or biased in an optimistic way, rather than being entirely realistic or rational. It also appears that the thinking of mildly depressed persons is more accurate in some specific ways than is the thinking of euthymic individuals. Beck conceives of bias as operating in either a positive or negative direction. According to his formulation, the nondepressed cognitive organization has a positive bias, as it shifts toward depression, the positive cognitive bias is neutralized, and as depression develops, a negative bias occurs. In bipolar cases, there is a pronounced swing into an exaggerated bias as the manic phase develops.

A negative bias in thinking is most likely to occur when data are not immediately present, are not concrete, are ambiguous, and are relevant to self-evaluation. An important feature of the cognitive bias in depression seems to be a perception that current negative circumstances cannot improve. Thus, a depressed person may perceive a situation accurately, but lack the persistence and creativity necessary to solve the problem.

IV. COGNITIVE RISK FACTORS IN SUICIDE

Research on suicide risk was a natural outgrowth of Beck's depression research, and his prospective studies have contributed to the understanding of psychological processes in suicide, particularly the role of hopelessness in predicting suicide. Hopelessness is conceived of as a relatively stable schema, incorporating negative expectations of the future.

Other researchers have identified additional cognitive risk factors for suicide that emerge even with the level of depression and degree of pathology controlled. They are low self-concept, dysfunctional assumptions, the absence of positive beliefs or reasons for living, cognitive rigidity, and poor problem-solving skills. The last two risk factors, cognitive rigidity and poor problem-solving skills, have received attention recently because of their pervasiveness in psychological disorders. Two examples of cognitive rigidity are dichotomous thinking and perfectionism. Evidence for the relationship between all-or-nothing thinking and suicidal behavior is long-standing. In addition, dichotomous thinking is found in a range of psychological disorders, including personality disorders. It is also characteristic of the thinking of normal adolescents.

Recent research also indicates a relationship between perfectionism and suicide risk. Among inpatients, for example, a perfectionistic attitude toward the self and sensitivity to social criticism have been found to be associated with suicide ideation independent of depression and hopelessness. Other research has found that a certain type of perfectionism—perceived expectations for the individual by society—is related to suicide ideation. The belief that the world holds unrealistic and unbending expectations for an individual represents a component of the cognitive triad, the negative view of the world.

Perfectionism may generally inhibit healthy functioning. Analysis of the data from the Treatment of Depression Collaborative Study, which compared the efficacies of pharmacotherapy, cognitive therapy, and interpersonal therapy, found that subjects who had perfectionistic attitudes had a significantly negative relationship to therapeutic outcome, regardless of the type of treatment modality they received. In contrast, subjects with relatively low levels of perfectionism were responsive to all forms of intervention. Perfectionism may be thought of as a risk factor for depression and suicide, and as a challenge to psychotherapy in general.

Problem-solving deficits are of interest not only because of their demonstrated relationships to depression and suicide, but also because social problem-solving is an important skill in general adjustment. Problem solving is being taught in schools as a way to reduce conflict and promote mental health.

Problem-solving deficits have been found in suicidal children, adolescents, and adults, and these deficits become compounded as problems become interpersonal in nature. Suicidal persons have difficulty accepting problems as a normal part of life and are not inclined to engage in problem solving. Once they engage in problem solving, their solutions show more avoidance, more negative affect, less relevance, less versatility, and less reference to the future than do the solutions of nonsuicidal persons.

An important aspect of problem solving among suicide ideators appears to be a tendency to focus on the potential negative consequences of implementing any solution. This feature reflects how pessimism affects motivation in depression and is congruent with the theory of helplessness depression.

A number of researchers have constructed and tested models of how various suicide risk factors might interact. It appears that hopelessness, problem-solving skills, and self-concept are independent risk factors. Beck's observations of patients hospitalized for suicidal ideation shed some light on how self-concept, problem-solving skills, and hopelessness may appear statelike for some patients and traitlike for others. One group studied was composed of depressed persons. Their hopelessness, suicidal ideation, self-concept, and problem-solving abilities improved when their depression remitted. The second group was composed of patients with alcoholism, personality disorders, and antisocial behavior problems. Their negative views of themselves were reinforced by society. This group was characterized by cognitive rigidity, impulsivity, and poor problem-solving skills, which persisted between suicidal crises. Indeed, these characteristics may have predisposed these patients to future suicidal episodes. Thus, for some, poor problem-solving is temporary; for others, it is more chronic. It appears that once suicide becomes an alternative, restricted problem-solving ability can establish it as a stereotyped response in a very limited behavioral repertoire.

V. COGNITIVE MODEL OF ANXIETY DISORDERS

Whereas the cognitive themes in depression are deprivation, defeat, and loss, the cognitive theme in anxiety disorders is danger. Following the continuity hypothesis, anxiety reactions are on a continuum with normal physiologic responses, but are exaggerated reactions to perceived threat. Cognitive therapy views anxiety from an evolutionary perspective, as originating in the flight, freeze, or fight responses apparent in animal behavior. These innate responses to physical danger became less adaptive in humans over the millenia as danger became less physical and more psychosocial in nature.

The cognitive model of anxiety emphasizes the roles of beliefs and interpretations of events in maintaining and escalating anxiety. Anxious cognitions reflect unrealistic perceptions of danger, catastrophic interpretations about loss of control, or perceived negative changes in a relationship. As in depression, there are underlying beliefs, such as, "the world is a dangerous place," which make one vulnerable to anxiety. Cognitive distortions support those underlying beliefs and contribute to the overestimation of the probability of a feared event, the overestimation of the severity of the event were it to happen, the underestimation of one's ability to cope with the feared event, and the underestimation of "rescue factors" such as the presence of people or environmental factors that could help or reduce risk.

The contribution of cognitions to anxiety is exemplified in the cognitive model of recurrent panic. In this case, the person's catastrophic misinterpretation of his or her own physiology escalates anxiety to the point of panic. The sequence is as follows: a variety of factors (e.g., mild anxiety, caffeine, exercise, excitement) create mild sensations that are interpreted as signs of internal disaster. Consequently, there is a marked increase in anxiety which leads to a further heightening of bodily sensations. This creates a vicious cycle, which culminates in a panic attack. Stress-induced hyperventilation may be part of this cycle if somatic sensations are interpreted as a sign of imminent danger. In the case of panic, the feared stimulus is one's own physiology. Once a person has had a panic attack, he or she becomes hypervigilant to any signs of physiological arousal. One's own physiology becomes the feared stimulus. Treatment, therefore, includes exposure to physical sensations.

Cognitive therapy, which uses cognitive techniques alone or in combination with behavioral techniques, can almost eliminate panic attacks after 12 to 16 weeks of treatment.

VI. COGNITIVE MODEL OF PERSONALITY DISORDERS

Cognitive therapy conceptualizes personality disorders as legacies of hominid evolution. They are seen as exaggerated expressions of primitive "strategies," which at one time influenced survival and reproductive success. For example, the adaptive strategy of attachment becomes exaggerated as "I am helpless" in the dependent personality.

In addition, the repetitive nature of maladaptive behaviors seen in personality disorders indicates the frequency with which maladaptive schemas are triggered. Beck and his associates have found that the maladaptive schemas in personality disorders are triggered in many if not most situations, have a compulsive quality, and are extremely difficult to modify or control. Compared with other people, the dysfunctional attitudes found in persons with personality disorders are rigid, overgeneralized, absolute, and resistant to change.

The dysfunctional beliefs in personality disorders are thought to be a result of the interaction between the person's genetic predisposition and exposure to specific undesirable or traumatic events. Maladaptive behavior patterns may result from reinforcement of such behaviors over a person's lifetime. Such maladaptive behaviors may arise from avoidance or from compensation or overcompensation for dysfunctional beliefs. For example, a person who fears abandonment might avoid relationships altogether, cling to partners and drive them away, or end relationships before they can be left by the other parties. Any of these behaviors can reinforce the dysfunctional belief that the person will inevitably be abandoned.

VII. WHAT DOES HEALTHY COGNITIVE FUNCTIONING LOOK LIKE?

Cognitive therapy is derived from research on clinical populations, particularly depressed patients. Characteristics of the diagnostic groups studied are assumed to be extreme manifestations of qualities that are also found in normal people. Among depressed patients, for example, thinking is characterized by cognitive distortions or errors in logic, by cognitive rigidity, and by maladaptive core beliefs. Does this mean that the thinking of nondepressed people is free of distortions or an accurate reflection of reality? It does not.

Considerable evidence from cognitive and social psychology testifies to the presence of illusion or a general, enduring pattern of error, bias, or both in the information processing of normal people. However, the bias in thinking is positively skewed. Experimental studies, typically done with college student volunteers, show that nondepressed thinking is characterized by unrealistically positive views of the self, exaggerated perceptions of control, and unrealistic optimism.

This is apparent in attributional or explanatory style. The explanatory style of depressed persons is to attribute causality of negative, uncontrollable events to internal, stable, and global causes. One fails a test because one is stupid, not because that particular test was especially difficult. Nondepressed people, who have positive illusions concerning control and self-perception, are better able to externalize failure and thus not damage their general sense of self-esteem.

It appears from several lines of evidence that mildly depressed people, those with low self-esteem, or both have more balanced self-perceptions, more evenhanded assessments of their future circumstances, and a more accurate sense of personal control than do nondepressed persons. In contrast, both clinically depressed and euthymic people have biased thinking.

It is not surprising that many of the same cognitive mechanisms operate in different mood states, but they operate to different ends. Studies in social cognition support many of the clinical observations on which cognitive therapy is based. In 1989, Janoff-Bulman wrote about the benefits of illusion for mental health. She describes how preverbal interactions with responsive caregivers establish supraordinate schemas that are positively biased and largely reflect reality at the time they are established. One need only substitute the experience of a child with unresponsive, neglectful, or depriving caregivers to arrive at maladaptive schemas. The early interactions among people receiving good care teach them that the world is benevolent and controllable, and that they are worthy of care. Although later experience may somewhat contradict or qualify these assumptions, they will remain fundamentally intact. Evidence that does not confirm positive assumptions can be ignored, dismissed, or reinterpreted to fit previously held beliefs. This process is the same as that in depression: cognitive distortions screen out positive information or distort neutral information to maintain negative schemas. Only traumatic negative events pose a serious challenge to the equilibrium of positive illusions.

Parallels between the cognitive processes in depression and those in well-being also appear in Taylor and Brown's theory of cognitive adaptation. They present a model of normal cognitive processing in which social and cognitive filters make information largely positive as opposed to the disproportionately negative bias that results from the mental filters operating in depression. These authors conclude that the mentally healthy person appears to have the capacity to distort reality in a direction that enhances self-esteem, maintains a sense of personal efficacy, and promotes an optimistic view of the future. This positive triad is in striking contrast to the cognitive triad in depression.

For both depressed and nondepressed people, biased thinking is most apparent in situations that are ambiguous and that are relevant to self-evaluation. For both negative and overly positive thinking, ambiguous information tends to be interpreted to fit with prior beliefs or schemas.

Just as the cognitive model of psychopathology might overemphasize the negative aspects of biased cognitive processing and thus appear to endorse rationality, models from cognitive and social psychology might overemphasize the benefits of positive illusion for mental health. Some researchers have addressed various types of illusions and the circumstances under which they appear helpful and not so helpful.

Taylor's research on cognitive adaptation to threatening events such as rape and cancer found that illusions of meaning, mastery, and self-esteem fostered positive adjustment. Individuals who made causal attributions that maintained a sense of personal control and who could construct some personal benefit from the negative experience fared better psychologically than those unable to use illusion. Taylor concludes that illusion is essential for normal cognitive functioning. She also argues that having an accurate self-perception should not be a criterion of mental health, as has been customarily believed.

It also appears from the work of others that illusions are only adaptive if they do not stray too far from the truth. Illusions that are too inflated may lead to self-defeating behavior. A small positive distortion of the truth, rather than unbridled optimism, seems optimal.

Janoff-Bulman proposes that positive illusions are most beneficial at the level of core beliefs or schemas. She sees conceptual (or cognitive) systems as hierarchically organized. Higher-order postulates represent one's most abstract, global, and generalized theories about oneself and the world. Lower-order postulates are narrow generalizations that relate to specific domains of life, such as one's abilities. These hierarchical distinctions are compatible with Beck's notions of core schemas and more accessible assumptions, respectively. Janoff-Bulman argues that higher-order postulates, which are least subject of all cognitions to empirical validation or invalidation, may contain positive inaccuracies without being problematic. However, inaccuracies and positive illusions at the level of lower-order postulates are maladaptive. In other words, it is not harmful to have a generally positive view of oneself as a competent person as long as one is aware of one's limitations in specific areas.

According to Janoff-Bulman's theory, the advantage of positive higher-order assumptions (or schemas) is that they enable a person to attempt to tackle new situations. Thus, positive illusion at this level benefits affect and motivation. One can see how such optimism might allow someone to engage in creative problem solving when faced with a novel situation.

Another benefit of generalized positive illusions about the self relates to efficacy in problem solving. People with high self-esteem appear better able to discriminate soluble from insoluble problems than are people with low self-esteem. They are more able than people with low self-esteem to know when to quit and to feel comfortable quitting. They may also choose to work only on problems that can be solved, thereby reinforcing their sense of self-efficacy.

In contrast to Taylor, Janoff-Bulman believes the healthiest people probably have a good sense of their strengths and weaknesses, their possibilities and limitations. The key appears to be maintaining positive illusions at the level of fundamental beliefs while aiming for and accepting accuracy at the level of everyday, specific interactions with the world. Healthy people can thus respond to environmental feedback and learn.

Healthy cognitive functioning is creative and flexible enough to reexamine strategies that no longer work. No doubt, healthy beliefs contain inaccuracies, but they are adaptive in that they allow one to maintain a sense of self-worth while trying to learn from one's experiences. Healthy functioning also recognizes emotions as important sources of information about the self and the environment. Cognitive therapy allows patients to reappraise and empirically test their lower-order postulates within the context of a caring and collaborative therapeutic relationship. Although schema change at the level of higher-order postulates is more difficult to achieve, longer term cognitive therapy may allow for these fundamental changes.

VIII. SOME DEVELOPMENTAL CONSIDERATIONS

Research in cognitive development, social cognition, and child psychology lends further insight into what healthy cognitive functioning looks like. The unrealistic optimism and self-confidence apparent in well-adjusted adults has also been found in healthy children. Studies have compared "helpless" and "mastery-oriented" children in their responses to failure. Mastery-oriented children are those who have a sense of control over an experimental task; helpless children have no such sense of control. Mastery-oriented children were less discouraged by failure than were helpless children. In fact, they did not seem to recognize that they had failed. Instead, they focused on how to overcome defeat. In addition, they expected success in the future and attributed success to their own ability. They exemplified the nondepressed explanatory style articulated by the learned helplessness model of depression. In contrast, the helpless children demonstrated an explanatory style that may be a cognitive vulnerability to depression.

The adaptive explanatory style may not be exclusive to confident children, but may be the rule for all very young children. Some developmental psychologists report that learned helplessness is relatively rare in very young children. They review studies that demonstrate that children around 3 years of age typically overestimate their skills on a wide variety of tasks and have unrealistically positive expectations for success. This may be highly adaptive for the same reason it is adaptive in adults: self-efficacy motivates further action. Unrealistic optimism gives young children the opportunity to try new skills and to practice them. Researchers hypothesize that ignorance of their limitations allows children to try more diverse and complex behaviors that exceed their grasp at the present time. This allows them to practice skills and may foster long-term cognitive benefits.

Kendall's research in cognitive–behavior therapy with children has identified two types of thinking errors in children, cognitive deficiencies and cognitive distortions. Cognitive deficiencies refer to an absence of thinking. Youngsters with such deficiencies lack careful information processing and often act without thinking. Impulsivity is a result of cognitive deficiencies. Cognitive distortions occur among those who engage in information processing, but who do so in a biased or dysfunctional way. Depressed and anxious children demonstrate cognitive distortions in their misperceptions of social and environmental situations and in their self-perceptions. Children with aggressive behavior demonstrate both cognitive deficiencies and cognitive distortions, because they overinterpret signs of hostility and react without careful thought. Targeting cognitive deficiencies in therapy requires stopping nonthoughtful activity and channeling activity into problem solving. Targeting cognitive distortions calls for the identification of faulty thinking and the correction of misperceptions, misattributions, and misinterpretations.

Both developmental theory and clinical studies support the notion that particular types of cognitive distortions are to be expected at certain stages of normal development. For example, dichotomous thinking and overgeneralization emerge in the preoperational stage of cognitive development. Dichotomous thinking is also viewed as characteristic of normal adolescent thinking. However, these natural proclivities may interact with maladaptive schemas and persist into adulthood.

IX. HOW DOES COGNITIVE THERAPY WORK?

Cognitive therapy combines behavioral and cognitive techniques in a collaborative effort with the patient to examine and test the validity and utility of the patient's maladaptive beliefs. The patient's beliefs and assumptions are viewed as hypotheses to be tested. In the course of therapy, alternative perspectives, interpretations of events, and solutions to problems are considered. Through logical examination of beliefs and behavioral experiments to test specific assumptions, the patient learns more adaptive ways of thinking.

Despite the demonstrated efficacy of cognitive therapy, the mechanisms by which it works have not yet been determined. Beck and others believe that cognitive therapy relies on empirical hypothesis testing to produce changes in beliefs. An explicit goal of the therapy is to teach patients this strategy so that they may apply it in the future, thereby preventing relapse. Some developmental psychologists explain change in cognitive therapy with Piagetian theory. In cognitive therapy, the presentation of contradictory evidence creates a cognitive imbalance or disequilibrium which can lead to a new and improved balance of knowledge.

There has been some debate as to whether cognitive therapy works by teaching compensatory skills to manage triggered schemas or whether schema change itself can be achieved. It may be that schema change is only possible with longer treatment, whereas compensatory skills operate early in therapy.

One cognitive feature that seems to change with cognitive therapy is explanatory style. Research has found that explanatory style and severity of depression improved together over a course of cognitive therapy and remained stable at follow-up. It has therefore been hypothesized that explanatory style is a mechanism of change for depressed patients receiving cognitive therapy. Undoing a pessimistic explanatory style may be an active ingredient in the therapy. If it is possible to reduce a pessimistic style, it may be possible to reduce the risk of future depressive episodes. Evidence for change in explanatory style among euthymic groups demonstrates that such training is feasible, so perhaps cognitive therapy can be used to prevent an initial depressive episode. For use with euthymic groups, such as business managers or students, cognitive therapy is modified slightly. There is less emphasis on behavioral activation strategies, which occur early in the treatment of depression, and greater emphasis on cognitive strategies to challange maladaptive thoughts and change explanatory style.

X. THE PREVENTION OF DEPRESSION

A number of outcome studies that examined the efficacy of cognitive therapy for depression found differential relapse rates among those treated with cognitive therapy, with or without medication, and those treated with medication alone. Specifically, it appears that cognitive therapy for depression prevents relapse. Currently, there is no evidence of a preventive effect after termination of antidepressant medication or any other psychotherapy. Interpersonal psychotherapy, another efficacious treatment for depression, appears to reduce risk only as long as it is continued.

As a result of these findings, there is interest in discerning whether cognitive therapy can truly prevent relapse and whether it can prevent a first episode of depression among populations at risk.

The Penn Prevention Program used a school-based, cognitive–behavioral intervention to prevent a first episode of depression in 10- to 13-year-old children. The children were identified as being at-risk for depression on the basis of depressive symptoms and their reports of parental conflict. The cognitive–behavioral techniques were designed to teach children coping strategies to use when confronted with negative life events, thereby increasing their sense of mastery and competence. In addition to preventing depressive symptoms, the intervention attempted to address problems associated with depression, such as academic difficulties, poor peer relations, low self-esteem, and behavior problems. [*See* Coping with Stress.]

The program consisted of a cognitive component, a social problem-solving component, and a coping skills component. The cognitive component taught flexible thinking and how to evaluate the accuracy of beliefs. It also included explanatory style training to foster more accurate, less pessimistic attributions. For situations in which an accurate interpretation of events was negative, children were taught to focus on solutions or on ways to cope with emotions. Coping techniques included decatastrophizing about potential outcomes of the problem, distraction, steps to distance oneself from stressful situations, relaxation training, and ways to seek social support. In this way, investigators tried to address both cognitive distortions and cognitive deficiencies. The cognitive interventions addressed dysfunctional thinking, and the problem-solving and coping skills components prevented impulsive actions.

Those children who received the intervention showed significant reductions in depressive symptoms and improved classroom behavior compared with controls. These differences persisted at 6-month follow-up. The decrease in depressive symptoms was greatest in the children most at risk for depression.

A controlled prevention trial was conducted by Munoz among adults at risk who comprised a multiethnic, low-income sample. This cognitive–behavioral intervention also resulted in a significantly lower incidence of depressive symptoms among those receiving treatment than those in the control group. In addition, there was a lower incidence rate of major depressive episodes in the treatment group, but the cases were too few to be statistically significant.

Prevention of actual depressive episodes was an outcome criterion in a study by Clarke and associates of adolescents at risk by virtue of their subclinical, depressive symptomotology. This 15-session, cognitive–behavioral intervention taught adolescents to identify and challenge negative or dysfunctional thoughts. Participants had a total incidence of unipolar depression of about half of that of the control group, and this persisted through a 12-month follow-up.

Other controlled trials of cognitive therapy and other modalities for the prevention of depression are underway. In the meantime, cognitive therapy skills are being used to promote general social adjustment in school settings. School-based programs nationwide are applying cognitive–behavioral techniques as part of interpersonal skills training and conflict resolution. Cognitive skills such as disputing negative self-talk and problem solving are part of programs that typically include emotional awareness, communication skills, and behavioral self-control strategies. These programs are an example of health promotion, because they are applied at the community level and decrease the likelihood of occurrence of a range of psychological problems. Although cognitive therapy was designed as a treatment for psychological disorders, it may be beneficial in the prevention of psychological distress and in the promotion of well-being.

BIBLIOGRAPHY

Beck, A. T. (1987). Cognitive models of depression. *Journal of Cognitive Psychotherapy: An International Quarterly, 1*(1), 5–37.

Beck, A. T. (1991). Cognitive therapy: A 30-year retrospective. *American Psychologist, 46*(4), 368–375.

Beck, A. T., Emery, G., & Greenberg, R. (1985). *Anxiety disorders and phobias: A cognitive perspective.* New York: Basic Books.

Beck, A. T., Freeman, A., & Associates (1990). *Cognitive therapy of personality disorders.* New York: Guilford Press.

Beck, A. T., Rush, A. J., Shaw, B. F., & Emery, G. (1979). *Cognitive therapy of depression.* New York: Guilford Press.

Clark, D. M., & Beck, A. T. (1988). Cognitive approaches. In C. G. Last & M. Hersen (Eds.), *Handbook of anxiety disorders.* New York: Pergamon.

Janoff-Bulman, R. (1989). The benefits of illusion, the threat of disillusionment, and the limitations of inaccuracy. *Journal of Social and Clinical Psychology, 8*(2), 159–175.

Salkovskis, P. M. (Ed.). (1996). *Frontiers of cognitive therapy.* New York: Guilford Press.

Seligman, M. E. P. (1991). *Learned optimism.* New York: Knopf.

Weishaar, M. E. (1993). *Aaron T. Beck.* London: Sage.

Community Mental Health

Edward Seidman and Sabine Elizabeth French

New York University

Deinstitutionalization The movement to reduce the number of patients kept in mental institutions by releasing them to the care of the community. The original intention of this movement was to maintain former patients in the community with a wide array of comprehensive and supportive services.

Inoculation Programs Programs that are designed to build and strengthen skills in groups of individuals in order to protect them from, and prepare them for, future difficulties.

Primary Prevention Programs that intervene with a population or setting to reduce the incidence, number of new cases, of one or more emotional disorders.

Promotion of Well-Being Programs that foster the development of healthy environments that encourage positive mental health; in turn, these programs reduce the incidence of one or more psychiatric disorders in the population or setting.

Restructuring The alteration of the unwritten rules of a setting in order to facilitate the development of new rules and an environment that facilitates positive mental health; indirectly, such a change reduces the incidence of disorder in the setting.

Risk and Protective Factors Circumstances in an individual's life, a population, or setting that either increase or decrease the chances of suffering from or manifesting problems-in-living. Stressful life events, for example, death of a parent or divorce, and daily hassles are common risk factors, while positive social support is a common protective factor.

Secondary Prevention Programs that identify early signs of a disorder and intervene quickly or at the point of a crisis to short-circuit the problem from developing into a full-blown mental health problem.

Tertiary Prevention Programs that intervene directly with patients to reduce the duration of their career as a patient, that is, to rehabilitate or treat them; thereby reducing the prevalence of psychiatric disorder in the community.

The confluence of two salient events in the early 1960s—efforts to deinstitutionalize the chronically mentally ill and legislation to create COMMUNITY MENTAL HEALTH centers across the nation—launched the community mental health movement. With the aide of a prevention framework adapted from the field of public health, this movement has continued to evolve and grow. Initial emphases on tertiary prevention, often in the form of alternative community-based methods of treatment for the severely mentally ill, were followed by efforts aimed at early detection and intervention (secondary prevention), for example, suicide prevention telephone "hotlines." In both tertiary and secondary forms of prevention, emotional and behavioral problems, or early antecedents thereof,

Copyright © 1998 by Academic Press.
All rights of reproduction in any form reserved.

continued to be identified at the level of the individual. Interventions were implemented within institutions in contrast to within communities. However, to reduce the incidence of disorder in the population, primary prevention programs aimed at communities, population groups, or settings were developed and implemented. The positive concept of promoting well-being was a further evolution from the notion of preventing disorder. This article describes, explains, and illustrates with exemplary programs the evolution from tertiary prevention to the promotion of well-being that has characterized the community mental health movement during the second half of the twentieth century.

I. ORIGINS OF THE COMMUNITY MENTAL HEALTH MOVEMENT IN TWENTIETH-CENTURY AMERICA

Widespread implementation of conceptions of community mental health did not begin in America until the early 1960s, even though these ideas and practices had numerous roots that originated both in previous centuries and in other nations. In fact, several scholars date the origins of interest in prevention as an alternative to treatment back to the twelfth-century Spanish philosopher Maimonides who spoke of "preventing poverty."

Returning to more recent history, in 1961, in response to a Congressional mandate the final report of the Joint Commission on Mental Illness and Health entitled *Action for Mental Health* was released. Among other things, it called for improved and expanded mental health services including: (a) improved care in small psychiatric hospitals of chronically mentally ill patients; (b) improved and expanded aftercare services, both partial hospitalization and rehabilitation in the community; (c) intensive care for acutely disturbed mental patients in mental health clinics in the community, general hospital psychiatric units, or in small intensive psychiatric centers; and (d) increased efforts at public education about both psychological disorders and the citizenry's inclination to reject the mentally ill.

President John F. Kennedy was extremely receptive to the *Action for Mental Health* report. In a message delivered in 1963, he stated:

> we must seek out the causes of mental illness . . . and eradicate them . . . For prevention is far more desirable . . . more economical and it is far more likely to be successful. Prevention will require both specific programs directed especially at known causes, and the general strengthening of our fundamental community, social welfare, and educational programs which can do much to eliminate or correct the harsh environmental conditions which are often associated with mental retardation and illness (p. 2).

Comprehensive care available to all people in their local communities was central to his clarion call for a "bold new approach." These concepts were enacted into legislation as part of the Community Mental Health Centers Act of 1963.

As a result of this legislation, some 1500 catchment areas (currently referred to as mental health service areas) with populations ranging from 75,000 to 200,000 people were created in the United States; each catchment area was eligible for federal construction and staffing funds for a community mental health center. These centers were mandated initially to offer inpatient care, outpatient care, emergency services, partial hospitalization, and consultation and education, and ultimately to include diagnostic services, rehabilitation services, precare and aftercare services, training, and research and evaluation.

Both implicitly and explicitly, the goals of the Joint Commission on Mental Illness and Health, the Kennedy Administration, and the Community Mental Health Centers Act were to provide more humane and effective rehabilitation to those who were severely mentally ill. Patients needed to be integrated into their local communities and smaller treatment settings in contrast to huge, anonymous state hospitals in remote physical locations. Most importantly, they needed continuity of care, as indicated by the array of services to be offered by the local community mental health center.

Several other factors converged with this more humane and progressive approach to the treatment of the chronically mentally ill that were critical to the implementation of this movement toward deinstitutionalization. The use of phenothiazines made it more feasible to return patients to their communities as they were less likely to engage in the extremes of deviant behavior. At the same time, deinstitutionalization was seen as a dramatic cost-saving device by fiscally conservative legislators. As we describe below, ultimately, these fiscal motives undermined the continuity of care and services in the community envisioned by its originators.

Other salient factors that drove the community mental health movement included well-publicized, analytic reports that indicated that the mental health needs of the population far outstripped the resources of trained personnel. Moreover, those that needed services the most, for example, urban and rural poor, children, adolescents, and the elderly, received them least often and, generally paid more for these services when they did receive them. If prevention was to fulfill its promise, hard-to-reach, unserved, and underserved populations needed to be reached.

The principles of comprehensive community-based treatment, prevention and the promotion of well-being inherent to the ideology of the community mental health movement have continued to hold sway among practitioners and scholars to the present time. However, presidential support, implementation mechanisms, and financial resources at the national level were seriously undermined during the Nixon and Reagan Administrations.

II. PRINCIPLES OF PREVENTION

As we have seen, the preceding policy initiatives in the area of community mental health were inextricably intertwined with the idea of prevention. In 1964, Gerald Caplan published his classic book entitled *The Principles of Preventive Psychiatry*. Using public health concepts, he described three types of prevention—tertiary, secondary, and primary—as they related to mental health and illness.

The overriding goal of prevention is to reduce the prevalence or number of cases of mental disorder(s) at a specified moment in time in the population or community. Prevalence is, however, a function of both the incidence (the number of new cases diagnosed during a specified time period) and duration (the time between the initial diagnoses and recovery) of a disorder. Reducing duration, incidence, or both, reduces prevalence. Tertiary prevention reduces prevalence by decreasing the duration of a disorder. Secondary prevention can reduce prevalence either by short-circuiting the duration of a disorder or by intervening in the developmental course of a disorder before it has become fully manifested (and so labeled) to decrease incidence. Primary prevention reduces prevalence solely by decreasing the incidence of disorder.

In tertiary prevention, the goal is to reduce the duration of an individual's career as a patient. Here, the patient has already been identified with a problem(s) in living. Thus, tertiary prevention is more appropriately referred to as rehabilitation. In secondary prevention, the goal is to identify early signs or antecedents of psychopathology in an individual so that intervention can be implemented promptly to alter the developmental course, duration, and/or severity of psychopathology. Here, short-circuiting a disorder's duration is the primary means of diminishing prevalence. Early treatment or crisis intervention represent the most common forms of secondary prevention or intervention.

In both tertiary and secondary prevention, problem identification and change take place at the level of an individual person. This distinguishes them from primary prevention. In primary prevention, the prevalence, and more specifically the incidence of a disorder, in a population or setting is reduced. Thus, primary prevention is mass in contrast to individually oriented. It also differs from tertiary and secondary prevention by occurring "before-the-fact." With regard to the nature/target of intervention, the distinction between tertiary/secondary and primary prevention is less clear. While most often the target of intervention in tertiary and secondary prevention is an individual, as we will see below, occasionally the target is the creation or alteration of a setting that a group of problem-identified individuals inhabit. However, based on the sharp differences in problem identification and the locus of change, some authors have suggested that referring to tertiary and secondary prevention as prevention makes the concept of prevention meaningless.

As early as 1964, Caplan offered a compelling definition of primary prevention:

> Primary prevention is a community concept. It involves lowering the rate of new cases of mental disorder in a population over a certain period by counteracting harmful circumstances before they have had a chance to produce illness. It does not seek to prevent a specific person from becoming sick. Instead, it seeks to reduce the risk for a whole population, so that, although some may become ill, their number will be reduced. It thus contrasts with individual patient-oriented psychiatry, which focuses on a single person and deals with general influences only insofar as they are combined in his unique experience (p. 26).

In primary prevention (or "true" prevention), the level of assessment or target of intervention is not an individual, but instead the reduction of the prevalence of disorder in an entire population or setting before it occurs. A vaccine can inoculate an entire population from contracting an illness before anyone has been affected, as exemplified by the polio vaccine or fluoride in water. Similarly, effective social policies can reduce the incidence and prevalence of unwanted problems in a society, as in the case of an effective gun control policy that reduces the homicide rate or a policy of availability and accessibility of condoms for sexually active adolescents that reduces unwanted pregnancies. An example specific to mental health is pellagra that is accompanied by psychotic-like symptoms. Pellagra is a disease that stems, in part, from a deficiency of niacin in the diet. Today, the disease is prevented with a dietary intake that includes a sufficient amount of niacin.

In an effort to reduce the prevalence of a disease, the progression from tertiary to primary prevention points the way toward the promotion of well-being. To the degree that interventions or policies can successfully promote well-being in the population, we will have succeeded in reducing the incidence and prevalence of a wide array of disorders and undesirable outcomes.

In the subsequent sections of this article, we will utilize the preceding principles and articulate more specific ones. These principles will be underscored with the use of exemplary programs in each area: tertiary, secondary, and primary prevention, and the promotion of well-being.

III. TERTIARY PREVENTION

Long-term hospitalization of the mentally ill seemed to do little more than guarantee a chronic pattern of institutionalization. Thus, with the ideology and resources behind the community mental health movement in the 1960s, we began to see the development of a variety of innovative, experimental alternatives to institutional treatment. The goals were to remove patients from state psychiatric or Veteran's hospitals and reintegrate them into local communities with the provision of a comprehensive and critical array of supportive services ranging from housing and employment to cooking, personal grooming, and treatment. These innovative community-based alternatives were not viewed as magical cures, but instead as the best means to provide patients with some semblance of "normal" lives, and at a minimum, a way to halt the well known iatrogenic effects of institutional treatment.

As a result of the Community Mental Health Movement, the number of state hospital beds were dramatically reduced over the years. Unfortunately, many of the patients who were deinstitutionalized did not receive the continuity of community-based services called for by the architects of this movement. Many patients would quickly return to the hospital for services. They would stay for a short period of time and, then again, be released to the community. This pattern would repeat itself; it came to be known as the "revolving door" phenomena.

Closing state hospitals and reducing the number of beds available did save money, but over time, fewer and fewer of these revenues were returned to local communities to provide for the continuum of services that were essential to community-based treatment. To date, this paradoxical pattern has not abated. Thus, an increasing number of people with serious problems in living are found roaming the streets; they lack access to a comprehensive array of essential residential and rehabilitative services.

While many in politics and the media have judged deinstitutionalization to have been a failure, this verdict is misleading. As envisioned by its architects, the policy of deinstitutionalization was never genuinely implemented since a continuum of comprehensive services tailored to the needs of individual patients was never put into place. However, though isolated, exciting and promising innovative experiments were implemented. Unfortunately, the results of these demonstration programs were ignored as fiscally minded politicians seized upon the opportunity to cut mental health budgets on the basis of the savings realized from the reduction in the number of hospital beds.

One such example of a successful demonstration program in the 1960s was developed by Fairweather and his colleagues; they created an innovative setting as an alternative to institutionalization, known as the community lodge program. Here, 8 to 10 long-term mental patients worked and lived in an autonomous unit outside the hospital. The "lodge" was often located on the border between a middle class and a poor neighborhood. In this way, the residents were able to create a small business and, at the same time, they were less likely to be rejected by their neighbors. The lodge residents shared household management and tasks ranging from cooking and cleaning to budgeting. They established a joint business, for example, a janitorial service, that enabled them to earn income and develop a sense of accomplishment. They ran their own "show" with leadership emerging from their ranks. Professional services, ranging from psychotherapy and medications to accounting, were available to them, but on an as needed basis, and after a time, only when the residents requested these services. Thus, unlike institutional treatment and many group homes that appear similar on the surface, patients no longer found themselves in the characteristic "one-down" relationship with the "doctor who knows best." Results demonstrated that they were able to remain in the community for a longer period than were patients who were assigned to traditional outpatient care upon their release from the hospital.

To prevent the negative effects of institutionalization a number of exemplary innovations were implemented at the point of psychiatric admission. For example, in the 1970s, the Stein, Test, and Marx group in Madison, Wisconsin, developed, implemented, and evaluated an intriguing program that occurred within 1 week of hospitalization. Patients with extensive histories of psychiatric hospitalization who were deemed "unreleasable" by hospital personnel were placed into independent living situations based on their individual resources and needs. The goal was for these patients to make it in the natural environment. In that vein, staff took on the roles of advocate, resource finder, and teacher. Initially available on a 24-hour basis, staff gradually phased themselves out. Staff endeavored to keep patients independent of the usual mental health system and to help them obtain the resources needed for daily living by prodding and supporting job finding, grooming and cooking skills, recreational and social activity, and so forth. Staff also encouraged others to view patients as responsible citizens, even if it meant allowing the patient to spend a day or two in jail for breaking the law. In research evaluating this program, as in the community lodge program, the experimental group of patients was far more successful at maintaining themselves in independent living arrangements than the control group, yet few differences in psychiatric symptomatology were demonstrated between the two groups of patients.

A dramatically different alternative to psychiatric hospitalization became more ascendant in the 1980s—self-help groups and mutual support organizations. Although self or mutual help groups often are viewed as adjuncts to traditional treatment, as illustrated in the next paragraph, mutual help organizations have greater potential as a true alternative, in that, beyond the weekly group meetings, there are many other ways that members engage themselves in each others' lives as prodders and supporters. Moreover, some of these organizations view themselves as an international community health movement.

GROW, a mutual help organization, came to the United States in the late 1970s. The organization was created in Australia in the late 1950s by a group of former mental patients seeking more appropriate ways to deal with their problems in living than what they were receiving within the state institutions. In part, they modeled their mutual help group meetings along the lines of Alcoholics Anonymous meetings, which some of them had attended. Over time they developed a far more elaborate structure and set of principles, both for the group meetings, per se, and for the larger and more encompassing "sharing and caring community" that they established for their members. The organization's most fundamental principle is not to do "to" or "for" people, but "with" people. Roles and niches are created, at whatever level of functioning people are at, where individuals can attain a sense of accomplishment and pride. In this way, their members can feel empowered and begin to grow. Members create friendship networks that provide support and assistance beyond the weekly group meetings. Local groups are organized into a regional network and they create other social functions; the regional network often establishes a small residential setting where they can tend to members at crisis times. Mutual help organizations clearly provide people with serious problems in living a social and psychological community in which to grow in contrast to institutional treatment and living.

Grassroots mutual help organizations such as GROW have a complete philosophy of treatment, offer a continuum of services, and operate relatively inexpensively. Because they are less dependent on outlays of financial resources from the government and, at the same time, are free of many bureaucratic constraints, they are more likely to be sustained and disseminated in contrast to many innovative demonstration programs that, most often, erode and disappear after the initial funds have been exhausted, no matter how effective they had been. The "catch 22" is that while mutual help organizations offer considerable therapeutic promise, their ascendance runs the risk of allowing governmental bodies to continue to rationalize their decreasing financial commitment to a continuum of mental health services.

As we have seen, several innovative treatment methods have been developed as alternatives to institutional treatment. They reduce the duration, and thus, the prevalence of serious problems in living. These alternatives are community-based and provide a continuum of supportive and residential services that keep people out of hospitals. Most often, these programs are characterized by a philosophy that dictates that they work *with* individual patients, in contrast to doing things to or for them. In essence, the traditional pattern of "one-up, one-down" role relationships between patients and service providers is restructured in these innovative and successful tertiary prevention programs. Nevertheless, these innovative methods provide rehabilitation to individuals constituting forms of tertiary prevention. They do not short-circuit problems, nor do they prevent groups/populations from developing mental health problems in the first place.

IV. SECONDARY PREVENTION

In secondary prevention, problem identification and intervention occur much earlier in the process than in tertiary prevention. The duration or magnitude of a mental health problem can be short-circuited by identifying and intervening early in the problem's developmental course, thus, reducing its prevalence. On the other hand, if a problem is identified early enough in its course that it is not even considered a mental health problem, its incidence and, in turn, its prevalence can be reduced. Here, the potential problem can be thought of as being "cut off at the pass." In both forms of secondary prevention, intervention occurs at the level of the individual; intervention is not mass-oriented as it is in primary prevention. However, in the latter form of secondary prevention, problem identification can occur at the level of a population or setting.

Once individuals enter the mental health system, they seem to become entrapped within it. From a secondary prevention perspective, we might want to examine gateways to the mental health system—how individuals enter the system. In some communities this gateway is the State's Attorney's Office, who must file a petition in order to legally involuntarily commit someone who appears disturbed. The State's Attorney is often asked to file petitions for involuntary commitment on persons who would profit more from other services, for example, short-term housing, a friendship network, help in finding employment, or intensive outpatient counseling regarding a recent family crisis. Unfortunately, given limited resources and options, involuntary commitment is too often the easiest and most expedient action for the legal system.

In the Midwest during the 1970s, Delaney, Seidman, and Willis developed and evaluated an innovative and successful crisis intervention program for individuals in jeopardy of being involuntarily committed to a psychiatric hospital. They negotiated an arrangement in which they would immediately be notified by the State's Attorney that they were considering filing a petition for involuntary commitment. Within 24 hours, the crisis intervention team would see the person in their natural environment, fully assess the problem, and develop a comprehensive plan of intervention, and set the plan into motion. State hospitalization was often deemed inappropriate or was used only as a last resort for a seriously disturbed individual. This program reduced the number of state hospitalizations in the area, provided persons with more appropriate services, thereby reducing many of the iatrogenic effects of hospitalization. (Were the focus of the program tertiary prevention, researchers would have aided the patients only *after* they had been involuntarily committed.)

Many secondary programs intervene with children since it is believed that the seeds of many problems are sown in childhood. Early detection and intervention is viewed as optimal. Since most children go to school, early identification programs often take place within schools, where populations of individuals can be screened.

One of the earliest exemplars of early detection and intervention programs was known as the Primary Mental Health Project developed by Cowen and his associates. Mass screening allowed early identification of children thought likely to manifest future adjustment problems. (This differs from a tertiary prevention program, which would focus on children that have already been identified as exhibiting problem behaviors.) The identified children were then assigned to minimally paid volunteer child aides (housewives or college students) to work one-on-one with them after school. These aides were trained and closely supervised by university personnel. By using paraprofessionals, the program extended the limited numbers and reach of mental health professionals.

Secondary prevention reduces incidence and prevalence by short-circuiting problems before they are fully realized. In this way it is clearly preferable to the rehabilitation strategies of tertiary prevention. However, intervention remains at the level of the individual and, thus, still runs the danger of stigmatizing and "blaming the victim."

V. PRIMARY PREVENTION

Primary prevention programs endeavor to reduce the incidence of disorder, or unwanted outcomes, in a population or setting, such as the school, the workplace, or the community. Problem identification occurs at the level of a population or setting, not at the level of an individual. In contrast to tertiary and secondary prevention, the population or setting's constituents have *not* been screened to determine if they have symptoms or problems.

Primary preventive interventions are mass-oriented; some programs are aimed at entire populations or communities, while others are aimed at population groups at high risk for negative outcomes. For example, poverty places some demographic groups at greater risk for maladaptive mental health outcomes. A variant of the high-risk approach is that a setting or transition can be considered "risky," where residing in a particular setting or making the particular transition is associated with a higher likelihood or negative outcomes. For example, the work environment of air traffic controllers is considered a risky setting because of the high rates of physical and psychological stress reactions controllers experience. Similarly, the movement from elementary to junior high school is often deemed a risky transition because of the concomitant and precipitous drops in self-esteem and academic performance. In these examples, the social and environmental organization and structure of these risky settings and transitions need to become the focus of primary preventive interventions.

Regardless of the scope of the preventive intervention, malleable risk and protective factors take on increased importance. Stressful life events, for example, the death of a parent or divorce, and daily hassles are common risk factors, while positive social support is a common protective factor. The immediate goal of many recent primary prevention programs has become the reduction of risk factors and/or the enhancement of existing protective factors with regard to a specific risk–disorder linkage. However, the relationship between a particular risk and disorder, by no means, manifests a one-to-one correspondence. The same risk may be linked to several outcomes. For example, the risk of parental discord is related to both conduct disorder and depression. Consequently, the reduction of a single risk (or enhancement of a specific protective) factor may lead to reductions in the prevalence of several disorders. Thus, primary preventive interventions may be most powerful when they target a broad range of disorders with a set of salient risk and protective factors.

When the focus of intervention is a population or subpopulation, "inoculation" methods are the most common type of preventive intervention. Such programs endeavor to provide individuals *directly* with the skills, resources, and know-how to cope with future stresses, strains, and interpersonal encounters that might lead to problems—that is, inoculate them beforehand. Such a repertoire is intended to make the individual stronger and better prepared to deal with whatever may occur in the future. Inoculation programs are often administered to entire classrooms as part of the educational curriculum. In this type of primary prevention program, individuals remain the agents of change, although they are less likely to feel "blamed" than in tertiary and secondary prevention programs since they have not been singled out; everyone is receiving the inoculation.

When the focus of an intervention is a setting, inoculation methods are not employed. Instead, the prevention strategy is more often to restructure the social regularities of the setting. The goal is to modify the setting to become more facilitative of positive mental health outcomes. Thus, strategies to restructure settings characterize efforts more aptly depicted as the promotion of well-being than primary prevention. *Indirectly* these strategies reduce the incidence of an array of disorders for members of the setting. A more detailed example is presented in the next section.

When one thinks of primary prevention, one generally envisions programs for children. However, there are many adult problems that cry out for preventive interventions. For example, unemployed workers often suffer from depression and diminished self-efficacy after a futile search for new employment. In true cyclic form, depression and diminished self-efficacy can make finding a job more difficult and thus lead to greater depression.

At the University of Michigan, the Jobs Project was designed by Price, Caplan, and Vinokur to inoculate a high-risk population of recently unemployed individuals from the sequelae of depression and to evaluate the program's success. Participants were recruited from the lines of the recently unemployed at the Michigan Employment Security Commission and randomly assigned to either an experimental or control group. The experimental group received an eight-session curriculum, while the control group received a brief booklet in the mail with general information about job seeking. The curriculum included topics such as dealing with obstacles to reemployment, handling emotions related to unemployment and job seeking, thinking like an employer, identifying sources of job leads, contacting potential employers, completing job applications, preparing a resume, conducting the information interview, rehearsing interviews, and evaluating a job offer. A second part of the intervention was participation in discussion and analysis of the unemployment situation; the researchers felt that when individuals felt empowered to solve their problems they would experience greater self-efficacy and be more committed to follow through and implement the strategies for seeking reemployment.

Participants in the program were assessed at 1 month and 4 months after the intervention program. At both times, program participants had a higher reemployment rate and reported a better quality of working life than the control group. Among those who were re-employed, program participants were more likely to report finding jobs in their main occupation and reported higher earnings. Participants who remained unemployed reported higher levels of job-search self-efficacy than the unemployed control group members. Even more importantly, long-term effects for the intervention were found in a follow-up approximately 3 years later. Program participants continued to report higher earnings and more stable employment than the control group. In addition, a cost-benefit analysis confirmed the utility of this program. Finally, central to our primary prevention focus, among participants deemed high risk for a depressive episode (based on their initial scores on depression, financial strain, and low social assertiveness), this intervention reduced both the incidence and prevalence of depressive symptoms. Had the researchers taken a secondary prevention perspective, they would have selected only individuals who manifested early signs of depression.

A different approach to primary prevention begins at the earliest point in human life—the unborn fetus. When carried by a poor, teenage mother, a baby is more likely to be delivered preterm and/or low in birth weight. As a result, these infants and children are at greater risk for physical and mental health problems. These poor, teenage mothers often do not get the necessary prenatal care to ensure a healthy and safe delivery. For many of these mothers, the lack of resources and social support often result in their dropping out of school and/or having difficulty maintaining stable employment; in turn, these negative outcomes further compound the negative effects and risk of disorder for their children.

To address these issues, David Olds and his colleagues developed the Prenatal/Early Infancy Project. It was designed as a population-level prevention program in which nurses went into the homes of teenagers in the early stages of their first pregnancy as well as during the first 2 years of the infant's life. Initially, the nurses educated the mothers about fetal and infant development and helped the women improve their diet and try to eliminate the use of cigarettes, alcohol and drugs, they identified signs of pregnancy complications, they encouraged rest and exercise, they prepared parents for labor and delivery and early care of the newborn, and they encouraged use of the health care system and future family planning. Once the infant was born, the nurses would visit the families weekly for the first 6 weeks, gradually reducing the frequency of their visits from every other week to every 6 weeks until the infant was 2 years of age. During these visits the nurses would improve parents' understanding of infant temperament, and they would promote socioemotional and cognitive development and the physical health of the child.

The Prenatal/Early Infancy Project focused on reducing the risk factors associated with being a teenage mother and provided the mothers-to-be with positive social support, a well-documented protective factor. The program promoted the involvement of family members in and around the mother's home in the development of the infant. The nurses also provided connections to other formal health and human services. Moreover, the nurses paid special attention to the culture and the norms of the family, and they were respectful if they differed from that of the nurse and the program. Once again, this program illustrates an inoculation design because it prevents maladaptive outcomes by preparing and educating the mothers.

Research on this intervention revealed that participants in the home visit program manifested many positive outcomes when compared with a control group who only received free transportation for regular prenatal and well-child visits. During pregnancy, program mothers made better use of formal services, reported greater informal social support, improved their diets, and reduced smoking more than the control group. As a result, among the very young teenagers in the program, the birth weight of their babies was higher, and they were less likely to have preterm deliveries. Among the program mothers at higher risk—poor, unmarried adolescents—their children were less likely to have bverified cases of child abuse and neglect and they had fewer emergency room visits. In a 15-year follow-up, program families had fewer subsequent pregnancies, approximately half the number of child abuse cases, and spent approximately half as long on welfare as the control group. Clearly, this primary prevention program was beneficial to the teenage mothers and their offspring. In a secondary prevention program, mothers would not have been targeted until after they had delivered a low birth-weight baby or had been accused of neglect.

In sum, primary prevention programs are generally targeted to populations or subpopulations before problems or even signs of problems are manifested. Individuals, per se, are not identified, but instead a population or group placed at increased risk for one or more disorders or unwanted outcomes, often on the basis of a developmental transition that members of the group experience. Inoculation programs are administered to these populations in order to reduce the incidence of one or more disorders. By providing skills and resources, individuals are able to cope more effectively with future stressful and problematic situations that they may encounter. On the other hand, because individuals are not singled out at the stage of problem identification, individuals are much less likely to be (or feel) blamed.

VI. PROMOTION OF WELL-BEING

There has been a recent movement to go beyond a prevention mindset to focus on promotion of well-being. Focusing on promotion of well-being leads us away from simply thinking in terms of defining problems, their negative outcomes, and ways to prevent them; instead we focus on methods for improving the lives of individuals, and making them healthier and more positive. Promotion of well-being interventions generally move beyond the population level and focus on the setting level, although they may target both or solely a population. To the degree that well-being is promoted, problems are inevitably, although indirectly, prevented.

In New Haven, Weissberg and his associates from Yale University joined together with the superintendent of schools, the Board of Education, parents, community leaders and school staff to develop an organized approach to the promotion of socio-emotional development in the public school system. A Department of Social Development was created with the central element being a comprehensive inoculation program. For every public school in the city, the Social Development Program was incorporated from kindergarten through twelfth grade. This program had from 25 to 50 hours of classroom instruction at each grade level, which focused on problem solving, self-monitoring, conflict resolution, communication skills, respect, responsibility, health, substance abuse, culture, and citizenship. Realizing that there was a need to provide children with activities and outlets outside of the school, and in order to reinforce lessons taught in the classroom, the program moved beyond mere classroom curricula and developed school and community activities. Students participated in mentoring, after-school clubs, an outdoor adventure class, peer mediation, and leadership groups. Finally, the new department took advantage of previously existing mental health teams in the schools (made up of mental health workers, school staff, and parents). These teams effectively restructured the nature and quality of communication patterns and relationships among the three groups in order to focus on the climate of the schools, needs of the community and the issues that pertained to the growth and development of the students. They ensured that additions to the program were implemented and supported by the school and community.

The majority of school personnel supported the comprehensive and integrative strategy. Lessons taught to the students about problem solving were not only implemented by the students, but actively used by teachers and other school staff. Rather than detaining children for fighting, children received peer mediation or discussed the issues in a life skills class. School hallways were filled with the Traffic Light diagrams illustrating the six problem-solving steps taught in the life skills component. This was not your typical primary prevention program because it did not focus on one problem or even a few problems; rather, it focused on promoting positive social and emotional development and it embraced the entire school day and system.

This comprehensive strategy had many positive outcomes, including reduced problem behaviors. Evaluation research with sixth graders indicated that the curriculum improved students' problem-solving skills, social relations with peers, and behavioral adjustment. Follow-up evaluations illustrated that students who received 2 versus 1 or no years of training had more durable improvements in problem-solving skills.

Often, enduring effects are also hindered by the unwritten social and organizational rules and procedures, or social regularities, that govern a setting. The best exemplars of programs that promote well-being challenge the social regularities of a setting and alter them so that they foster positive development and mental health. An excellent example of a promotion of well-being program is one that altered the social regularities involved in the transition from junior to senior high school.

Normative school transitions may be disruptive and negatively impact adolescents' self-esteem and academic achievement. Often, adolescents make a transition into a more chaotic, more impersonal, less nurturing, and larger school where they have to contend with new routines and demands, numerous different teachers for short periods of time, and a completely different set of peers in each class. In these situations, the social regularities of the new school setting are critical to student well-being.

In the School Transitional Environment Program (STEP), Felner and his colleagues sought to reduce the chaos and flux upon entry into an inner-city high school. STEP students from each homeroom class took all their primary subjects together as a group. The homeroom teachers also taught the students one of their primary classes so they saw their homeroom students at least twice a day. In addition, the five STEP classrooms were in close proximity to each other in order to reduce the distance students traveled, and to keep them close to each other and in less contact with older, perhaps more intimidating students. STEP students experienced a very different environment than their peers, despite being in the same school.

The program was designed to provide adolescents with greater social support from school staff. Homeroom teachers served as the primary liaisons between the students and their parents and the school. Students received a counseling session with their homeroom teachers once every 4 to 5 weeks to discuss any school or personal problems. The homeroom teachers contacted parents of students during the summer before the transition to explain the purpose of the program and that they wanted to be accessible to the parents. Whenever a student was absent, the homeroom teacher would contact the family and follow-up on excuses. The teachers had regular meetings to discuss the students and the program. If a particular student was having a problem, all the STEP teachers were aware of it and tried to work together to help the student.

Research findings revealed that by the end of the first marking period, a comparison group of students declined in academic achievement and increased in absenteeism, whereas STEP students remained stable. By the end of the first year, 19% of comparison students dropped out compared to 4% of STEP students. In terms of academic achievement and absenteeism, the STEP students had significantly higher grades and lower absenteeism than the comparison group in both the first and second years of high school. Moreover, STEP students perceived the school environment to be more stable, well-organized, and supportive than the comparison group.

Although the STEP program was only in place for the incoming freshmen, the researchers felt that this program should have a long-term effect on the students because the transitional year is often the most vulnerable year for students. The researchers followed up their study of the original cohort by examining their school records after they should have graduated from high school. The most impressive finding was the difference in drop-out rates between the STEP students and the comparison students. The drop-out rate was 43% for the comparison group, which was similar to the drop-out rate of other students from the school in previous years. However, the drop-out rate was only 21% for the STEP students. The STEP program has been replicated in many sites, both at the senior high school level and the junior high (and middle) school level. The results are generally consistent across sites. This program illustrates an ideal promotion of well-being program that targets the school environment and makes it less chaotic, rather than a prevention program, which would most likely try to prevent school drop-out by targeting all students and providing them with extra help or supportive services to deal with the school transition.

VII. CONCLUSIONS

The evolution of the Community Mental Health Movement from tertiary prevention to the promotion of well-being demonstrates the field's growth, development and increased knowledge of mental health and the factors necessary to promote positive mental health. Although tertiary (rehabilitative) and secondary (early intervention) programs are still necessary and very much in practice today, it is clear that to incorporate prevention in their names is a misnomer. True prevention can only be through primary prevention and promotion of well-being programs. These types of programs, especially promotion of well-being are the present and future of the development and maintenance of positive mental health. Healthy, positive behavior in the individual cannot be maintained in a negative or chaotic environment. We must move away from solely targeting individuals to targeting the environments in which people live, work and learn.

BIBLIOGRAPHY

Albee, G. W., & Gullotta, T. P. (Eds.). (1996). *Primary prevention works.* Thousand Oaks, CA: Sage.

Bloom, B. L. (1984). *Community mental health: A general introduction.* (2nd ed.). Monterey, CA: Brooks/Cole.

Caplan, G. (1964). *Principles of preventive psychiatry.* New York: Basic Books.

Price, R. H., Cowen, E. L., Lorion, R. P., & Ramos-McKay, J. (1988). *14 ounces of prevention: A casebook for practitioners.* Washington, DC: American Psychological Association.

Salem, D. A., Seidman, E., & Rappaport, J. (1988). Community treatment of the mentally ill: The promise of mutual help organizations. *Social Work,* **33,** 403–408.

Constructivist Psychotherapies

Robert A. Neimeyer and Alan E. Stewart

University of Memphis

Constructivism An epistemological position that emphasizes the personal and collective processes of meaning-making and their implications for psychotherapy. Human beings are viewed as active creators of constructions that vary in the extent to which they help a person adjust to life's challenges.

Narrative Therapeutic Approaches A way of thinking about psychotherapy that views the client's life as a story or text. The life-as-narrative metaphor suggests that problems in living result from gaps, incongruities, or problematic passages in one's life story. Narrative therapeutic approaches seek to restore the client as an active narrator of his/her life by helping the person re-author aspects of experience to give events greater meaning or the plot structure of life new direction.

Postmodernism A philosophical position, deriving in part from constructivism, that acknowledges the multiplicity of constructions that can be developed for people, things, ideas, or institutions. Postmodernism assumes that no definition, characteristic, or attribute of something is fixed and invariant across either time or context. Adherents of postmodernism recognize that efforts to understand the "truth" or "essence" of an experience ultimately lead instead to constructions about those experiences.

Social Constructionism An epistemological approach that emphasizes the socially shared meanings developed between people about phenomena experienced by a culture or society. In contrast to constructivism this approach emphasizes the ambient meanings that exist prior to any individual and that serve as the basis for people's identity and forms of relating.

Systemic Approaches A general psychotherapeutic approach common to family therapy that emphasizes the ways in which one's embeddedness in a network of interpersonal relationships (which can encompass family, community, and organization) affects the experiences and behavior of persons in the system as well as the functioning of the system as a whole.

CONSTRUCTIVISM, a philosophical position that emphasizes the human penchant for meaning making in understanding both psychological distress and therapeutic intervention, has influenced several current traditions of psychotherapy. Following a review of the historical contributions to this approach, we consider two critical issues: the relationship between language and reality and the construction of the self, as viewed from both constructivist and related social constructionist perspectives. We then trace the implications of constructivism for the practicing therapist, reviewing four traditions that are characterized by a central concern with the person as interpreter of experience: personal construct therapy, developmental cognitive therapies, narrative approaches, and sys-

Copyright © 1998 by Academic Press.
All rights of reproduction in any form reserved.

temic orientations. We conclude that constructivism is making a robust contribution to the further development of psychotherapy, both in terms of research and practice.

I. INTRODUCTION

In both popular and professional writing, many schools of therapy are distinguished by their concrete clinical procedures, the fund of therapeutic techniques most closely associated with particular traditions. Thus, psychoanalysis is characterized by its historical preference for free association and dream reporting on the part of the client, and the interpretation of transference and defense by the therapist. For its own part, cognitive therapy is linked with various methods for evaluating, monitoring and disputing dysfunctional thoughts or beliefs both in and between therapy sessions (e.g., homework assignments). Likewise, behavior therapy is associated with counterconditioning procedures (such as systematic desensitization), and contingency management (through the manipulation of reinforcement to increase or decrease desired or undesired behavior). Even family therapy is associated with a distinctive set of procedures, ranging from the use of paradoxical interventions to the challenging of dysfunctional coalitions or boundaries among family members. In each case, these approaches to therapy are linked in the popular and professional imagination with a preferred set of techniques, which govern the pattern of therapeutic interaction in a way that sets them apart from others. [*See* BEHAVIOR THERAPY; COGNITIVE THERAPY.]

In contrast, constructivist psychotherapy is characterized by the distinctive *mind-set* that guides it, more than by any particular set of procedures that distinguish it from other clinical traditions. Of course, the unique philosophical position that informs constructivist practice does subtly encourage some ways of working with clients, while constraining others, as we shall see below. But to understand the evolution of this form of practice, it is helpful to view it against the backdrop of what constructivist therapists *believe,* in order to gain a deeper appreciation of what they *do.* This will then allow us to consider variations in the constructivist tradition, which has begun to permeate traditional schools of therapy, ranging from the psychodynamic and behavioral to the humanistic and systemic. As the "family" of constructivist therapies has grown, so too has the repertory of clinical strategies associated with them, and the body of qualitative and quantitative research emanating from them. While a thorough review of the theoretical, empirical, and applied literature associated with this perspective is clearly beyond the scope of this article, the present article provides an initial point of entry into this burgeoning contemporary therapeutic tradition, and offers some leads for the reader interested in pursuing its implications for clinical scholarship, research, and practice in greater detail.

We begin with an examination of the philosophical heritage of constructivism and discuss the emergence of psychological theory from constructivist epistemology, the study of knowledge. We then consider two current issues pertaining to constructivist theory and therapy: first, the relationship between language and reality, and second, the construction of the self. Next, we compare and contrast four traditions of constructivist psychotherapy, including personal construct theory, narrative approaches, family systemic orientations, and developmental perspectives. Finally, we conclude by considering the implications of constructivism for psychotherapy research, and offer a critical evaluation of the current status of constructivist practice.

II. PHILOSOPHICAL HERITAGE OF CONSTRUCTIVIST ASSUMPTIONS

A. Constructivist Epistemology

Although most constructivist scholars and practitioners acknowledge that a real, ontologically substantial world exists, they are much more interested in understanding the nuances of the person's construction of the world than in evaluating the extent to which it accurately "represents" some external "reality." Constructivists emphasize the development of a viable or workable construction of people, things, and events over the attainment of a singularly "true" rendering of one's surrounds. This suggests that multiple meanings can be developed for the events in one's life, and that each may have some utility in helping the person understand his or her experience and respond creatively and adaptively to it.

The idea that people actively and continuously engage in meaning-making processes, that is, construction, dates at least to the ancient Greek philosopher Epictetus who maintained people were more perturbed by their views of reality than by reality itself. But it was the Italian rhetorician Vico (1668–1744) who systematized the rudiments of a truly constructivist philosophy, tracing the origins of human mentation to the gradual acquisition of the power to transcend immediate experience. Vico argued that the origins of human thought lay in the attempt to understand the mysteries of the external world by projecting upon it the structures of human motives and actions in the form of myths and fables. This tendency to order experience through the application of such "imaginative universals" was eventually displaced, he thought, by the development of linguistic abstractions that permitted categorization of events and objects on the basis of single characteristics.

The work of Kant (1724–1804) also contributed significantly to a conception of the human mind as an active, form-giving structure. Specifically, Kant believed that experience and sensation were not passively written into the person, but that the mind transforms and coordinates the multiplicity of sense data into integrated thought. Because human beings can come to "know" only those phenomena that conform to the structures of the human mind, with its penchant for organizing the world in three-dimensional terms and imputing causality to events, humans are forever barred from contacting the "thing in itself," a "noumenal" reality uncontaminated by human knowing.

At the threshold of the twentieth century, the German analytic philosopher, Vaihinger (1852–1933), embraced constructivist epistemology in asserting that people develop impressions of the real world and create *workable fictions* that help them to adjust and to meaningfully respond to people and events. Conceptual "artifices" (e.g., of mathematical infinity or of a "reasonable man"), while having no exemplars in reality, performed a heuristic function in helping the person organize and integrate disparate pieces of knowledge or sensory data. Vaihinger categorized his *Philosophy of 'As If'* as a kind of "idealistic positivism," to acknowledge the dual reliance upon hard data and impressions received by the sensory system along with a purposive, form-giving activity of the mind to create useful constructions.

Avenarius (1843–1896) and Mach (1838–1916) espoused a unique form of impressionistic positivism, known as empiriocriticism, that also contributed to the history of constructivist epistemology. Contemporaries of Vaihinger, Avenarius and Mach placed heavier emphasis on raw sensory data as the beginning point for human knowing processes. While maintaining that people constructed an understanding of the world based upon sensory data, their principles of economy and parsimony maintained that sense data were minimally embellished by activities of the mind. Despite this more empirical emphasis, these two authors, working separately, both recognized an active, organizing role of mental processes in rendering sense data more holistically.

Within this century, the work of Vaihinger, Mach, Avenarius, and others influenced Korzybski's development of general semantics. Korzybski (1879–1950), a Polish intellectual working independently of established academic circles, essentially criticized the use of the verb "to be" and its conjugations because it tended to identify people or things, in an Aristotelian sense, with qualities or characteristics that often were meant only to describe them (e.g., "Terry is lazy"). Such identity, Korzybski maintained, de-emphasized the multiplicity of meanings and modes of existence that characterize most phenomena, living or inanimate, and obscured the role of the speaker in attributing meaning to events. Korzybski's negation of the use of "to be" makes it possible for people or things to be construed in different ways and provides a linguistic basis for a constructivist epistemology. Korzybski developed an approach to language usage, known as E′ (E-prime), that recommended persons use conjugations of "to be" sparingly or not at all in written or spoken language. The idea behind E-prime is that the map (in this case, language) is not the territory (other persons or things in the world).

B. Constructivist Psychologies

Constructivist epistemology provided a conceptual basis for three distinct psychologies in this century. First, the British researcher, Bartlett (1886–1979), applied constructivist concepts in his investigations of human memory processes. In his classic work on remembering, Bartlett maintained that memories were reconstructed out of bits and pieces of recollected information. That is, memories did not consist of stored, complete representations of past events that were recalled *in toto.* Bartlett viewed memories as past information unified by *schemas,* the threads of constructive processes that exist at the time information is remembered.

The Swiss genetic epistemologist Piaget (1896–1980) was the second psychologist to establish a coherent theory founded on a constructivist basis. As a developmental psychologist with interests in children's forms of knowing, Piaget chronicled how children's meaning-making capacities changed as a function of both physical growth and active adaptation upon exposure to a succession of conceptually challenging experiences. Piaget contended that rather than representing a smooth "learning curve" over time, cognitive development was punctuated at critical points by qualitative transformations in the very style and form of thinking, permitting the eventual emergence of abstract, formal thought having a level of plasticity unavailable earlier in childhood. Subsequent developmentalists in the Piagetian tradition have extended this model into adult life, when still more subtle dialectical forms of thinking emerge to permit more adequate accommodation to the complexities of social life.

Finally, the American clinical psychologist, Kelly (1905–1967), became the first to develop a personality theory and psychotherapeutic interventions based upon a constructivist epistemology. Influenced by both Korzybski and the psychodramatist, Moreno, Kelly's psychotherapeutic system exemplified constructivist thinking in that he viewed people as incipient scientists, striving to both anticipate and to control events they experienced through developing an integrated hierarchy of personal constructs. As will be discussed in a later section, Kelly viewed psychological intervention as a collaborative effort of the therapist and client to help the latter revise or replace personal constructions that were no longer viable. By making the reconstruction of personal belief systems the focus of psychotherapy, Kelly anticipated the work of later cognitive theorists and therapists. More generally, Kelly's position that multiple, viable constructions can be developed for a given phenomenon and that no single version of reality is prepotent over others heralded the arrival of postmodern critiques of the humanities and social sciences.

Although overshadowed by psychology's embrace of information processing perspectives on human mentation in the 1960s and 1970s, constructivist approaches experienced a strong resurgence of interest in the 1980s with the founding of *The International Journal of Personal Construct Psychology* in 1988. This forum was renamed *Journal of Constructivist Psychology* in 1994 to accommodate the growing diversity of constructivist scholarship beyond Kelly's personal construct psychology. Increasing interest in constructivist theory, research, and practice in both individual and family therapy has enriched the field, spawning the diversity of constructivist perspectives outlined below.

A common thread among various constructivist scholars is that human psychological processes are proactive and form generating. Thus, rather than viewing people's behavior as a mere reaction to the "stimuli" of the "real world," constructivists view humans as actively imposing their own order on experience and shaping their behavior to conform to their expectations. Thus, a fundamental concern of constructivist psychotherapists becomes the study of the personal and communal *meanings* by which people order their experience, meanings that must be transformed if clients are to envision new (inter)personal realities in which to live. While most members of the broad family of constructivist approaches would endorse this basic position, they differ significantly in the emphasis they place on the individuality or communality of meaning making, and their corresponding emphasis on private interpretations of experience as opposed to broad linguistic and cultural processes that shape human action. For this reason, it is useful to examine two central issues in constructivist epistemology from the standpoints of both (personal) constructivist and social constructionist positions, to lay a groundwork for understanding the different foci and methods of the various "schools" of constructivist therapy that follow.

III. CURRENT ISSUES IN CONSTRUCTIVIST THEORY

Two areas in which there has been continuing elaboration of constructivist ideas involve first, the relationship between language and reality, and second, the construction of the self. The former issue bears directly on constructivist epistemology and the central role of language in ordering experience. The latter issue relates to the structural aspects of meaning systems and how they function together in creating temporally or situationally coherent identities. Each of these issues also carries direct implications for psychotherapy, although with different nuances in the case of constructivist versus social constructionist accounts.

A. Language and Reality

1. Constructivist Perspective

Perhaps the pivotal concept in a constructivist account of human nature concerns the relationship between human knowledge and reality. Specifically, constructivists reject or at least suspend the implicit epistemology of the modern social sciences, which assumes that one's understanding of the world, especially the world of complex and dynamic interpersonal systems, can be considered "true" or justified to the extent that it corresponds to a reality external to the person's knowing system. Instead, they posit that human knowers have no direct confirmatory access to a world beyond their grasp, no firm contact with a bedrock of reality that would provide a secure foundation for their constructions.

This posture of epistemological humility, for most constructivists, stops short of an "anything goes" relativism, insofar as the development of personal knowledge is constrained by the need for varying degrees of internal coherence, on the one hand, and the quest for consensual validation of our private constructions on the other. While the resulting meaning systems cannot be strictly "validated" in the sense of matching some objective criterion independent of the observer, they can nonetheless be judged more or less viable as guides to organizing our anticipations regarding our activities in and our accounts of our experiential world.

Language, in this constructivist view, represents a medium for articulating private discriminations, enabling us both to manipulate them symbolically and to inject them into the medium of public discourse. Using language as a straightforward instrument of "communication" is viewed as problematic insofar as commonality of construing becomes more of an aspiration than an assumption. This view of meaning as resident primarily in individual construction systems, which are bonded together by the thin substantiality of language, is most evident in "cognitive constructivist" accounts like Kelly's that consider persons as agents capable of making choices and creating original, personal constructions with minimal interference by larger social systems or structures.

2. Social Constructionist Perspective

Social constructionists largely agree with cognitive constructivists in rejecting objectivist epistemologies that a real world exists and can be discovered by establishing a correspondence between the knower and the phenomenon to be known. Social constructionists, however, differ with constructivists regarding the centrality accorded to individually constructed experiences. That is, constructions of people, things, or events in the world arise from negotiations between persons rather than within them. The implication of this sociocentric view is that individuals' constructions both derive from and contribute to the social and cultural contexts with which they are associated.

Given their attention to collective, rather than individual experience, language and linguistic processes occupy an even more central role for social constructionists than for constructivists. This increased emphasis is also reflected in social constructionists' broader definitions of language to include all manner of semantic, semiotic, and symbolic methods of negotiating and disseminating meaning, rather than restricting it to the spoken or written word alone.

As a form of collective meaning making and coordinated social action, language can be used to create cultural tales that become repositories of socially constructed meanings from the past or from other societies or cultures. The availability of ready-made meanings that embody the local "truths" of one's place and time implies that cultural narratives may "author" people, rather than vice versa, in the sense that they constitute prefabricated and socially validated patterns to which individual identities are expected to conform. Thus, in this constructionist view, language and culture predate the experience of any particular individual, and provide the ineluctable scaffolding for constructing one's identity in relation to others.

B. The Construction of the Self

1. Constructivist Perspective

The personal quest for coherent and socially warranted knowledge carries with it clear implications for an image of the *self*. Like the "world," the "self" is relativized and problematized in constructivist accounts, stripped of stable traits or enduring features that define its essence. Instead, selves are constructed as a by-product of our immersion in language and practical activity, as one strives for personally significant ways of thematizing, organizing, and narrating experiences. Stated differently, *people are their constructs,* so that at least in a distributed sense, selfhood consists of an entire repertory of shifting and provisional patterns for understanding, engaging, and "storying" the world and other people. Because the majority of these patterns are tacit, only rarely articulated in symbolic or explicit ways for either for the person or for others, clear limits are imposed upon self-knowledge. At best, efforts to "know oneself" represent an attempt to impose an explicit order on the relatively abstract and durable themes that punctuate one's lived engagement in the world.

Viewing self-development as oscillating between an extension of our forms of concrete activity in the world and the effort after an abstract reflexivity toward the self poses major challenges to modernist goals associated with an essentialized image of human nature. In particular, the loss of a fixed and "real" self erodes the value of "genuineness" or "congruence" in one's relationships to others. That is, the multiplicity of selves that exists for each of us across time and contexts precludes the discovery of a primary or essentialized self, just as it undermines the quest to discover who a person "really is." Thus, this postmodern conception emphasizes narrative elaboration over authenticity, and self-explanation over self-actualization.

2. Social Constructionist Perspective

Social constructionists and constructivists agree in rejecting the concept of a single, essentialized self. The social constructionist critique, however, runs deeper to challenge the very category of "self" as an individually based construct, viewing it instead as an historically circumscribed concept arising only fairly recently in Western culture, with its pervasive emphasis on individuality, autonomy, and personal responsibility. In contrast to this cultural trend, social constructionists view discussions of the "self" as merely one possible form of *discourse,* one that may be insufficiently attentive to the numerous ways in which our sense of identity is penetrated by relationships to significant others and even impersonal media, especially in the electronic age. In making this critique, social constructionists emphasize the fragmentation and incoherence of self in divergent social contexts rather than embracing the idea of an integrated agent whose coherence transcends such divergent social realities. In this view, therefore, characteristics of the self such as responsibility, purpose, agency, and so forth are seen as fictions derived from society's construction of the individual, rather than as universal "facts" or ideals that generalize across different times and settings.

As might be expected in view of these differences, constructivism and social constructionism also differ in their endorsement of self-knowledge as a goal of life in general, or psychotherapy in particular. Whereas constructivists encourage the conscious elaboration of a multifaceted "self" and reflexive recognition of this process, social constructionists focus more upon the implicit ways in which practical engagement in specific contexts shapes one's mode of self-presentation, with or without one's conscious awareness or "choice." This divergence contributes to a differential use of self-reflective versus social-conversational methods in various traditions of constructivist therapy, a topic to which we shall now turn.

IV. CONSTRUCTIVIST PSYCHOTHERAPIES

A. General Orientation

Just as constructivists are suspicious of a psychological science that pursues a universal set of factual observations concerning human nature, they also distrust "scientific" forms of psychotherapy that establish highly standardized and manualized procedures for modifying human behavior. In addition, the growing family of constructivist interventions eschews methods that simply supply clients with supposedly more "functional" or "adaptive" ways of existing, thinking, or feeling rather than helping persons or families find their own unique way to adaptive meaning making. This suggests that at the level of clinical practice, constructivists accord both therapist and client an "expert" role in understanding what changes are necessary in the assumptive foundation of the client's life.

Consistent with this emphasis, constructivists reject pathologizing diagnostic systems that focus on client deficits and deviations from supposedly "normal" patterns of behavior. Accordingly, they resist the common practice of applying universal categories of disorders that fail to capture the richness and subtlety of any given individual's way of interpreting the social world and constructing relationships with others. For instance, a diagnostic category such as "major depression" merely describes a presumably maladaptive "mood disorder," without conveying any information about the way the person's meaning-making processes have ceased to be viable for construing life's experiences. In contrast, constructivists prefer assessment techniques and working conceptualizations that are idiographic or tailored to each use, which examine both the positive and negative implications (from the client's, family's, or society's standpoint) of clients' ways of construing their lives and problems.

Because both therapist and client lack access to a straightforward "truth" beyond their constructions, neither can define hard and fast criteria for distinguishing "healthy" or "rational" beliefs or actions from those that are "disordered" or "irrational." Given this "level playing field," the therapist is left with the somewhat daunting task of building an empathic bridge into the lived experience of the client by attempting to construe his or her process of meaning making. Establishing this connection will help the therapist to understand the entailments of the client's constructions of events and help negotiate their possible deconstruction and elaboration. The personalism of this encounter requires that the therapist have a sensitive attunement to the unspoken nuances in the client's conversation, and skill in using evocative and metaphorically rich language to help sculpt their mutual meaning making toward fresh possibilities. To be successful, such "structural coupling" between client and therapist systems must ultimately move beyond bland generalizations about the nature of the "working alliance" and banal prescriptions for "effective interventions," and instead foster a unique "shared epistemology" irreducible to the individual systems of either partner in the therapeutic relationship.

What "outcomes" might be valued in this constructivist approach to the counseling process? While the specific aims of psychotherapy are necessarily defined by the participants, at an abstract level, the goals of constructivist therapies include adopting a "language of hypothesis" by recognizing that one's constructions are at best working fictions rather than established facts. As such, they are amenable to therapeutic deconstruction (e.g., through subjecting the same events to alternative "readings") and reconstruction (e.g., through acting upon alternative interpretations to realize their effects).

Although enhanced reflexivity toward the "self" may be a legitimate aim of this work, it is ultimately subordinated in importance to the aim of constructing a self with sufficient narrative coherence to be recognizable, but sufficient fluidity to permit continued tailoring to the varied social ecologies the client inhabits. Because new and tentative reconstructions of the self require social support, therapy typically also fosters a deepened engagement with selected others who can function as "validating agents" for the growing edges of the client's provisional attempts at meaning making.

B. Distinctive Traditions

The last 10 to 20 years have witnessed a growing diversity of psychotherapeutic approaches that have embraced a constructivist epistemology. There is no single or unique constructivist psychotherapy, no single "approved" set of techniques that define constructivist interventions. Instead, a constructivist mind-set has percolated into most major traditions of therapy, from the psychoanalytic to the cognitive-behavioral, producing novel ways of conceptualizing therapeutic practice as well as a broad variety of associated change strategies or techniques. Our goal in this section will be to survey some of these developments, concentrating on four discernible therapeutic traditions within constructivism that make somewhat different assumptions about human change processes, and carry distinct implications for the role of the therapist.

1. Personal Construct Theory

The first tradition we will consider is Kelly's personal construct psychology, which despite its status as the first consistent expression of clinical constructivism, continues to attract fresh adherents and generate new therapeutic strategies. Kelly's psychotherapeutic approach derived from his unique conception of personality. Kelly employed the metaphor of the "person-as-scientist" to characterize the ways in which people attempt to formulate personal theories to both anticipate regularities in their environments and to channel their behavior in relation to them. Central to Kelly's theory is the idea that people create constructs, or basic dimensions of contrast, that help them to discover relevant similarities and differences arising from the people, situations, and events with which they interact.

More than other forms of constructivist intervention, personal construct therapy emphasizes the hierarchical nature of the person's construct system. That is, some constructs are more central to the person's meaning-making processes than other, more peripheral and subordinate constructs. For example, one person may evaluate all others primarily in terms of whether they are likely to form accepting, close relationships with him or her, or are likely to reject and abandon the person without warning. Moreover, the construing of another on either the "accepting" or "abandoning" pole of this construct is likely to carry sweeping implications for the person, resulting in a global appraisal of the other as an individual and the prospect of constructing a meaningful relationship with him or her. Another person may employ this construct in a much less central way, perhaps to understand the behavior of potential dating partners, and may see it as carrying fewer implications for the other's personality or the relationship as a whole. Key to Kelly's theory is that such constructs ultimately say more about the individual who formulates them, than about the person to whom they are applied.

Systems of personal constructs operating as an organized whole affect what phenomena a person can construe as well as how these phenomena will be interpreted. Continuing with the example above, the person who views others in "close versus rejecting" terms may not be able to understand the behavior of a person who wishes to form a friendly, but casual relationship. An implication of this, again echoing the sentiments of Epictetus, is that people are not victims of problems in reality as much as they suffer from the constraints and limitations of their construct systems.

Personal construct therapists believe that psychological problems stem from anomalies in the structure or operation of the person's construct system. More specifically, a disorder consists of any personal construction that is used continually despite its repeated invalidation. Given this general conception of problems in living, various kinds of problematic experiences can be predicted.

Threat, for instance, results when the individual feels on the brink of an imminent, comprehensive change in core identity constructs, as when marital discord reaches a crisis point, and the threatened spouse recoils from the awful recognition that divorce will mean a wholesale reworking of his or her view of the self and world. *Anxiety* arises with the awareness that critical events are outside of the range of the person's current constructs, that one confronts experiences that cannot be meaningfully construed or anticipated. Another problematic experience, *hostility,* results when the person continues to garner or even force support for one or more constructs after they have repeatedly led to unsuccessful predictions. For example, a husband who maintains that his wife should assume a subservient, domestic role and not seek employment, and who uses verbal or physical threats or abuse to keep her in the role he has constructed for her would be manifesting hostility in Kelly's sense. Finally, personal construct therapists view the experience of *guilt* as stemming from the client's awareness that he or she has been dislodged from central value commitments, as defined idiosyncratically within his or her construct system.

At a general level personal construct therapy helps the client examine his or her repertory of constructs and to find more meaningful constructions with which to face life challenges. In particular, the therapist first may help the client articulate constructs of significant others through use of the repertory grid or laddering techniques. In the former exercise the client may be asked to consider two or more persons he or she knows and then describe how the people differ. In this way the client's basic dimensions of meaning are articulated as successively different groups of people are considered. The laddering technique helps the person examine the implications of systems of constructs as they are applied to some real life problem.

The therapist may then help the client expand the construct system so that a wider or more diverse range of people or events may be construed without the person experiencing fear or anxiety. The therapist may also help the client to create new constructions that revise or replace previous constructs. Therapy may also help to "tighten" a construct by requiring the client to examine its concrete, specific implications for the people and events encountered in life. Alternatively, it may be therapeutic for the client to "loosen" certain constructs so they become more flexible and are applied provisionally to a wider range of experiences. In the case of the person who perceived all relationships in terms of acceptance or rejection, therapy may help the person to apply this construct more selectively and discriminately than before. In summary, from this general perspective the therapist helps the client identify interesting problems that derive from his or her view of life, gather evidence in daily life about their viability or utility, and experiment with new or revised constructs. Thus, the role of the personal construct therapist is analogous to that of a *co-investigator*, with the important questions to be researched being defined by the unique affordances and limitations of the client's personal meaning system, rather than the therapist's.

A specific technique pioneered by Kelly and modified by subsequent personal construct therapists is the fixed role technique. This technique was based upon Kelly's observation that the dramatic license to portray a role sometimes led to the actor retaining some of the mannerisms and modes of thinking associated with the role after he or she stepped out of it. That is, temporarily assuming the role helped the person to develop or elaborate his or her construct system in useful and enduring ways.

The technique begins with the client writing a self-characterization sketch that the therapist then uses in drafting a new role for the client to enact. The new role may help the person to construe a wider range of people or events, to revise old constructs, or to help create new constructs. To be useful, the exercise must allow the client to enact a rather different—although not simply opposite—way of approaching life for a fixed period of time. As the therapist and client practice relating to an increasingly intimate set of figures from the client's life in therapeutic role plays, and then experiment with generalizing the new role to real-life situations, the client may come to realize that "personality" is itself a construction, one that can (with effort) be reconstructed as one evolves. Thus, at the end of a time-limited period (typically only a few weeks), the client explicitly relinquishes the new role and considers its implications for his or her ongoing engagement with social life.

Despite its appearance more than 40 years ago, personal construct theory and therapy continue to attract the interests of new generations of researchers and clinicians. Repertory grid methodology has been used to review clients' life histories, their vocational interests and preferences, and their construal of group members' behavior, among other uses. Recent work on personal construct therapy has focused upon death and loss issues, agoraphobia, marriage and family interventions, and life-span development. This level of continued interest by researchers and clinicians underscores the enduring heuristic value of Kelly's original vision, while permitting accommodation of the theory as it comes into contact with more recent additions to the constructivist family of approaches described below.

2. Developmental Perspectives

A second tradition in constructivist therapy includes a "fuzzy set" of approaches that share a focal concern with psychological development, and especially the development of self. Like personal construct theory, they view the evolution of personal meaning systems as the individual's progressive attempts to create "working models" of self and significant others, but they place greater stress than does personal construct theory on the origin of these models in childhood attachment relationships. In keeping with constructivist epistemology, determining the authenticity of reported childhood events (e.g., whether the client as a child was or was not incestuously abused by a stepfather) is less critical than the conclusions the client has drawn about herself and others (e.g., that she must always accede to others' needs, or that others cannot be trusted). In this sense, therapy consists of a sensitive search for the *narrative truth* of the client's life, rather than detective work to "uncover" the literal events that supposedly shaped the client's personality. By focusing attention on the domain of meanings, the therapist also is sensitized to the considerable range of personal reactions to any given "objective" event, as when childhood sexual involvement with a parent is viewed by one client as a shameful secret to be maintained, and by another as indisputable evidence for the contemptability of the opposite sex. Still a third client may view such involvement as an emotionally complicated but essential haven from the still more painful abuses of the other parent. In developmental perspective, these highly individualized themes are viewed as core ordering principles that shape much of the person's subsequent experience of reality, identity, emotionality, and control.

In developmental therapies of this type, the therapist functions as a kind of *psychohistorian*, prompting the client to link current distress to problematic experiences from the recent or more distant past, and explore them more deeply. Theoretically, this involves helping the client subtly shift between two aspects of him- or herself, the experiencing "I," which engages life in all of its emotional immediacy, and the explaining "me," which attempts to give a coherent account of these experiences in rational terms. Because the tacit experience of events tends to precede the ability to articulate and evaluate them, the therapist frequently must assist the client to focus closely on problematic events, reliving them in "slow motion" in all of their emotional intensity in the session, to provide the "raw material" for interpreting the experiences in more useful ways. For example, a confused and self-critical client might trace her recent seemingly inexplicable loss of initiative to her sense of discomfort following an interaction with a male employer. The therapist might then encourage her to "unpack" the interaction in all of its sensory detail, discovering that the client experienced heightened anxiety at the point that her employer rolled his eyes during her presentation, in a way that was reminiscent of her father's silent dismissal of her as a child. This might lead to further exploration of more remote scenarios, and to the thematization of her sense of insufficiency, especially in relation to men.

Among the specialized techniques that are compatible with this developmental perspective is the life-review procedure, which involves attempting to piece together a more continuous sense of one's biography by organizing one's own memories by year, noting significant events, feelings, and developments in one's self understanding on a chronological series of index cards that are added to over the course of therapy. Other forms of reflective writing (e.g., exploring one's changed sense of self after a major early loss) are also frequently used by developmental therapists, either as an adjunct to formal therapy or a means of ongoing self-exploration. More than any specific outcome, the goal of such work is to develop the ability to transition between delicate attention to the nuances of one's engagement in life, and the attempt to interpret them in a way that promotes ongoing reconstruction of one's sense of self.

3. Narrative Approaches

The third tradition, the narrative approach, views life as organized by personal, familial, and cultural themes, and regards therapy as an intimate form of collaboration in editing the client's life story. Narrative perspectives have burgeoned over the last 15 years as clinicians have found the generative and integrative characteristics of stories to be apt metaphors for individuals' meaning-making processes. Most narrative therapeutic perspectives share the common view of the person as both author and hero of a life story that invariably includes an unexpected (and often unchosen) cast of characters, events, and twists on the temporal and situational plots of one's life. In this way narratives lend coherence and integrity to one's past as well as contribute to the way one anticipates the outcomes of a life story in the future.

Clinicians working in the narrative vein view emotional distress as resulting from or marked by a break, failure, or gap in one's ongoing autobiography. Such narrative suspension leaves the person with a diminished capacity to emplot experienced events or subjected to unanticipated subplots that are markedly discrepant with what the person expected from life. For instance, the traumatic loss of a spouse later in one's life removes a highly valued figure from the partner's life story and necessitates the tragically painful revision of the partner's storied role as companion, friend, caretaker, and lover, among others.

Most narrative therapeutic approaches share the goal of weaving painful, negative, or other unexpected events into the client's dominant life narrative. That is, the client and therapist collaborate to help the person both live and author an active, integrated story. Here, the therapist functions as an *editor or co-author* in attempting revisions of the client's life narrative. For instance, treatment for the bereaved spouse might focus on grieving the loss of the partner by examining how the person dealt with previous losses and the way these were integrated or interpreted in the larger framework of meaning that informs the person's life. Emphasis also may be placed upon developing further roles with children, other family, and friends as a way to emplot a new life "chapter" without the deceased spouse.

Given the goals of narrative repair and reconstruction, therapists working from this perspective may employ a variety of literary techniques. Developing metaphors to help clients more clearly define problems, tease out the meanings of significant struggles and emotional experiences, and find solutions may provide benefits at all phases of therapy. Structured reminiscence may help the client identify salient events, people, and plots in their own stories over the course of their lives. Reminiscence for the grieving spouse may reveal how emotions of sadness, anger, or betrayal from previous losses were incorporated into the life narrative. Writing assignments, such as a letter to the deceased partner, journals, and dialogues may help to both bring problems into greater relief and to help transform them so they may be integrated with existing life stories. Other written documents exchanged between the client and therapist such as certificates of "readiness for change" or "completion of therapy" may help to document and certify real changes in the client's life story.

In summary, narrative approaches to therapy include a rich and growing collection of constructivist methods for acknowledging and creating change in clients' lives. As exemplified by the recent growth in both the number and types of books and scholarly articles on narrative themes, this field of endeavor appears to be among the most rapidly growing areas of constructivism.

4. Systemic Approaches

The fourth set of approaches includes variants of systemic family therapy, which generally reflect a social constructionist concern with "languaging" and its role in shaping the family's definition of the problem. From this perspective, "psychological disorders" are not viewed as syndromes or symptoms that attach themselves to persons, but instead are defined in language through the interaction of those persons—including the identified "client"—engaged in the problem. For example, whether a woman's depressive withdrawal after the death of her stillborn child is considered "normal" or "pathological" is very much a matter for social negotiation, especially within the family context. Problems arise and are sustained in language when they are conferred a "reality" by individuals, family members, and the broader society, and particularly when they are attributed to deficiencies, deficits, or diseases in one individual. Therapy, in this perspective, consists of creatively helping participants in a problem system "language away" the difficulty by reframing it in a way that it is either viewed as no longer problematic (e.g., the mother's continuing sadness is reconstrued as an attempt to maintain her connection to her deceased child) or becomes amenable to solution (e.g., her sense of loss might be validated by a shared family ritual acknowledging the place of the child in their collective lives).

In this approach to therapy, the therapist assumes the role of *conversation manager*, artfully eliciting divergent views of the problem within the family system and exploring their implications for each member. Because family members are often engaged in interlocking patterns of recursive validation (e.g., when the bereaved father's confused withdrawal from his wife is viewed by her as emotional abandonment, and her resulting tearfulness is construed by him as further evidence for her "falling apart"), the therapist must often find ways of exposing the hidden premises of each family member's view, and prompting them to view their interaction, at least temporarily, in novel terms. Among the many techniques for accomplishing this are the use of circular questions, which inquire about perceptions among family members (e.g., "Who is most convinced that mom is suffering from major depression? Who is least convinced that this is what is going on?") and their relationships to one another (e.g., "Who in the family is next most depressed? Next? Least?").

Systemic therapists who operate from a constructivist standpoint also make use of novel therapy formats, such as the reflecting team, in which a group of clinicians observes a family therapy session, and then joins the therapist and family to share divergent, but provocative interpretations of the family's difficulty. The aim of such interventions is not to determine the single "correct" interpretation of the complaint, but to dislodge both therapist and clients from habitual ways of thinking about the problem in a way that contributes to its maintenance. As the systemic therapies have continued to evolve, they have become increasingly open to "importing" concepts from more individual constructivist approaches (e.g., personal construct and narrative models) that help reveal the "selves" within the system, and that provide a means of tacking back and forth between individual and family level work across the course of a given therapy.

V. IMPLICATIONS OF CONSTRUCTIVISM FOR PSYCHOTHERAPY RESEARCH

Constructivism and the epistemological approach that undergirds it possess profound implications for guiding inquiry in science in general and for the social and psychological sciences in particular. Work in all science is essentially a human enterprise because people formulate hypotheses, devise working models, conduct experiments, interpret data, and prepare scientific papers and reports. To the extent that the constructivist image of human nature questions our degree of contact with either a knowable world or a knowable self, it shakes the foundations of modern psychological science conceived as the cataloging of factual observations and their systematization into unified theories in the natural, physical, or social sciences.

Constructivists view science instead as continuous with other forms of knowing, yielding inherently partial and positional perspectives reliant on the models and metaphors of a particular place and time, even when it formulates general "laws" of human functioning. This implies that the theories and "laws" that have been developed in all of the sciences represent complex and organized constructions that have been elaborated to varying degrees. Each field also may enjoy different amounts of coherence among theoretical constructions.

Conceptualizing science in this manner may raise fundamental and provocative questions for some about whether observing the same results about a thing, event, or a person with different methods or at different times reveals successively more "accurate" or "real" characteristics or just reflects a coherent system of constructions that function somewhat equivalently. The former position seems to assume a realist or objectivist position that reality can be known and that science incrementally advances by developing more accurate or realistic knowledge through successive approximations of theories and their research paradigms. The latter position of constructivism deemphasizes "knowing reality" by focusing instead on coherent, viable, and workable constructions of relevant phenomena. A question that follows from the constructivist perspective concerns the methods and criteria for determining how construction systems are viable and workable. When and under what conditions is a construction system viable and when does it appear to lose its ability for meaning making?

Within psychology, tensions exist between realist/objectivist positions and those that assume a more constructivist stance. These tensions can, in part, be traced to the long-standing dialectical relationship between nomothetic and idiographic perspectives on psychological inquiry. Typically the experimental psychologies (social, cognitive, biological, and so forth) have attempted to catalog observations about human nature that are invariant over time and place, that is, to use a nomothetic approach. In focusing more on the life phenomena of individuals, the clinical sciences have developed a more idiographic approach to their field of inquiry. While nomothetic and even quantifiable generalizations about human behavior may be attempted at the level of abstract theory, constructivists ultimately contend that the lived particulars of the person's knowing systems can be best understood through adopting an idiographic and qualitative approach to the study of concrete individuals in their unique social ecologies.

The differing foci of constructivist and realist/objectivist approaches in psychology presents a dilemma for how these methods of inquiry may interface with each other and how the fruits of each paradigm may be incorporated by the other. How can generalizations about the "average anorexic" from the nomothetic perspective be of use to the therapist engaging this *particular* client and the way she constructs her role in life? Similarly, what is the utility of individual constructions, no matter how rich and clinically informative, when trying to discover and articulate fundamental principles of human behavior? At a more general level, what would psychological science look like if all research were conducted at the idiographic and qualitative level associated with constructivist inquiry?

Such questions face those who study psychotherapy outcome. In trying to document the "real world" effects of therapeutic interventions, researchers may use instrumentation and assessment techniques that fail to capture the subtle nuances of human change. Yet, persons may report greater happiness, adjustment, or ability to proceed with life despite producing unremarkable profiles on standard instruments. How does the realist/objectivist outcome researcher account for this phenomenon? Constructivists would propose using idiographic and ipsative measures that are uniquely tailored to the work that is being undertaken in psychotherapy. Methods such as goal-attainment scaling, content analysis procedures, and repertory grids may both help trace the client's level of achieved change and permit the outcome researcher to compare the extent to which clients as a group received benefits.

Beyond these issues in the assessment of therapeutic outcome, lie the questions of what constructivism has contributed to psychotherapy research, and what psychotherapy research has revealed about the nature of constructivist psychotherapy. As implied above, constructivists have actively pursued the development of both qualitative and quantitative procedures for tracking human change processes, particularly at the level of meanings that reflect one's evolving appraisal of the self, life problems, and significant relationships over the course of therapy. While such procedures add refinement to nomothetic measures of personal change, they essentially operate within the traditional paradigm for the study of psychotherapy.

A bolder contribution being made by some constructivists is the development of new paradigms for research on psychotherapy process, which attempt to identify "markers" of significant in-session change episodes (e.g., points of sensed internal conflict or confusion) and then pinpoint the processes that facilitate their positive resolution (e.g., therapist initiated confrontation of the inner "split," or use of metaphor to place experiences in a new perspective). At a more general level, constructivists have also pioneered the development of models of research that actively involve clients as co-investigators and interpreters of a study's results, and that foster deep-going reflection on the part of investigators about shifts in their methodological and conceptual commitments across the course of their research programs.

What has research taught us in turn about the distinctive processes or outcomes of constructivist therapies? In a sense, a definitive answer awaits further study. As fairly recent contenders in the psychotherapy arena, the approaches described in this article have yet to receive the empirical attention given to more "mature" therapeutic traditions. In addition, the abstract and philosophic nature of constructivist theory has discouraged more traditionally trained investigators, who are understandably drawn to simpler models that work with a limited range of concepts and techniques. However, the preliminary research that has been conducted on these novel forms of practice suggests that they are often more acceptable to clients than more regimented, prescriptive alternatives, that they can be effective for even quite discrete problems such as speech disfluencies, phobias, and social anxieties, and that they are adaptable to a range of formats including individual, group, and family therapy. With recent and ongoing efforts to examine their efficacy in the treatment of eating disorders, sexual abuse, and other serious clinical problems, we are optimistic that they will continue to contribute to the refinement of both psychotherapy research and practice.

BIBLIOGRAPHY

Mahoney, M. J. (1991). *Human change processes.* New York: Basic Books.

McNamee, S. & Gergen, K. J. (Eds.). (1992). *Therapy as social construction.* Newbury Park, CA: Sage.

Neimeyer, R. A., & Mahoney, M. J. (Eds.). (1995). *Constructivism in psychotherapy.* Washington, DC: American Psychological Association.

Rosen, H., & Kuehlwein, K. T. (Eds.). (1996). *Constructing reality: Meaning-making perspectives for psychotherapists.* San Francisco, CA: Jossey-Bass.

Journal of Constructivist Psychology, published quarterly. Philadelphia, PA: Taylor and Francis.

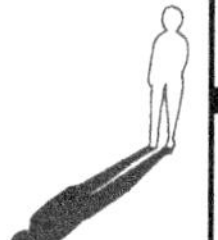

Coping with Stress

Anita DeLongis and Sarah Newth
University of British Columbia

Coping Cognitive and behavioral efforts to manage stress.
Emotion-Focused Coping Coping responses that are geared toward managing one's emotions during stressful episodes.
Problem-Focused Coping Coping responses that are geared toward directly changing some aspect of the stressful situation.
Relationship-Focused Coping Coping responses that are geared toward managing and maintaining one's social relationships during stressful episodes.
Stress Situations that the person cognitively appraises as taxing or exceeding his or her resources.

COPING refers to a person's cognitive and behavioral responses to a stressful situation. This article reviews literature on coping with stressful experiences. It discusses the antecedents and consequences of various strategies for coping with stress, including the role of coping in health and well-being. It describes three functions of coping: problem-focused, emotion-focused, and relationship-focused.

I. CONCEPT OF COPING

In common parlance, "coping" is often used to suggest that individuals are handling stress well or that they have the situation under control. However, most health psychologists who study stress and coping would define coping broadly to include all thoughts and behaviors that occur in response to a stressful experience, whether the person is handling the situation well or poorly. Coping includes what we do and think in response to a stressor, even if we are unaware of why or what we are doing. This broad definition is important for two reasons. First, if we limit the definition of coping to thoughts and behaviors that the individual purposefully and intentionally engages in as a way of handling the stressful situation, we may exclude a wide array of responses that typically remain outside of awareness. These can include, for example, believing in unrealistically positive illusions, escaping through the use of alcohol and other drugs, or fleeing from stress in one area of life (e.g., family) by immersing oneself in some unrelated activity (e.g., work). Second, this definition of coping does not assume a priori that some forms of coping are bad and others are good. *All* of the person's responses to the stressor are considered coping, whether or not they help to resolve the situation. This is important, as in recent years researchers have found that many forms of coping that have traditionally been considered bad coping, such as escape-avoidance, may actually have beneficial effects when coping with certain types of stressors under specific circumstances.

A. Why Is Coping Important for Mental Health?

Many disorders of mental health are either directly caused by stress or their expression is triggered by

Copyright © 1998 by Academic Press.
All rights of reproduction in any form reserved.

stress. In cases where a person is already experiencing poor health, stress can exacerbate and maintain the problems. However, there are wide individual differences in the effects of stress, and these are thought to be largely due to individual differences in coping with stress. Therefore, many health psychologists have turned their attention in recent years to trying to understand the antecedents and consequences of various ways of coping with stress.

B. Historical Overview

In early models, certain forms of coping (and people who used them) were viewed as immature, dysfunctional, or maladaptive. Many emotion-focused strategies were not even considered forms of coping, but merely defenses. These models lost favor as evidence accumulated that many forms of coping previously assumed to be maladaptive could sometimes have positive effects, at least in certain circumstances. Researchers such as Lazarus conceptualized coping as a process in constant flux, responsive to changes in situational demands. The focus on situational factors as primary determinants of coping responses was welcomed as a correction of previous tendencies to treat coping in trait terms. Claims made by Mischel in 1968 that personality traits are poor predictors of behavior were also influential. Furthermore, the findings of a number of studies suggest that in general, situational factors play a larger role in determining responses to stress than do personality traits. Thus, earlier notions of rigid "styles" of coping have been replaced by an understanding that coping is best conceived in process terms. Given this new understanding of coping that emerged during the 1970s and 1980s, the role of personality in coping was given scant attention during those years. Recently, it has been acknowledged that although personality may not be the single most important determinant of coping responses to stress, its role is nonetheless quite important. In the past few years, health psychologists have again turned their attention to examining personality factors that might determine how people cope with stress. Currently, most researchers in the field would agree that how a person copes with stress will shift over time depending on an array of factors that can be broken down into two broad categories: person and situation.

II. DETERMINANTS OF COPING RESPONSES

A. Personality Characteristics as Determinants of Coping

Clinicians and researchers alike have examined the role of personality in coping in an attempt to predict and explain which individuals are at risk for experiencing psychological maladjustment. The underlying assumption is that personality can influence how one copes with stress, and coping determines whether stress will have deleterious effects on health and well-being. A consistent set of personality traits have emerged as significant predictors of the ways in which people cope and the impact coping has on their health. The following is a brief summary of the various personality traits that have been empirically related to coping.

The last 50 years have seen a growing interest in the role of personality as measured by the big five personality traits of neuroticism, extraversion, openness to experience, agreeableness, and conscientiousness. These five factors are believed by many personality researchers to be the five basic underlying dimensions of personality. Researchers have tended to find that neuroticism (the tendency to experience negative affect) is related to maladaptive coping efforts and poor psychological well-being. In comparison, researchers have tended to find that extraversion (the tendency to be gregarious and to experience positive affect) is related to adaptive coping and better psychological well-being. Individuals high on openness (the tendency to be creative and open to feelings and experiences) remain strong in the face of adversity and are more able to engage in coping that is sensitive to the needs of others. Given that two defining features of openness to experience are originality and creativity, future research may show individuals high on openness to be particularly effective and flexible copers. Those individuals high on agreeableness (the tendency to be good-natured) also appear to cope in an adaptive manner that is sensitive to the needs of others. Individuals high on agreeableness tend to engage in less negative interpersonal coping strategies (e.g., confronting others), more positive interpersonal coping (e.g., seeking social support), and lower levels of maladaptive emotion-focused coping (e.g., escape avoidance). Individuals high on agreeableness may seek to avoid additional conflict and distress when coping. Finally, those individuals high on conscientiousness (the tendency to be careful and reliable) have been found to engage in lower levels of maladaptive emotion-focused coping (e.g., escape avoidance) and higher use of problem-focused coping. Individuals high in conscientiousness may seek to engage in the most responsible and constructive forms of coping.

The way in which one anticipates future events has also been established to have an impact on well-being. The tendency to anticipate positive outcomes for the future is referred to as optimism. Carver, Scheier, and others have reported this trait to be associated with both adaptive coping and good mental health. High levels of optimism may lead to higher levels of constructive coping, which in turn reduce distress, making positive expectations highly adaptive. In contrast, pessimistic individuals (those who do not generally anticipate positive future outcomes) tend to use more maladaptive coping strategies, which in turn are related to higher levels of both anxiety and depression.

An internal locus of control (i.e., feeling a sense of personal control) over the events and experiences in one's life is often positively related to psychological well-being, whereas an external sense of control (i.e., lacking a sense of personal control and feeling that control over events is external to oneself) is often negatively related to mental health criteria. Research examining locus of control as a stable personality trait has identified several ways in which this trait influences both coping and psychological adjustment. For example, studies have found that an internal locus of control is related to greater use of problem-focused coping. It appears that a belief in one's ability to impact or change events is related to constructive attempts to alter or change aspects of the environment or oneself under times of duress. Given that such problem-focused coping efforts are generally associated with better psychological outcomes, at least when used with stressors that are controllable, an internal locus of control can have beneficial effects upon mental health.

B. Situational Specificity in Coping

Currently, there is much interest among researchers in studying the factors within a given situation that determine how an individual will cope, how the chosen coping strategies influence mental health, and how this process varies from situation to situation. In 1984, Lazarus and Folkman identified a number of dimensions of stressful situations that are important determinants of the stress and coping process. Novelty (has the individual coped with this type of stressor in the past?), predictability (are there signs that will alert an individual to the onset of the stressful event/situation?), event uncertainty (how likely is it that the situation will occur?), imminence (is the event likely to occur in the near future?), duration (how long will the experience last?), and temporal uncertainty (is it possible to identify whether the event will occur?) all impact affective, cognitive, and behavioral reactions to stress. That is, these situational factors play a role in determining the extent to which a person experiences a situation as stressful, and in turn, how he or she copes with the stressful situation.

Several researchers have conducted studies that explore a variety of situational determinants of coping. Consistent with the hypothesis that situational factors do influence the coping process, researchers have tended to find that different situations elicit different forms of coping, and similar situations elicit similar modes of coping. In addition, similar coping strategies have been found to have different effects across different situations, in that the effectiveness of any one coping strategy and its impact on well-being varies from situation to situation. This points to the importance of a match between a chosen coping strategy and the situationally specific demands of a stressor to maximize emotional adjustment and minimize ongoing struggles. Thus, the particular characteristics of a stressful situation determine both coping choice and coping effectiveness. For example, positive reappraisal is generally an effective coping strategy related to psychological well-being. However, in 1991, Wethington and Kessler noted that when the stressful situation calls for some form of action to be taken, the use of positive reappraisal alone is related to psychological maladjustment. Likewise, in 1994, Aldwin pointed out that emotion focused coping is more effective when coping with a situation that is perceived as involving loss, whereas problem-focused coping is more effective when coping with a situation that is appraised as a threat or challenge. Therefore, one must be cautious in making generalizations about the relation of specific coping strategies to mental health, as this relation will vary according to the situational demands.

Empirical evidence supports the hypothesis that individuals will vary their coping efforts and choices systematically to fit a given stressor. General coping styles aggregated over time tend to be poorly correlated with the ways in which one copes in a specific situation. That is, researchers or clinicians cannot accurately predict how an individual will cope with any one specific stressor by relying on the average way in which the same individual copes across a variety of situations over time. To illustrate, an individual may engage in moderately high levels of a particular coping strategy over time but not use this particular strategy at all when coping with a certain type of stressor. Averaging coping responses across multiple situations, therefore, obscures important information about how coping is related to well-being under specific and well-defined circumstances.

Researchers such as Wethington and Kessler have identified several ways in which coping varies from situation to situation. First, the ways in which individuals cope with an acute but short-term stressor often differs from the ways in which they cope with an ongoing chronic stressor. Second, the ways in which individuals cope can also be influenced by the coping responses of others around them. Third, individuals tend to use different strategies depending on the role domain in which stress occurs. Fourth, situations are defined by a multitude of demands and therefore any one stressor may demand multiple coping strategies in order to be resolved effectively. Those with the highest psychological well-being may well be those individuals who can successfully engage in a variety of coping strategies. Rigid adherence to a small set of coping strategies geared toward direct resolution of the stressor, at the expense of those that might help to reduce stress-related negative emotions, could be maladaptive in many circumstances.

Researchers have begun to examine the ways in which situational factors interact with person factors in determining how people cope with stress. Existing evidence suggests that coping varies as a function of both the situation and the person. For example, in 1986, Parkes found that individuals low in neuroticism varied their use of direct action according to the level of work demands. In comparison, those individuals high in neuroticism did not vary their use of direct action in response to changing levels of work demands. Furthermore, although situational factors play a larger role overall in determining coping responses, the more ambiguous a stressful situation is, the greater the influence of person factors on the coping process.

III. WAYS OF COPING

Historically, coping has been seen as serving two basic functions: problem-focused (active attempts to alter and resolve the stressful situation) and emotion-focused (efforts to regulate one's emotions). Recently, a third function that concerns relationship-focused coping (efforts to manage and maintain social relationships during stressful periods) has been studied as well.

A. Problem-Focused Coping

Problem-focused coping includes those forms of coping that are geared directly toward solving the problem or changing the stressful situation. Most of the research examining problem-focused coping has been on planful problem-solving. Coping strategies based on planful problem-solving involve conscious attempts to determine and execute the most appropriate course of action needed to directly prevent, eliminate, or significantly improve a stressful situation. Making a plan of action and following it is an example of the sort of cool deliberate strategy that typifies this form of coping. Although the primary effect of problem-focused modes of coping is to change or eliminate the stressful environment, it is not unusual for such coping to result inadvertently in a reduction in negative affect and/or an increase in positive affect (e.g., devising and carrying out a plan to finish a task that one has felt pressured to complete). The increase in positive affect following the use of planful problem-solving may be the result of an improvement both in the way one perceives the stressful situation and in the direct changes in the stressful situation itself. In general, planful problem-solving tends to be associated with less negative emotion, more positive emotion, positive reappraisals of the stressful situation, and satisfactory outcomes.

Important moderators of this strategy and its influence on psychological well-being have been documented. First, it appears that individuals engage in a higher use of planful problem-solving when they perceive a situation or encounter as one in which something can be changed for the better. Furthermore, the use of this strategy in uncontrollable or unchangeable situations seems to have a negative impact on psychological health. It appears that pursuing a futile course of action can interfere with the adaptive function of accepting those things that cannot be changed or altered. Second, when a loved one has something to lose in a stressful situation, individuals tend to use lower amounts of planful problem-solving than when a loved one does not have something to lose. Individuals seem to experience difficulty formulating a plan of action when coping with the added emotional distress invoked by concern for a loved one's well-being. Third, when the stress occurs at work, individuals tend to use higher levels of planful problem-solving. In this context, many forms of emotion-focused coping strategies may be viewed as ineffective and socially inappropriate.

In summary, in situations that require a course of action to minimize or reduce stress, the individual may be better off engaging in planful problem-solving efforts rather than in emotion-focused strategies such as denial. Such efforts will more likely improve the interactions between an individual and their environment, and have a positive impact on well-being.

B. Emotion-Focused Coping

Emotion-focused modes of coping include those forms of coping that are geared toward managing one's emotions during stressful periods. A larger number of studies have examined emotion-focused modes of coping than either problem- or relationship-focused modes of coping. All of the many forms of emotion-focused coping that have been described in the literature cannot possibly be discussed here. Instead, we focus on those forms that have received the most attention in the scholarly literature.

1. Emotional Expression

Emotional expression is the active expression of one's thoughts and feelings about an experience or event, and is a common way to cope with stress. The expression can take place through a variety of interpersonal, verbal, and artistic means, including talking or corresponding with someone, keeping a diary, and drawing or painting.

Pennebaker reviews the historical relation of emotional expression to mental health, as reflected in Maslow's notion of self-expression and Freud's concept of emotional catharsis. However, modern researchers studying this phenomenon have construed emotional expression as more than simply the venting of emotions. Pennebaker and his colleagues suggest that it is the active expression of both thoughts and feelings surrounding experiences that makes emotional expression a beneficial form of coping with stress. Pennebaker suggests that this expression can aid in deriving a sense of meaning, insight, and resolution by initiating a process in which facts, feelings, thoughts, and options can be organized effectively.

Pennebaker and colleagues have found across several studies that emotional expression is positively related to both psychological and physical well-being. These studies used a variety of modes of emotional expression, such as writing essays about one's experiences, talking out loud into a tape recorder, or talking to another individual. In comparison, active inhibition (i.e., the deliberate and conscious nonexpression of one's thoughts and feelings) has been found to be negatively related to psychological well-being. In addition, emotional expression that is inappropriately disclosing (e.g., telling a nonreceptive stranger), overly self-absorbed (i.e., disengaging and isolating the listener), overly intellectualized (i.e., lacking acknowledgment and expression of one's feelings), or done in the presence of an unsupportive and critical person, is less likely to have beneficial effects.

There are individual differences in people's ability and desire to engage in emotional expression. For example, some people tend to engage in high levels of emotional expression, whereas others do not. This area of research suggests that the degree of emotional expression may reflect a general personality trait. Gender differences in emotional expression have also been found as women tend to report higher levels of emotional expression than men.

There are a variety of contexts in which individuals coping with stress may engage in emotional expression. As Pennebaker points out, support groups, self-help programs (e.g., Alcoholics Anonymous), telephone crisis lines, psychotherapy, pastoral counseling, and even internet discussions all provide a context in which emotional expression is supported, if not actively encouraged. Evidence suggests that emotional expression has a disease-preventative effect.

2. Seeking Social Support

Another common way of coping with stress is to seek some form of social support. The social support sought may be informational support (e.g., an individual recently diagnosed with HIV contacting a support group to find out more about the virus), tangible support (e.g., a grieving widow asking a friend to help baby-sit her children for an afternoon), or emotional support (e.g., a recently laid-off worker accepting sympathy and understanding from a friend). In general, higher levels of social support are associated with better psychological and physical well-being. However, the quality of available social support is more important to well-being than the absolute amount of available social support. To illustrate, an individual who has a few constructively supportive friends and family members may receive better social support and experience greater health benefits than an individual who has many friends and family members but who do not provide constructive social support. In this context, constructive social support consists of support provision that meets the needs of the individual seeking such support.

In 1988, Fisher and colleagues differentiated between solicited versus unsolicited social support. There are times when members of one's social support network provide unsolicited social support. Unsolicited support tends to occur when the stressor is highly visible and there exist social norms as to how members of the social network should behave (e.g., a death in the family, loss of a child, dissolution of a marriage). However, individuals often have to cope with stressors that are not readily apparent to those around them. During such times, an individual must actively seek social support in order to receive it. Furthermore, a variety of factors seem to play a role in the extent to which individuals will seek social support as part of their coping with such stressors. For example, if individuals blame themselves for the occurrence of a stigmatizing stressor (e.g., contracting HIV after having unprotected sex), they may be less likely to seek social support because of the potential for embarrassment, stigmatization, judgment, and further blame. Given that nondisclosure of stressful experiences has been associated with threats to psychological well-being, not seeking social support may result in an increase risk for disorders of health and well-being.

Individuals may also resist seeking social support when the support available has the potential to add stress to an already stressful situation. Social support would be feared when the support provider delivers social support in an excessive or inappropriate manner. To illustrate, an individual suffering from a chronic, debilitating illness such as rheumatoid arthritis (RA) may avoid seeking social support if doing so threatens their independence (e.g., a support provider insists on doing everything for the individual with RA rather than simply facilitating the sufferer's own coping efforts).

In addition, individual differences have been found in both the extent to which individuals will seek social support and the degree to which they perceive seeking social support to be an effective coping strategy. For example, Thoits, in 1991, found that women engage in higher levels of support seeking than men and perceive seeking social support as a more effective coping strategy than do men. Personality differences also influence the extent to which seeking social support is an effective coping strategy. Recent research has indicated that certain personality traits may explain some of the individual differences in the seeking and receiving of social support. To illustrate, individuals high in neuroticism may tend to elicit negative reactions from others when they seek social support, whereas individuals low in neuroticism may tend to elicit positive reactions. Therefore, different individuals may seek social support to varying degrees and invoke different reactions from others depending on their particular personality and interpersonal style. This suggests that the very individuals most likely to experience threats to their psychological well-being (e.g., those high in neuroticism) and therefore most in need of social support may be those individuals least likely to seek and receive social support in a way that is beneficial to their mental health.

3. Escape-Avoidance

There are times when individuals fail to cope actively with a stressful situation and instead engage in efforts to avoid confronting the stressor. Attempts at escape and avoidance can take a variety of cognitive or behavioral forms, such as wishful thinking, distancing, denial, or engaging in distracting activities. For example, an individual may attempt to repress thoughts of a recently deceased spouse as a cognitive means of escape-avoidance. Likewise, one could immerse oneself in cleaning the house as a way of avoiding a stressful task such as paying bills. As Aldwin noted, certain ways of coping can serve as avoidant coping strategies on one occasion despite serving as approach coping strategies on another. As an example, Aldwin suggests that cognitive reappraisal may function as a constructive approach strategy when used to view a stressful situation more positively and when acting as a catalyst for further action. Conversely, cognitive reappraisal may serve as an avoidant coping strategy when used to rationalize a lack of action or justify engaging in actions that lead to further avoidance (e.g., drinking to make oneself feel better).

Avoidant coping strategies are often a response to the negative affect that results from a stressful situation. For example, some individuals may initially deny that a stressful situation has occurred in an effort to minimize their distress (e.g., not accepting the possibility that a lump in one's breast may be cancer). Researchers such as Lazarus have suggested that in the early stages of a stressor, such avoidant type strategies may be adaptive in that minimizing distress levels allows one time to adapt and to gather one's resources. By decreasing levels of distress, short-term escape-avoidance may increase one's ability to engage in active problem-focused coping. Similarly, the use of escape-avoidance may minimize negative affect while one is waiting for a potentially short-term stressor to pass (e.g., reading a magazine to relieve anxiety while waiting to hear the results of an important medical test).

Despite the positive short-term effectiveness of escape-avoidance in reducing psychological distress, the long-term use of escape-avoidance is generally associated with lowered psychological well-being. For example, although distraction is useful when coping with short-term stressors (e.g., medical and dental procedures), long-term use of distraction with an ongoing stressor (e.g., coping with unemployment) is associated with maladjustment. The negative association between the use of escape-avoidance strategies and well-being may result from the lack of constructive action that the continued use of escape-avoidance can entail. That is, when avoiding thoughts or behaviors that are directed at a stressor, one also tends to avoid engaging in constructive efforts that could potentially reduce both the source and degree of one's distress. In extreme situations, the use of prolonged escape-avoidance can backfire by amplifying a stressful situation and creating added emotional distress (e.g., avoiding obtaining medical attention until it is too late to receive basic treatment).

4. Positive Illusion

Historically, it has been assumed that reality-based perceptions are essential to the maintenance of mental health and psychological well-being. However, in 1988, Taylor and Brown suggested that "positive illusions" (i.e., unrealistically positive perceptions) are related to several common criteria of mental health, such as feelings of contentment and the ability to care for others. They argue that a positive misconstrual of experiences over time is beneficial to the psychological adjustment of the individual engaging in such perceptions. Research suggests that more positive views of the self are associated with lower levels of distress, and Taylor and Brown have argued that a relatively unbiased and balanced perception of the self tends to be related to higher levels of distress. Given that distress tends to be related to less constructive forms of coping, a positive view of the self may have beneficial effects through an increase in constructive coping efforts, even if the positive self-view is illusory. For example, individuals fighting life-threatening illnesses such as diabetes may perceive themselves to be higher in personal strength than others, which in turn may lead to more persistent and effective attempts to cope with their disease.

In a similar vein, Taylor reviews research that establishes a positive relation between illusory perceptions of control and mental health. For example, depressed individuals have been found to have perceptions of control closer to reality than nondepressed individuals. Research assessing control has also demonstrated that when coping with a stressful experience, those individuals who feel a greater sense of control will tend to experience better psychological well-being, even when the sense of control is overestimated. For example, a patient dying of AIDS may experience better psychological well-being by choosing to use alternative medicine, thus obtaining some sense of personal control over the treatment of a disease that remains incurable.

Various mechanisms may explain the relation between positive illusions and mental health when individuals are faced with coping with stress in their lives. For example, Taylor hypothesizes that positive illusions are related to positive mood, which in turn is related to social bonding, which in turn is related to higher levels of well-being. Given the adaptive role that constructive social support plays in the coping process, the potential ability of positive illusions to increase social bonding could be highly beneficial. Taylor also suggests that illusions may enhance creative functioning, motivation, persistence, and performance. Higher levels of all of these factors may lead to more effective coping and better well-being (e.g., higher levels of motivation and creativity could increase one's ability to develop an unusual but highly effective coping strategy).

Recently it has been suggested that conclusions regarding the relation between positive illusions and mental health are an artifact of methodological problems inherent to this area of study. Specifically, Colvin, Block, and Funder, in 1991, argued that previous research has not used valid criteria for establishing objective reality. Without such criteria, it is difficult to verify which individuals are truly engaging in positive illusions. Therefore, conclusions regarding the relation between positive illusions and psychological adjustment may have been premature. These researchers found empirical evidence suggesting that positive illusions can have negative influences on both short-term and long-term mental health.

5. Social Comparison

In 1954, Festinger suggested that individuals are driven to compare themselves to others as a means of obtaining information about oneself and the world during times of threat or ambiguity (i.e., stress). Although the patterns of findings are diverse and sometimes complex, most research in this field suggests that social comparison processes have important implications for psychological well-being. In fact, several researchers have proposed that social comparisons play a central role in the way in which people cope with stressful experiences. For example, social comparisons can help individuals evaluate their resources and provide information relevant to managing emotional reactions to stress. However, the underlying motivation and purpose that each individual has for engaging in this type of coping and the resultant psychological outcomes can be diverse.

In 1989, Wood described three classes of motivational factors that drive a person to engage in social comparisons: self-evaluation, self-improvement, and self-enhancement. All three purposes can be relevant to coping with stress and may aid the individual in striving toward an adaptive outcome. Self-evaluation motivations to engage in social comparison stem from an individual's desire to obtain information regarding his or her standing on a particular skill or attribute. Self-improvement motivations to engage in social comparison suggest that individuals are interested in deriving information regarding another's standing on a particular skill or attribute in order to improve their own standing on the same dimension. Self-enhancement motivations to engage in social comparison stem from a need to see oneself in a more positive manner; that is, the results of the social comparison are used to make one feel better about one's own standing on a particular skill or attribute relative to others.

When an individual seeks a social comparison target as a means of coping with an ambiguous or threatening situation, several options are available. One can select an individual who has a higher or more positive standing than oneself on the dimension in question (i.e., an "upward social comparison"). Alternatively, one can select an individual who has a lower or more negative standing than oneself on the relevant dimension (i.e., a "downward social comparison"). Presumably, comparisons against others who differ from oneself produce distinctive and discriminating information that has immediate and practical implications for the individual when engaging in coping efforts.

In general, research suggests that when people engage in downward comparisons, they feel more positive and less negative about themselves than when they engage in upward comparisons. Individuals engaging in downward social comparisons because of self-enhancement motivations tend to experience reduced levels of negative affect and feel better about themselves in both field and experimental studies. For example, in their 1985 study of women coping with breast cancer, Wood and her colleagues found that downward comparisons appeared to help women feel better about how they were dealing with their illness by yielding positive evaluations relative to women who were not coping as effectively. However, research has also demonstrated that when individuals are motivated by self-improvement or self-evaluation needs, there is a clear preference for upward comparison information. Under these circumstances, comparisons may help determine what kinds of interventions or efforts are both possible and necessary to cope more effectively with a particular stressor.

Collins proposed in 1996 that the outcomes of social comparisons are not predetermined by the direction in which one makes a comparison. Instead, evidence supports the notion that both upward and downward comparisons can have both positive and negative impacts on psychological well-being. First, upward comparisons can generate negative psychological outcomes through a contrast effect (i.e., one feels inferior to the comparison target). Second, upward comparisons may also yield positive effects through the inspiration and hope they generate. These types of comparisons may be especially helpful for problem-solving activities, as they can provide constructive information that suggests specific coping strategies. Third, downward comparisons can lead to positive outcomes presumably because they allow one to focus on ways in which one is doing well relative to others. Such comparisons may be especially helpful in regulating negative emotions. Finally, downward comparisons can lead to negative outcomes from the fear that one will "sink" to the lower level of the comparison target at some future point in time. Such comparisons may have special significance for individuals coping with illness, where it is feasible that their disease will progress negatively. Given that both downward and upward comparisons contain both positive and negative information relevant to the self, the particular aspect the individual focuses on while coping will determine the valence of the outcome.

A growing number of moderating variables are being identified as important factors in determining the impact social comparison will have as a coping strategy during times of stress, threat, or ambiguity. For example, it appears that individuals with high self-esteem have a greater tendency to derive positive outcomes from either upward or downward social comparisons than individuals with low self-esteem. Other researchers have also noted the important role played by perceived control. Individuals with high degrees of perceived control over the dimension in question may be less likely to experience negative reactions to social comparisons in contrast to those with low levels of control. Individual differences in familiarity with a stressor may also moderate the process of social comparison. For example, an individual who has just discovered they have HIV (unfamiliar dimension) may select different comparison targets for coping than an individual who has been living with the illness for some time (familiar dimension). Presumably, the type of information one needs in order to adapt to threats will vary according to how long one has been dealing with the threat. In addition to individual differences, it appears that the situational context in which the social comparison process takes place is an important determinant of the impact of the comparison itself. For example, different contexts vary in terms of the potential social comparison targets they provide.

At times, individuals will actively self-select when to engage in social comparison and with whom they wish to compare themselves. However, as Collins noted, social comparisons can sometimes be forced on the individual. For example, researchers have found that someone who needs health care services for a serious condition may have no choice but to sit in a waiting room with other individuals who also have the same condition, making social comparisons unavoidable. Such comparisons most likely make it difficult for an individual to avoid the possibility that his or her own illness and condition could get worse. In addition, researchers have suggested that the impact of forced comparisons can be particularly aversive when the comparison target is someone with whom the individual is interdependent (e.g., close friend, co-worker). This suggests that individuals may sometimes have to cope with the stressful nature of the social comparison itself.

Regardless of whether or not one chooses to engage in social comparison, once the social comparison process is underway (i.e., target is compared against), there are some active strategies that individuals can use to maximize the probability of obtaining a positive outcome. First, peripheral dimensions can be used to moderate comparison outcomes. If a comparison produces an unfavorable outcome (e.g., an upward comparison that leaves one feeling inferior), one can always attribute the lower standing to differences between oneself and the target on other related variables (e.g., sex, ethnicity, duration of stressor). Alternatively, as previously discussed, individuals can actively distort information to maintain a more positive perception of reality.

In summary, social comparison processes provide valuable information that individuals can use for a variety of purposes when coping with stress, threat, or ambiguity. The target selected, the situation or context in which the comparison is made, and the unique traits of both the individual and the comparison target have an impact on the outcome of the comparison process. As a result, social comparison may have a positive impact on well-being for particular individuals in certain situations, and a negative impact on well-being for other individuals in different situations. Research has demonstrated the relevance of social comparison to coping with a variety of stressors such as illness and marital problems.

C. Relationship-Focused Coping

Relationship-focused coping refers to the various attempts made by the individual to manage, regulate, or preserve relationships when coping with stress. Recently, there has been growing interest in the interpersonal dimensions of coping as distinct from the intrapersonal dimensions of emotion- and problem-focused coping.

1. Empathic Responding

Empathic coping is one such form of relationship-focused coping. The use of empathy has been related to positive social behaviors such as providing social support and caring for others. Recently, O'Brien and DeLongis have suggested that empathic coping includes the following elements: (a) attempts to see the situation from another's point of view, (b) efforts to experience personally the emotions felt by the other person, (c) attempts to read between the lines in order to decipher the meaning underlying the other person's verbal and nonverbal behavior to reach a better understanding of the other person's experience, (d) attempts to respond in a way that conveys sensitivity and understanding, and (e) efforts to validate and accept the person and their experience while avoiding passing judgment. One may engage in empathic coping either verbally (e.g., telling a spouse that you understand what they are feeling) or nonverbally (e.g., tenderly holding someone's hand as they talk).

Empathic coping can play a significant role in coping with stress, particularly stress caused by interpersonal problems. Research suggests that empathic coping is related to a decrease in distress caused by interpersonal tension and an increase in relationship satisfaction. The increased understanding gained from empathic coping may result in more appropriate and well-considered coping choices that will maximize the benefits for all involved. Empathic coping may also lead to further benefits for psychological adjustment because of its impact on concurrent or subsequent use of problem- and emotion-focused coping. For example, in 1993, Kramer found that caregivers who engaged in empathic coping strategies were more likely to engage in planful problem-solving than caregivers who did not engage in empathic coping. The greater use of these strategies was related to greater caregiver satisfaction with the caregiving role. In the same study, lower use of empathic coping was related to more maladaptive emotion-focused coping efforts, which were in turn related to depression.

Individuals vary in how often and how effectively they use empathic coping. For example, O'Brien and DeLongis have found that when a close other is involved in a stressful situation, those high in neuroticism are less able to use empathic coping than are those low in neuroticism.

2. Active Engagement and Protective Buffering

In addition to empathic coping, other forms of relationship-focused coping are also receiving attention. In 1991, Coyne and Smith identified active engagement (e.g., discussing the situation with involved others) and protective buffering (e.g., attempting to hide worries and concerns from involved others) as two forms of relationship-focused coping. They found that higher degrees of protective, relationship-focused coping (e.g., not conveying fears to one's spouse) among wives of myocardial infarction patients was related to higher degrees of distress among the wives. Note that this is consistent with research suggesting that suppression of emotional expression is related to lowered psychological well-being. However, wives' use of protective buffering was positively related to self-efficacy among their husbands. It appears that the wives were coping with the stress of their spouse's illness in a way that maximized the benefits for their sick husbands (i.e., interpersonally adaptive) yet threatened their own well-being (i.e., intrapersonally maladaptive). Such results point to the need to include interpersonal dimensions of coping in addition to the traditional intrapsychic dimensions of coping in order to understand the relation of coping and health outcomes.

IV. FINAL COMMENTS

In conclusion, there is no one "good" way to cope with stress. Stress takes on many forms, and likewise, so must coping. The most adaptive way to cope with any given stressor depends on both the personality of the stressed individual and the characteristics of the stressful situation. Dimensions of the stressful situation that must be considered in determining the best way to cope with a given stressor include (a) whether others are involved in the situation, how they are coping, and the relationship of these people to the stressed individual; (b) the timing of the stressor and the degree to which it is anticipated or controllable; (c) the types of specific demands inherent to the stressful situation, the duration of such demands, and one's prior experience with similar stressors; and (d) what is at stake in the stressful situation. Perhaps the key to good coping is flexibility. That is, the ability to vary one's coping depending on the demands of the situation. What is clear is that no one form of coping will be effective in dealing with all stressors. There are times when attempts at problem-focused coping will be a waste of time and energy that could be better spent engaged in emotion- and relationship-focused coping. At other times, when something can be done directly to prevent or alter the stressful demands, energy may be better spent doing something concrete to solve the problem rather than concentrating on emotion management. Perhaps it is the wisdom to know the difference, and then to act on that knowledge, that is essential to successful coping.

BIBLIOGRAPHY

Aldwin, C. (1994). *Stress, coping, and development: An integrative perspective.* New York: Guilford Press.

Collins, R. (1996). For better or for worse: The impact of upward social comparison on self-evaluations. *Psychological Bulletin, 119,* 51–69.

Eckenrode, J. (Ed.). (1991). *The social context of coping.* New York: Plenum Press.

Gottlieb, B. (Ed.). (1997). *Coping with chronic stress.* New York: Plenum Press.

Lazarus, R. S., & Folkman, S. (1984). *Stress, appraisal, and coping.* New York: Springer.

Goldberger, L., & Breznitz, S. (Eds.). (1993). *Handbook of stress: Theoretical and clinical aspects.* New York: Free Press.

O'Brien, T. B., & DeLongis, A. (1996). The interactional context of problem-, emotion-, and relationship-focused coping: The role of the Big Five personality factors. *Journal of Personality, 64,* 775–813.

Pennebaker, J. W. (1990). *Opening up: The healing power of confiding in others.* New York: William Morrow.

Taylor, S. E. (1989). *Positive illusions: Creative self-deception and the healthy mind.* New York: Basic Books.

Zeidner, M., & Endler, N. S. (Eds.). (1996). *Handbook of coping: Theory, research, applications.* New York: John Wiley & Sons.

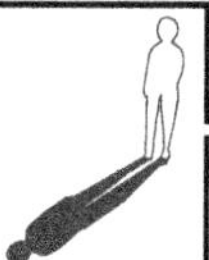

Couples Therapy

Kieran T. Sullivan
Santa Clara University

Andrew Christensen
University of California, Los Angeles

Differentiation The degree to which a person (or a couple) is able to differentiate between his or her *emotional system* (i.e., instinctual reactions) and his or her *intellectual system* (i.e., the ability to use reason and to communicate complex ideas).

Emotional Joining around the Problem Focusing partners on the pain each is experiencing rather than on the blame each deserves.

Negative Attributions Distressed partners' tendencies to attribute each other's negative behavior to unchangeable characteristic of the partner rather than to temporary, external circumstances.

Problem–Solution Loop Attempted solutions that partners use to control or alleviate the problem that actually make the problem persist.

Projective Identification One partner projects onto the other his or her repressed objects or aspects of the self.

Securing the Frame The therapist outlines the parameters for therapy, including setting the fee and scheduling the sessions, which creates a safe and stable environment for partners.

Selective Inattention Distressed partners' tendencies to remember negative relationship events with great clarity, but to have little recall of positive events.

This article presents five major approaches to COUPLES THERAPY and discusses their relative effectiveness in treating relationship distress. Each of these approaches is based on a theory of the development of relationship distress and uses specific therapeutic techniques to help alleviate this distress. In addition, two recent integrative approaches are presented that combine elements of the previous approaches in an attempt to increase the effectiveness of the intervention. Interventions for couples with psychiatric disorders and alternative interventions, such as group couples therapy and prevention, are also discussed.

I. INTRODUCTION

Joe and Diane have both been feeling very unhappy lately with their marriage. Diane feels that Joe spends too much time at work and has been neglecting his responsibilities at home, particularly child care with their daughter. She is lonely and angry at him. Joe thinks that Diane is too demanding and feels overwhelmed when he comes home to her criticism and nagging. They seem to be fighting more and more, and their sex life has diminished considerably. Unable to work these problems out on their own, they seek the help of a couples therapist.

When faced with a distressed couple like Diane and Joe, there are many different ways to conceptualize and treat their problems. Some therapists might focus on the couple's negative interactions, for example,

Copyright © 1998 by Academic Press.
All rights of reproduction in any form reserved.

when Diane becomes very angry at Joe and Joe withdraws from Diane. Others might emphasize the problems in the family system, exploring Diane's relatively stronger alliance with their daughter compared with Joe. Still others might explore Diane's and Joe's relationships with their own families of origin and try to discover how those relationships have affected their marriage.

Over the last two decades, many models have emerged to explain and treat relationship distress. This article begins with a history of the development of couple's therapy and then presents five empirically validated therapeutic approaches to treating couples in distress, using the preceding example to illustrate each type of intervention. It is important to note that these approaches may not correspond with approaches typically practiced in the community. They are theoretically based models of couples therapy, most of which have been subject to controlled clinical trials in order to evaluate their effectiveness. The results of these outcome trials are presented after the description of each approach.

In an attempt to provide optimal treatment for couples, couples researchers have begun to develop interventions that integrate effective aspects of different theories into one general approach. Two of these integrative models are briefly described after the five core models. The term *marital therapy* is avoided in favor of *couples therapy* (except in historical contexts) to reflect the recent shift away from a marriage bias to include all types of couples who seek treatment.

II. HISTORY OF COUPLES THERAPY

The identification of couples and families as a system for which psychological intervention is appropriate and even advantageous is a relatively recent phenomenon. In this section, we highlight important movements, historical developments, and influential contributors to the development of couples therapy from the post-World War I era to the present.

In the period after World War I, professionals from various disciplines began to promote human sexuality as a legitimate area of scientific study and to call for public education regarding sexual and reproductive issues. Spearheaded by Hirschfield in Germany, Ellis in Great Britain, and Kautsky in Austria, public centers were founded throughout Europe to promote awareness and knowledge of these issues. In these centers, advice was given on contraception, eugenics, and psychological and relational issues. Concurrent with the rise of Nazi Germany, however, the focus of the centers became increasing eugenic. As noted by Kopp in 1938, "In the United States of America marriage counselling to date has in the main been concerned with the solution of the problems related to the psychology and physiology of sex, reproduction, family and social relationships. In Europe, on the other hand, the main objectives are the betterment of the biological stock" (p. 154).

Although the idealistic vision of sexual reformers was impeded in Europe, the development of couples and family therapy continued in the United States. Social workers emphasized the need to expand interventions to include the family. Educators implemented home economics courses in high schools nationwide. Workshops addressing family and marital issues were offered through churches and universities. Finally, new psychoanalytic theories (such as object relations theory) opened the door for psychological interventions beyond just one individual.

Emerging from such varied fields, the marriage counseling movement was both eclectic and pragmatic. Early couples counseling was mainly conducted as a secondary profession by college professors, physicians, and gynecologists. In the early 1930s, the first institutes were opened whose primary function was to provide couples therapy. These institutes included the American Institute of Family Relations in Los Angeles, an ecumenical marriage center in New York and the Marriage Council of Philadelphia.

The American Association of Marriage Counselors (AAMC) was established in 1945 for establishing standards, exchanging information, and helping in the development of interest in marriage counseling. Of the professionals who initially formed the AAMC, "no less than fifty percent came primarily from the medical specialties, while the rest represented such fields as social work, psychology, and sociology" (p. 433). During the 1950s and early 1960s, centers for marriage counseling were opened across the country, marriage counseling textbooks were produced for a general professional audience, standards were proposed for marriage counselors, and training centers were accredited. Despite this progress, however, the new profession of marital counseling had yet to establish a clear sense of professional identity. Marriage counseling continued to be a secondary profession for most practitioners, leaving the status of marriage counseling as a profession marginal.

In the late 1960s and early 1970s, the profession matured. Perhaps the most important development during this period was the establishment of a common journal, the *Journal of Marital and Family Counseling* (now the *Journal of Marriage and Family Therapy*). It was also during this period that varying approaches to conjoint therapy were developed and proposed by marital therapists and researchers. In 1970, the AAMC changed its name to the American Association for Marriage and Family Counselors (AAMFC) to reflect the convergence of marriage and family counseling during this period.

In the last two decades, many marital and family therapists have worked for the recognition of their profession as autonomous and distinct. In 1992, regulations in the Federal Register officially declared marriage and family therapy to be the fifth core mental health profession (along with psychiatry, psychology, social work, and psychiatric nursing). By 1993, 31 states had implemented licensing procedures for marital and family therapists. The struggle for an autonomous profession is not without controversy, however. Proponents of marital and family therapy remaining within an established profession (e.g., psychology, psychiatry, etc.) have specific advantages, such as ease in obtaining funding and reimbursement for research and clinical work. Today, marital and family therapy "is partially established as a major profession, but its status in the broader society remains frustratingly marginal" (Shields et al., 1994). [*See* FAMILY THERAPY.]

III. THEORETICAL APPROACHES IN CONDUCTING COUPLES THERAPY

A. Behavioral Couples Therapy

1. Theory of Distress

Behavioral couples therapy (BCT) emphasizes the behaviors that partners exchange and the antecedents and consequences of those behaviors. Although behaviorists acknowledge the role of affect and cognition in the development and maintenance of distress, they target the external determinants of behavior as the point of intervention for distressed couples. Therapists help couples to define their problems in behaviorally specific terms and to gain control over them by manipulating the conditions that precede the problematic behavior and those that are consequent to it. By teaching couples various communication and problem-solving skills, therapists help couples minimize distressing exchanges and maximize rewarding exchanges. [*See* BEHAVIOR THERAPY.]

2. Development of Dissatisfactions

According to behavior theory, people select mates based on the actual and anticipated reinforcers received in the relationship (e.g., sexual pleasure, emotional intimacy, wealth, etc.). Couples who are initially satisfied with these reinforcers may become less satisfied over time because reinforcements become habitual and routine or because greater contact and/or life changes may expose important incompatibilities that were not apparent to the couple during the courtship phase of their relationship. When faced with important incompatibilities, partners may cease previously rewarding behaviors and engage in coercive techniques in an effort to get their own way. When one partner gives in to such aversive techniques, his or her partner is reinforced for using these techniques and will therefore be more likely to use them in the future. For example, Diane may nag Joe to complete his share of the housework. When Joe finally gives in to her nagging, her nagging is reinforced. The partner who gives in is also reinforced by the removal of the aversive stimulus. Thus, Joe is more likely to give in to the nagging in the future, because it is reinforcing for him to have the nagging stop. As partners become habituated to these aversive stimuli, the coercing partner must use them in greater amounts. Also, the coerced partner may engage in coercion to achieve his or her own goals. Thus, an initially satisfied couple may develop negative interaction patterns that cause them both distress, but which they are unable to stop.

3. Intervention

The emphasis in BCT is on behavioral change, specifically, behaviors that contribute to a partner's satisfaction and distress. The techniques most frequently used to promote these changes are behavior exchange and communication/problem-solving strategies. In behavior exchange, the therapist helps the couple to identify behaviors that are reinforcing and through various strategies directs them to increase these reinforcing behaviors. This exchange of behaviors provides some immediate relief of distress and paves the way for more difficult negotiations which require communication and problem-solving strategies. The therapist then teaches the couples noncoercive ways of discussing and resolving conflicts and practices these skills with the couple using conflicts that the couple is currently experiencing. The final goal is for the couple to learn to apply these skills on their own whenever a new conflict arises.

4. Specific Therapeutic Techniques

In behavior exchange, therapists guide partners in the selection of reinforcing behaviors, direct them to increase the frequency of these behaviors, and debrief their experiences with these change efforts. Ideally, couples select behaviors that are maximally reinforcing to the receiver and of minimal cost to the giver. Typically, low-cost behaviors are behaviors that are not a current source of conflict, do not require the learning of new skills, and are positive. Therapists may directly assign partners to increase the overall frequencies of the selected behaviors or direct each partner to increase the target behavior within a certain time frame, as in "love days" or "caring days." Finally, therapists debrief these behavior change experiences. In these sessions, receivers are encouraged to acknowledge and positively reinforce the increase in positive behavior by the giver.

In communication/problem solving training, couples are taught to approach problem solving in two distinct steps, problem definition and problem solution. The distinction between these two steps is made to avoid premature problem solving. During the problem definition phase, partners are encouraged to begin by acknowledging some positive part of the problem. They are then encouraged to state their problems in specific behavioral terms, to express their feelings, to acknowledge their own role in the problem, and to devise a brief summary statement of the problem. For Joe and Diane, one problem might be that Joe frequently comes home late from work and is criticized for his lateness when he comes home. Diane would be encouraged to acknowledge that her criticism may be part of the reason why Joe comes home late and to discuss how she feels when he is late. Joe would be encouraged to acknowledge his lateness and to discuss his feelings in response to Diane's criticism. During the problem–solution phase, the couple begins by brainstorming all possible solutions, without further elaborating on the problem. Then, the couple evaluates these solutions based on a cost–benefit analysis. Finally, a specific agreement is reached, which is often set in writing. Throughout the discussion, couples are instructed to address only one problem at a time, to focus on their own views without presupposing what their partner's views are, and to paraphrase what their partner just said to ensure listening and to avoid interruptions.

5. Efficacy of Treatment Approach

More controlled, clinical trials have been conducted on BCT than on any other modality. The results have been mixed. Although about two thirds of couples who receive BCT show an increase in satisfaction at the end of therapy, long-term follow-up data suggest that about 30% of couples who were successfully treated relapse after 2 years. Thus about one half of couples treated with BCT experience lasting improvement in their relationships.

B. Cognitive Behavioral Couples Therapy

Cognitive behavioral couples therapy (CBCT) emerged in response to a number of studies that revealed the importance of cognitions in the development and maintenance of couples' distress. It uses the same basic structure and therapeutic strategies as BCT, but it also includes assessment of and intervention in partners' maladaptive cognitions. The following description focuses solely on the cognitive components of CBCT, as the behavioral components have been described previously.

1. Theory of Distress

Researchers have identified five areas of cognition that are related to distress. *Selective inattention* refers to distressed partners' tendencies to remember negative relationship events with great clarity, but to have little recall of positive events. *Negative attributions* occur when distressed partners attribute each other's negative behavior to unchangeable characteristic of the partner rather than to temporary, external circumstances. Partners may also have unrealistic *expectancies* about the future and *assumptions* about how relationships operate that contribute to their distress.

Finally, partners' *standards* about what a relationship should be like often interfere with their ability to be satisfied with their current relationship.

2. Development of Distress

The conceptualization of the development of distress in CBCT is similar to the conceptualization used in BCT. One difference is that maladaptive cognitions are seen as contributing to the behaviors that lead to distress as well as to the distress itself.

3. Intervention

The structure of the sessions in CBCT is flexible to allow for varying focus on behavior, cognition, and emotion. Therapists address maladaptive cognitions when they emerge as the main problem or when they are clearly interfering with behavioral skills training. The therapist's role is active and directive. When assessing or evaluating cognitions, the focus is on the content of the cognitions rather than on the process that is occurring between the partners. This is done to get a clear understanding of problematic cognitions. Couples are taught about cognitions and how they can influence behavior and emotions. Over the course of therapy, couples learn how to become more aware of cognitions, how to evaluate them, and how to challenge them when necessary.

4. Specific Therapeutic Techniques

One technique that CBCT therapists frequently use to help partners become more aware of selective inattention, unrealistic expectancies, assumptions, and standards, and maladaptive attributions is the use of daily logs. Couples write down their automatic thoughts as they occur and this material is used for later evaluation. For example, when Joe does not come home in time to say good night to their daughter, Diane might think "He doesn't love her," or "He is a very selfish person." During actual sessions, therapists use open-ended questions, coaching, and direct questions to uncover relationship standards and beliefs that are difficult to access. To modify cognitions, partners learn to challenge their own cognitions as they make them, evaluating whether their inferences make sense logically. They are also trained to identify alternative, relationship-enhancing attributions. Diane would be encouraged to rethink her automatic attribution that Joe is late because he does not love her daughter and instead attribute Joe's lateness to his temporary and stressful project at work. Finally, therapists teach couples about specific types of distortions (e.g., personalization, overgeneralization) so that they can be aware of them when they occur. Therapists also help to uncover deeply held relationship standards and assumptions and to evaluate the advantages and disadvantages of maintaining these standards.

5. Efficacy of Treatment Approach

A series of clinically controlled outcome studies have consistently shown that CBCT is equally effective in treating marital distress when compared to other treatment strategies, including BCT. In addition, CBCT has been shown to affect partners' actual cognitions. Baucom, Epstein, and Rankin (1995) have identified several reasons why CBCT has not been shown to be more effective than BCT alone. First, couples were randomly assigned to either BCT or CBCT. Because the need for cognition restructuring varies in couples, matching couples to treatment is necessary to determine whether CBCT will be more effective in helping those couples with distorted and maladaptive cognitions. Second, the interventions (skills training and cognitive restructuring) were separated in time rather than integrated. This is inconsistent with a naturalistic intervention, which would use cognitive restructuring when needed by the couple, not when dictated by the protocol. Finally, the cognitive restructuring phase was often very brief (about 3 weeks), which is probably insufficient. For these reasons, it remains unclear whether adding cognitive components to BCT increases the effectiveness of BCT.

C. Systemic Couples Therapy: Bowen Family Systems Therapy

Several distinct approaches for couples therapy have been developed based on systems theory. One of the most prominent and widely practiced is Bowen Family Systems Therapy (BFST). This section begins with a general overview of systems theory followed by a more in-depth description of BFST. The systems approach emphasizes the organization of the family as a whole and the patterns of interaction that the family engages in. The family, or in this case the couple, is seen as made up of elements that are organized by the consistent nature of the relationship between them.

Systems theory states that all systems work to maintain balance and stabilization. Each part of the system plays an important role in maintaining that balance. For families and couples, mechanisms can be identified whose primary purpose is the maintenance of an acceptable behavioral balance within the family. Families tend to establish a behavioral balance and to resist any change from that predetermined level of stability.

1. Theory of Distress

In BFST, a key concept in understanding couples distress is *differentiation,* which refers both to individuals and to couples. Differentiation is the degree to which a person (or a couple) is able to differentiate between his or her emotional system (i.e., instinctual reactions) and his or her intellectual system (i.e., the ability to use reason and to communicate complex ideas). Persons or couples who are unable to make this differentiation consistently respond to their environment using the emotional system, which makes them vulnerable to distress. In contrast, persons and couples who are able to regulate their behavior using their intellectual system are less likely to develop symptoms of couples' distress. Symptoms of distress appear when a couple encounters anxiety; these symptoms include emotional distancing, conflict, development of dysfunction in one partner, and, in the case of families, projection of the problem onto a child.

2. Development of Dissatisfaction

The BFST approach relies on an intergenerational theory that suggests that degrees of differentiation do not change much from generation to generation. This is based on two assumptions. The first is that parental differentiation affects how well children are able to separate emotionally from their parents. Adult children of undifferentiated parents will experience unresolved emotional attachment to parents that will prevent them from becoming differentiated themselves. Second, people pick marital partners who have similar levels of differentiation. When undifferentiated partners marry, they tend to be overly dependent on one another and are very vulnerable to the development of distress when anxiety is encountered. Differentiated adults, in contrast, tend to have a strong sense of self within their own marriages, and their functioning is less dependent on the behavior of their partner. They are able to tolerate the anxiety that is generated when inevitable differences appear.

3. Intervention

The overall goal of BFST is not to relieve the immediate symptoms, but to increase the level of differentiation of the members and of the unit. Symptom relief without increased differentiation leaves the couple vulnerable to developing new symptoms when additional anxiety is encountered. In BFST, the therapist functions as a coach who creates a climate in which each individual can reach their highest potential level of differentiation and in which the relationship can assist the individuals to develop further than they might have alone. The couple or family system is viewed as the patient, and the therapist attempts to interact with the system to enhance its own natural restorative processes. This is accomplished by focusing not on the content presented during therapy, but on the emotional processes of the couple over time. In particular, the therapist wants to prevent the couple from engaging in an *emotional chain reaction* of instinctive, emotionally laden reactions to one another. To accomplish this, it is critical for the clinician to understand and control his or her own emotional reactivity to provide a safe environment in which the couple can discuss emotionally charged issues. The therapist must remain emotionally neutral, unembroiled in the family system, and maintain his or her own differentiation.

4. Specific Therapeutic Techniques

The BFST therapist begins with a thorough history of the immediate and extended family to formulate a picture of the family emotional system. The survey should give the therapist a working knowledge of the current symptoms as well as the mechanisms that the couple uses to manage anxiety and to keep the relationship stable. Bowen (1978) identified four main functions of the clinician. First, the clinician defines and clarifies the emotional processes between partners. Because partners are preferentially sensitive to one another, each behavior is perceived, interpreted, and reacted to by the other. These reactions are often based in the emotional system in distressed couples, guided more by feeling than by thinking, with each reaction generating its own counterreaction. The therapist's goal is to get couples to become more aware of and to think about this process (i.e., use their intellectual system) rather than simply to enact it. Thus, when Joe feels nagged by Diane to do housework, he becomes aware that he is having this feeling and is more able to discuss this with Diane, rather than to react by withdrawing and neglecting the housework. Second, it is critical for the clinician to remain detriangulated from the emotional process. "Conflict between two people will resolve automatically if both remain in emotional contact with a third person who can relate actively to both without taking sides with either." (Bowen 1978, p. 224). Third, the therapist teaches the couple about the emotional system. Fourth, the therapist models differentiation of self for the couple. To do so, the therapist must be aware of his or her own viewpoint and values, and how he or she typically responds to a variety of situations. The usual format is for the therapist to talk with one person while the other listens, using low-key questions aimed at clarifying the emotional reactivity of the person and the chain reaction between partners. Overall, the questions are used to elicit thinking and to tone down emotional responses.

5. Efficacy of Treatment Approach

To date, there are no controlled outcome studies examining the efficacy of the Bowenian approach with couples or with families. There have been studies examining other family systems approaches; a review of the few *controlled* outcome studies found that family therapy, compared with no treatment and alternative treatments, did have positive effects. Because the studies varied in the type of family therapy and in the type of alternative therapy, it remains unclear how effective a systems approach is in treating couples' distress.

D. Psychoanalytic Couples Therapy

1. Theory of Distress

Psychoanalytic theories of marriage emphasize the interplay of unconscious wishes, fears, and fantasies between spouses. According to object relations theory, all adult individuals have "lost" parts of themselves which were "split off" and repressed into the unconscious during infancy. This happened as a result of the inevitable gap between the infant feeling a need and the satisfaction of that need. This gap leads to feelings of frustration in the infant and to the perception of the mother (the object) as rejecting. Because the infant is unable to tolerate the ambiguity of a giving mother who is sometimes rejecting, it splits off the image of the rejecting mother from the image of the ideal mother and represses it into the unconscious (as the rejecting object), along with the part of the self that related to the rejecting mother. When individuals choose a mate, they do so at both a conscious and an unconscious level. Unconsciously, they are attracted to mates whose unconscious objects and selves are complementary to their own. Ideally, this complementarity helps partners to regain lost parts of themselves in relation to their partner. When the unconscious interplay between partners causes partners to repress further rather than reintegrate lost parts of the selves, distress can occur.

2. Development of Dissatisfaction

Partners' unconscious communication takes place through a process called *projective identification.* In projective identification, one partner (e.g., the wife) projects onto her husband her repressed objects or aspects of the self. Ideally, her husband is able to identify temporarily with and embody these projections. Through this process, the projection is modified and "detoxified" for the wife, who can then consciously assimilate this new view of herself. As a result, she is better able to distinguish herself from her husband and to love him for who he is and not for what she projects onto him. This process takes place simultaneously for both partners. Thus, through the complementarity of unconscious objects, partners facilitate growth and reintegration in one another. When partners' projective identification is not mutually gratifying and objects are more firmly repressed rather than modified, distress occurs.

3. Intervention

The main focus in intervention is the unconscious projections that each person is making and the partners' responses to these projections. The overall goal of therapy is to increase partners' abilities to contain, modify, and reintegrate aspects of the self that they project onto one another. Through this reintegration, the partners become more able to give and receive genuine love. This is accomplished through careful observation of partners' defenses and anxieties and through creating an environment in which these anxieties can be worked through. Psychoanalytic couples therapy is ideally a long-term, in-depth enterprise, which typically requires a period of 1 to 2 years.

4. Specific Therapeutic Techniques

The techniques used in psychoanalytic couples therapy are more attitudinal than behavioral. The therapist typically engages in careful, undirected listening and, later, in interpretations. The therapist begins with a period of assessment that allows the couple to understand the nature of the undertaking so that they may freely choose to enter into psychoanalytic couples therapy. In this assessment process, called *securing the frame*, the therapist outlines the parameters for therapy, including setting the fee and scheduling the sessions, which creates a safe and stable environment for the partners. It is also the first opportunity for partners to attempt to gratify unconscious wishes by encroaching on the frame, which provides insight into the unconscious difficulties affecting the marriage. For example, Joe might object to the therapist's policy that he must attend therapy every week and that he must pay the therapist her usual fee if he misses an appointment. He may feel infantalized and "nagged" to attend therapy regularly. This feeling gives the therapist some insight into Joe's unconscious processes and the current difficulties in the marriage. As mentioned previously, the therapist attempts to listen primarily to the unconscious and to make use of countertransference (the therapist's feelings regarding the couple) for clues into the unconscious. The therapist maintains a neutral position and uses his or her own self as a "holding place" where the couple can recognize and modify their own dysfunctional unconscious patterns. The therapist is able to create this holding place based on the intimate knowledge of his or her own unconscious attained through rigorous training, supervision, and personal psychotherapy. As the therapist begins to understand the unconscious dynamics between the partners, he or she begins to offer interpretations to help the couple gain insight into their process of projective identification. Termination is initiated once the couple is able to "internalize" the therapist and create their own holding space within which to work through anxieties and defenses. Ideally, the couple will also have recognized, modified, and taken back much of their projective identifications, although usually this process must continue even after therapy has ended.

5. Efficacy of Treatment Approach

In the first controlled outcome study comparing a variant of psychoanalytic couples therapy (Insight-Oriented Marital Therapy, IOMT) with BCT, Snyder and colleagues found IOMT and BCT equally effective at termination and at a 6-month follow-up. Four years after treatment, however, a significantly larger percentage of couples had divorced when treated with BCT (38%) than when treated with IOMT (3%). These findings have been disputed, with critics questioning whether therapists using the BCT intervention used state-of-the-art behavioral interventions. Nevertheless, Snyder et al. have provided at least preliminary evidence that psychoanalytic couples therapy may have more long-term effectiveness than behavioral approaches. [*See* PSYCHOANALYSIS.]

E. Brief Problem-Focused Couples Therapy

Short-term, problem-focused couples therapy was developed in response to the difficulties that arise in treating two individuals who may have different agendas and intentions for entering into therapy as well as for the current difficulties in receiving reimbursement for couples treatment from insurance companies. Two major models of brief couples therapy have been developed and evaluated in the last three decades. Brief problem-focused therapy was developed at the Mental Research Institute (MRI) in the late 1960s and early 1970s. The model was further developed at the Brief Family Therapy Center in Milwaukee, Wisconsin (the Milwaukee model), as brief solution-focused therapy beginning in the late 1970s.

1. Theory of Distress

Brief couples therapy was developed to be as efficient and parsimonious as possible. The goal of brief couples therapy is to address and provide relief for the presenting complaint. Therapists do not probe for underlying emotional or unconscious issues, they do not seek to promote personal growth in their clients, nor do they spend time teaching communication or problem-solving skills. Consistent with these goals, brief couples therapy offers no developed theory regarding couples distress or its development. Instead, it takes couples' complaints at face value and works for the relief of those complaints through lessening the behaviors related to the presenting problem (the MRI model) or through finding alternative solutions for the presenting problem (the Milwaukee model).

2. Development of Distress

Although brief couples therapy offers no theory about the development of distress, it does focus on the perception of distress. A couple has a problem when they perceive a problem, and the problem is alleviated when the couple perceives such alleviation. Brief couples therapy makes no attempt to objectively define dysfunction or normality in marriage. Furthermore, brief couples therapy does not seek to understand the origin of the particular presenting problem, but rather to identify and alter the behaviors of both partners that serve to maintain the current problem.

3. Intervention

In brief problem-focused couples therapy, the clinician works with the couple to identify the presenting problem and the interactional patterns that are perpetuating the problem. Usually, the attempted solutions that partners use to control or alleviate the problem are the very behaviors that make the problem persist (this phenomena is called the problem–solution loop). For example, Diane's solution to Joe's lateness is to nag him to come home on time. However, it is her nagging that causes him to dread coming home and to want to work longer. Likewise, it is his hiding at work that motivates Diane to nag him. Once problem-maintaining behaviors are identified, the therapist encourages the couple to lessen those behaviors. For Diane and Joe, this would mean less nagging from Diane and less lateness from Joe. Because the continuance of the problem is contingent on the problem-maintaining attempted solutions, once these are eliminated the problem itself should be alleviated. In brief solution-focused therapy, the emphasis in intervention is on identifying exceptions to the problem and encouraging the couple to increase those behaviors that are effective solutions to the problem. Here, the therapist would ask Diane and Joe to remember times when Joe did come home from work early and they shared a pleasant evening together. This approach is more cognitive than the MRI approach, assuming that behaviors will change once the couple perceives the problem differently. Clinicians attempt to reframe the problem as not so overwhelming and the solution as something the couple already has in their behavioral repertoire. The clinician's main goal is to increase the couple's sense of mastery over the presenting complaint.

4. Specific Therapeutic Techniques

Therapy in the MRI approach begins with a thorough behavioral understanding of the presenting complaint and the related behaviors that contribute to its perseverance. Through this formulation, the therapist identifies specific problem-maintaining behaviors that should be lessened in specific situations. The therapist then communicates this to the client using three important principles. First, the change is prescribed in a way that is consistent with the client's own goals and views of the relationship. Second, the therapist works with the customer by targeting the person most concerned about the problem. In fact, therapists will often work individually with a concerned person whose partner is resistant to therapy. Theoretically, intervention with even one partner's maladaptive solutions should have an impact on the problem–solution loop. Third, the therapist maintains maneuverability by avoiding premature commitments to therapeutic strategies. Overall, the therapist consistently reminds couples that change takes time and encourages them to make small changes at a slow rate. In contrast, therapists using the Milwaukee approach bypass examination of the problem relatively quickly and instead ask questions designed to influence the client's view of the problem in a manner that leads to solutions. An example is miracle questions. Clients are asked what their relationship would look like if a miracle occurred and the problem disappeared overnight. The therapist also asks about times in the past when the problem has not occurred or when they have dealt with it successfully. The therapist may also probe the degree of distress and commitment to change (scaling questions), how well the couple is managing given their difficulties (coping questions), and what changes have they already made before therapy began (questions about presession change). These questions are designed to challenge feelings of hopelessness by highlighting the small, positive changes that couples have managed on their own. Therapists also use tasks to help couples recognize possible solutions that they are already using. For example, couples are asked at the end of their first session to observe things about their relationship that they would like to have *continue*. Throughout therapy, the therapist provides ample praise for positive changes and continually inquires about and highlights use of constructive solutions whenever they occur.

5. Efficacy of Treatment Approach

Both centers have conducted follow-ups on many of their cases to find out whether a complaint has been resolved. The MRI team has called clients 3 and 12 months posttreatment and evaluates "success" based on whether the treatment goal was attained, whether the complaint has been resolved, other areas of improvement in the relationship, and the emergence of new problems. For the first 97 cases, 40% were deemed successful, 32% significantly improved, and 28% failures. Two recent studies by Shoham and colleagues reported outcome rates of 44%, 24%, and 32%, respectively, and a success rate of 86% at an 18-month follow-up, with an average of 4.6 sessions. However, there are several reasons to interpret these numbers with caution. These include the lack of detail in describing follow-up procedures, which prevents analysis of reliability or validity of the results, and the fact that the same clinical team was used to conduct therapy and to conduct follow-up interviews. To date, no controlled clinical outcome trials have been conducted on either approach.

IV. INTEGRATIVE APPROACHES TO COUPLES THERAPY

A. Integrative Behavior Couples Therapy

Integrative Behavior Couples Therapy (IBCT) was developed by Andrew Christensen and Neil Jacobson to increase the power and effectiveness of Behavior Couples Therapy. It is strongly rooted in behavior theory and uses many of the same treatment strategies as BCT. It does not, however, focus on promoting behavioral change exclusively, but gives equal emphasis to *acceptance* of partners' behavior the way it is. This shift in focus has both theoretical and practical implications for therapy. First, IBCT targets major controlling variables for change, rather than derivative variables. In BCT, because of the exclusive emphasis on discrete, currently observable behavior, functional analysis often focuses on variables only indirectly related to partners' dissatisfaction, for example, Diane's complaint that Joe comes home late from work. The IBCT therapist would attempt to uncover the underlying controlling variable, that is, the wife's desire for more closeness with her husband. The IBCT therapist looks for affect (especially "softer" feelings such as sadness or fear) and themes in couples' interactions to help uncover the crucial variables for the couple.

Once the crucial variables are identified, IBCT therapists work simultaneously for change and emotional acceptance. Emotional acceptance is a shift in the way a partner reacts to the problematic behavior. Behaviors that were once seen as intolerable and blameworthy are now seen as tolerable or even desirable. For example, Joe may begin to perceive Diane's "nagging" as a desire to be more closely involved with him, and Diane might see Joe's intense work involvement as his desire to provide material comforts for the family. Change and acceptance are mutually facilitative, with greater change leading to greater levels of acceptance, and greater levels of acceptance leading to more spontaneous and long-lasting change.

The IBCT therapists use several strategies to promote acceptance. They facilitate an emotional joining around the problem, focusing partners on the pain each is experiencing rather than on the blame each deserves. Therapists promote this by reformulating recurring problems as differences between partners to which each person has an understandable emotional reaction. Therapists also encourage partners to talk about their own feelings and emphasize "soft" disclosures which make each partner appear more vulnerable and thus more acceptable and less blameworthy. They encourage partners to see the problem as a common external enemy to facilitate emotional acceptance through unified detachment of the problem. In emotional acceptance through tolerance building, therapists use a number of techniques designed to increase partners' tolerance for negative interactions, such as role playing, faked incidences of negative behavior, and emphasizing the positive features of negative behavior. Finally, therapists encourage emotional acceptance through greater self-care by helping partners to identify alternative methods of getting their needs met and additional options when faced with a partner's negative behavior.

Preliminary data from a clinical trial that compared IBCT to BCT has provided some promising support for IBCT and suggests its superiority over BCT.

B. Emotionally Focused Couples Therapy

In Emotionally Focused Couples Therapy (EFT), Susan Johnson and Leslie Greenberg integrate psychoanalytic theory, specifically attachment theory, with recent research on negative behavioral interactions to formulate an intervention for distressed relationships. According to EFT, couples' adjustment involves both the intrapsychic emotional experiences of each partner and the couples' interpersonal interaction patterns. These processes are mutually determined and both are targeted for intervention in BFT.

Intrapsychic emotional experiences are rooted in partners' internal models of attachment, learned from past attachment experiences, particularly the infant's attachment to the mother. These working models affect how partners respond emotionally to negative interpersonal experiences and are in turn affected by these experiences as well. Distressed relationships are insecure bonds in which the attachment needs of one or both partners are not met because of rigid interaction patterns that block emotional engagement. The core problem in these relationships is partners' inaccessibility and inability to respond to or engage the partner. Therapists target both the underlying emotions and the rigid, negative interaction patterns in order to restore accessibility and form a new, secure bond between partners where each can have his or her innate needs for protection, security, and connectedness met.

The core of EFT is the accessing and reprocessing of the emotions underlying negative interaction patterns and the enactment of new patterns in which partners are affiliative and engaged. Distress is alleviated, not through new skills or new insights, but through the *experience* of new aspects of the self and new interaction patterns that take place in the therapy sessions. Thus, when Diane begins to nag Joe in therapy, the therapist helps Diane to focus on the underlying sadness she feels at not being close to Joe. Joe is better able to respond to her feeling of sadness than to her nagging, and the two experience a moment of closeness and understanding. The EFT therapist uses several general techniques to create this experience for the couples. First, a strong positive alliance is established with both partners. This alliance is critical if the couple is to feel safe enough to express and process their underlying emotions. Second, the therapist focuses on the moment-by-moment experience of the clients to help them reshape interactions and emotional experiences as they occur. Third, as interactions are tracked and emotions restructured, the therapist encourages the clients to replay their interactions to create new, more positive relationship events.

Initial studies have indicated that EFT is more effective than a waiting period of no therapy and at least as effective as CBCT and BCT. In comparing EFT, CBCT, and BCT, EFT was found to be more effective than BCT on marital adjustment, intimacy, and target complaint level.

V. COUPLES THERAPY FOR SPECIFIC PSYCHIATRIC DISORDERS

Couples and family therapists have developed specialized interventions for a wide variety of psychiatric disorders, including depression, alcohol, and a variety of anxiety disorders. Outcome studies have generally found that intervening with couples and families (rather than individuals) leads to lower drop-out rates and higher treatment success rates. Behavioral and cognitive couples treatments for depression have been found to reduce depression and increase satisfaction when the depressed person is in a distressed relationship. Behavioral Couples Therapy has also been shown to reduce alcoholism and to improve couples' satisfaction. Finally, spousal involvement has been shown to increase the effectiveness of behavioral treatments for agoraphobia.

VI. ALTERNATIVE APPROACHES TO COUPLES TREATMENT

Alternative treatments for distressed couples have been developed to improve the success rates of more traditional couples treatments as well as to provide less costly interventions. Two prevalent alternative approaches are group couples therapy and prevention/enrichment programs. In group couples therapy, couples help each other as firsthand observers of couples' conflict and provide perspective on the problems each couple is experiencing. The group process provides an arena where couples can learn from one another, obtain insight, experience support, and receive feedback. Preliminary descriptive data on the outcome of group therapy indicates that most couples experience improvement at termination in areas as diverse as communication, reframing problems, appreciating each other more as individuals, and feeling more acceptance toward the partner's family of origin.

Premarital programs designed to prevent future marital distress and programs designed to enrich couples' relationships attempt to spare the couple and their children from the negative consequences of distress. Like traditional couples therapy, these programs vary theoretically and methodologically, with some programs focusing on teaching communication and problem-solving skills and others promoting awareness of underlying emotional or unconscious factors that might make a couple vulnerable to the development of distress. A review of 85 controlled outcome studies found that the average participant in one of these programs improved more than did 67% of those in corresponding control groups at termination. A recent longitudinal study of a behavior intervention program (PREP) demonstrated that couples who received the intervention had significantly higher relationship satisfaction than the control couples 18 months after the intervention and reported significantly higher sexual satisfaction, less intense marital problems, and higher relationship satisfaction than control couples at the 3-year follow-up. Because prevention spares couples (and their children) from the detrimental effects of distress that many couples experience before they seek couples therapy, prevention models may prove more efficient and effective than treatment models of already distressed couples.

VII. CONCLUSION

The need for effective treatments for couple distress has grown in the last few decades for several reasons: the United States has the highest divorce rate of any major industrialized country, there has been a sharp increase in divorce rates from 1960 to 1980, and there is unambiguous evidence that marital distress and divorce have harmful consequences for spouses and children. As a result, couples therapists and researchers have developed therapies that appear to be effective, at least in the short run. The comparative effectiveness of the different types of therapeutic approaches remains unclear, however. Further study is needed to clarify the comparative effectiveness of different approaches and to begin to understand how approaches and techniques might be matched to couples to maximize the effectiveness of the intervention for each couple that seeks treatment.

BIBLIOGRAPHY

Baucom, D. H., & Epstein, N. (1990). *Cognitive-behavioral marital therapy*. New York: Brunner-Mazel.

Bowen, M. (1978). *Family therapy in clinical practice*. Northvale, NY: Aronson.

Giblin, P., Sprenkle, D. H., & Sheehan, R. (1985). Enrichment outcome research: A meta-analysis of premarital, marital, and family interventions. *Journal of Marital and Family Therapy, 16*, 257–271.

Gurman, A. S., & Kniskern, D. P. (Eds.). *Handbook of family therapy*. New York: Brunner-Mazel.

Jacobson, N. S., & Christensen, A. (in press). *Integrative couple therapy*. New York: Norton.

Jacobson, N. S., & Gurman, A. S. (Eds.). (1995). *Clinical handbook of couple therapy*. New York: Guilford Press.

Johnson, S. M., & Greenberg, L. S. (1985b). Differential effects of experiential and problem-solving interventions in resolving marital conflict. *Journal of Consulting and Clinical Psychology, 53*, 175–184.

Lebow, J. L., & Gurman, A. S. (1995). Research assessing couple and family therapy. *Annual Review of Psychology, 46*, 27–57.

Sheilds, C. G., Wynne, L. C., McDaniel, S. H., & Gawinski, B. A. (1994). The marginalization of family therapy: A historical and continuing problem. *Journal of Marital and Family Therapy, 20*, 117–138.

Snyder, D. K., Wills, R. M., & Grady-Fletcher, A. (1991). Long-term effectiveness of behavioral versus insight-oriented marital therapy: A four-year follow-up study. *Journal of Consulting and Clinical Psychology, 59*, 138–141.

Depression—Applied Aspects

Ricardo F. Muñoz
University of California, San Francisco

Depressed Mood A feeling state consisting of dejection, sadness, and demoralization, usually accompanied by diminished reaction to pleasurable events.
Depressive Disorder A condition in which an individual exhibits a specified number of depressive symptoms of enough severity and duration to meet well-delineated and widely accepted diagnostic criteria.
Emotion A noticeable subjective feeling, usually lasting on the order of minutes, in reaction to internal or external stimuli.
Mood A relatively persistent feeling state, lasting for hours or days.

The term DEPRESSION can be used in a number of ways. As commonly used, it refers to a normative, usually transient and generally dejected, dispirited, or sad mood state. It can also be a symptom related to several emotional or physical disorders. It can refer to a syndrome (a collection of symptoms that usually occur together) and is also used as the official name for a specific mental disorder in the current psychiatric nomenclature. As the latter, depression is considered to be a psychopathological entity hypothesized to have distinctive etiological mechanisms, prognosis, and treatment implications. This entry describes these types of depression, discusses the prevalence of the more common types studied, and presents prevention, treatment, and maintenance interventions currently suggested for persons with depression. The final section examines the concept of healthy mood management from a developmental perspective.

I. TYPES OF DEPRESSION

A. Depressed Mood

Depressed mood states appear to be a normal part of human subjective experience. Most individuals have a personal understanding of depressed mood, in contrast with, say, psychotic experiences or addictions. Depressed mood states usually involve the emotion of sadness, a subjective lack of energy, reduced motivation to engage in formerly pleasant activities, reduced desire to have positive interactions with other people, and a belief that one's lot in life is difficult. Such states color one's reactions to external events, but they can themselves be modified by such events. Normal states of depressed mood last hours or days. Once they become more chronic and start affecting one's ability to function, they are often conceptualized as part of a pathological process, which can ultimately meet criteria for a diagnosis of a clinical depressive disorder.

It is useful to examine the relationship between emotions, such as sadness, and mood states. Emotion researchers generally conceptualize emotions as rela-

Copyright © 1998 by Academic Press.
All rights of reproduction in any form reserved.

tively short-lived reactions to external or internal stimuli. These reactions appear to be relatively autonomous, that is, not ordinarily subject to conscious planning. They have physiological, expressive, and subjective elements. They usually occur within seconds of the triggering stimulus and last on the order of minutes. As the subjective feeling which is part of an emotional response lasts longer, it can become a mood state. Alternatively, the emotion can fade away or change into a different emotion; for example, in response to being surprised, one can exhibit a startle response, then fear, anger, and finally amusement and relief. The trigger for these kinds of changes can be external (the availability of new information) as well as internal (the subjective interpretation of the new information).

Although, under normal circumstances, the initial emotional response to specific triggers appears to be too quick to be under conscious control, once the emotion begins to develop, the modulation of the emotional response does seem to be amenable to planned influences. Part of the developmental process in humans involves the regulation of emotion. Maturity is judged in part on the individual's ability to control his or her emotional responses.

The role of mood states in the development of psychopathology has yet to be adequately elucidated. It is well known that prior to having a major depressive episode, there is usually a period of gradually increasing depressed mood and symptoms. If these symptoms develop into a major depressive episode, they are retrospectively considered a prodrome of the clinical episode. However, most individuals with high depressive symptoms do not go on to a clinical episode of depression. It may be that naturally occurring events in daily life may increase or decrease the probability of pathological depression. Or perhaps different coping mechanisms, when put into practice, afford differential degrees of protectiveness. Alternatively, it may be that those who are predisposed, because of genetic or other biological factors, are the ones who are most likely to fall prey to the pathological process. As of now, the answers to these questions are not yet in. [*See* Coping with Stress.]

B. Depression as a Symptom

Depression can be viewed as a dichotomous concept: it is present or it is not. It can also be conceptualized as a continuum: one can be more or less depressed. The former conceptualization is compatible with the disorder view of depression, and is covered later. The latter concept has been much used in epidemiologic studies and in clinical studies, particularly in those focused on treatment outcome. The general strategy for measuring the level of depression that an individual is experiencing has been to construct a questionnaire or a structured interview that inquires about several aspects of the depressive state, usually focus ing on duration and/or intensity of several symptoms of depression. The questionnaire or interview is then scored, yielding a single continuous variable. Higher scores reflect a greater level of depression. Depression symptom scales have been useful in providing normative data on the experience of depression in community samples and in helping to evaluate the effect of treatment on level of depression. Depression symptom scales are usually not intended to diagnose depression.

Epidemiological studies provide evidence that depressive symptoms are prevalent in the general population. High levels of depressive symptomatology, as measured by self-report symptom scales, have sometimes been referred to as demoralization. Demoralization appears to be more prevalent in low-income minority populations than in white middle-class samples. It is unclear whether the difference is due primarily to ethnicity or to social class, but the preponderance of the evidence indicates that when controls are implemented for socioeconomic factors, the differences in depression levels diminish or disappear.

The interpretation of similar differences in depression scores showing higher levels for women has also been controversial. Disentangling the role of socioeconomic issues between men and women is much harder, because married women, especially those who do not have a paying job outside the home, are generally assigned their husband's social class, even though they may not have the same type of independence or control over resources that their husbands do.

The relationship between age and depressive symptoms is not clear. Most studies have found no difference, others have found higher rates in younger persons, and still others found higher rates in older persons.

There is a relatively clear connection between depressed symptoms and substance abuse. Studies of national samples have found that individuals with negative mood states, including depression, are more likely to use cigarettes and alcohol. They are also less likely to quit smoking, and if they quit, are more likely to relapse. The direction of causality is not easy to disentangle, however. Use of drugs, including alcohol, can increase the likelihood of depressed states. The physiological effects of drugs on the nervous system is probably implicated in this process, but it is also true that the disruption to the individual's life caused by drug abuse probably produces significant psychological stress.

C. Depression as a Syndrome

Major depressive episode is the most common depressive syndrome. A syndrome is a configuration of symptoms that often occur together and constitute a recognizable condition. Although the presence of a major depressive syndrome is a necessary characteristic of major depressive disorder, it is not sufficient. The syndrome can occur for other reasons. For example, medications or drugs of abuse, as well as general medical conditions, can have direct physiological effects which can trigger the symptoms of a major depressive episode. Similarly, the loss of a loved one can result in this configuration of symptoms. In the latter case, unless the symptoms persist for longer than 2 months, or produce marked functional impairment, suicidality, or psychosis, they are considered to be part of the normal course of bereavement.

The implication is that major depressive syndrome is much more prevalent than major depressive disorder. Currently, major depressive disorder is conceptualized as a clinical entity that may have genetic, other biological, and psychosocial sources, much like a specific illness. Major depressive syndrome is a condition that may be triggered by specific life events or by physical influences on the body, but it does not necessarily imply an underlying psychopathological process. These assumptions reflect a basic dilemma in the mental health field, namely, whether there is a qualitative difference between "normal" conditions (such as depressed mood or major depressive syndrome) and the officially recognized mental disorders (such as major depressive disorder), or whether the latter are merely quantitatively more intense and longer lasting manifestations of normal mood fluctuations.

D. Depressive Disorders

The most commonly used diagnostic system in the United States is the Diagnostic and Statistical Manual of Mental Disorders, fourth edition (*DSM-IV*). Depression is implicated primarily in what are termed the mood disorders. The mood disorders are themselves divided into two major categories: the depressive disorders and the bipolar disorders. The depressive disorders are sometimes referred to as unipolar depressions, that is, mood disorders in which changes from normal mood occur in only one direction, toward depressed mood. Bipolar disorders exhibit bidirectional fluctuations, either to depressed mood or to abnormally euphoric (manic) mood states. It is recognized that mood disorders can be the result of general medical conditions as well as the result of the use or abuse of drugs and other substances. Mood disorders caused by drug use or abuse are not considered primary mood disorders. In the following section, the *DSM-IV* diagnostic criteria for the more common mood disorders are presented.

II. DEPRESSION AS A DISORDER

A. Major Depression

Major depression is the most common of the mood disorders. The key diagnostic criterion for major depressive *disorder* is the presence of a major depressive *episode*.

There are nine symptoms that define a major depressive episode. Of the nine, at least five must have been present during a 2-week period. They must represent a change from previous functioning and they must cause significant impairment in daily functioning. At least one of the five symptoms must be either the first or the second symptom in the following list:

1. Depressed mood most of the day, nearly every day
2. Reduced interest or pleasure in all or almost all activities
3. Significant weight loss or weight gain, or a significant decrease or increase in appetite
4. Trouble sleeping or sleeping too much
5. Psychomotor agitation or retardation
6. Fatigue or loss of energy
7. Feeling worthless or guilty in an excessive or inappropriate manner

8. Problems in thinking, concentrating, or making decisions
9. Recurrent thoughts of death, suicidal ideation, specific suicidal plan, or a suicide attempt

B. Dysthymia

Dysthymia differs from major depression in that it is generally more chronic and is defined by fewer symptoms. The *DSM-IV* criteria for dysthymic disorder include a depressed mood for most days for at least 2 years in adults or at least 1 year in children and adolescents. In addition, two or more of the following six symptoms must be present: poor appetite or overeating, trouble sleeping or sleeping too much, low energy or fatigue, low self-esteem, poor concentration or difficulty making decisions, and feelings of hopelessness. The initial 2-year period must not have included a major depressive episode and the 2-year period of depression must not have been broken by a period of normal mood lasting more than 2 months.

C. Bipolar Disorder

Depressed mood and a major depressive episode may be part of bipolar disorders. However, what characterizes bipolar disorders is the occurrence of one or more manic episodes. The *DSM-IV* criteria for manic episode include a period of abnormally elevated, expansive, or irritable mood lasting at least 1 week, plus three or more of the following seven symptoms:

1. Inflated self-esteem or grandiosity
2. Decreased need for sleep
3. More talkative than usual or pressured to keep talking
4. Flight of ideas or racing thoughts
5. Distractibility
6. Marked increased in goal-directed activity or psychomotor agitation
7. Excessive involvement in pleasurable activities with a high potential for painful consequences

There are two subtypes of bipolar disorders: Bipolar I involves full-blown manic episodes, and Bipolar II involves less intense, manic-like episodes, known as hypomanic episodes. There is also a bipolar disorder that parallels dysthymia, called cyclothymia. It is a chronic disorder that is characterized by the presence of both hypomanic periods and depressive periods most of the time for at least 2 years. Both depressive and bipolar disorders include residual categories called, respectively, "depressive disorder not otherwise specified" and "bipolar disorder not otherwise specified." In both cases, the disorders do not meet the full criteria for either depressive or bipolar diagnoses.

III. PREVENTION OF DEPRESSION

In its major 1994 report, *Reducing Risks for Mental Disorders,* the Institute of Medicine put forward a framework for mental health interventions that has three major levels: prevention, treatment, and maintenance. The most commonly known level of intervention is the treatment of acute cases of mental disorders. The Institute of Medicine also wanted to highlight the need for interventions that occur before the onset of the disorder, namely, preventive interventions, and interventions that occur after an acute episode has ended, that is, "maintenance" interventions intended to reduce relapse or recurrence or to help the individual regain the highest possible level of functioning. Each of these three levels is divided into the following subcategories.

A. Levels of Preventive Intervention

1. Universal Preventive Interventions

Universal preventive interventions for mental disorders are targeted to the general public or to a whole population group that has not been identified on the basis of individual risk. These interventions are believed to have a preventive effect on the population as a whole, and are believed to be protective of several types of psychological disorders. In general, such interventions should be of relatively low cost and easily disseminated.

2. Selective Preventive Interventions

Selective preventive interventions for mental disorders are targeted to subgroups of the population whose risk of developing mental disorders is significantly higher than average. Risks factors used to identify these groups may be biological, psychological, or social. The important factor is that they are associated with the onset of a mental disorder. Selective interventions could include interventions targeted to widows, people who are getting married for the first time, children going into the school system or graduating from the school system, individuals who have been laid off from work, women about to have their first child, or victims of trauma.

3. Indicated Preventive Interventions

Indicated preventive interventions are targeted to high-risk individuals who are identified as having minimum but detectable signs or symptoms foreshadowing a mental disorder or who have biological markers indicating predisposition for mental disorders. As in all of the preventive interventions, the individuals or groups targeted do not meet the full diagnostic criteria for the particular disorder being prevented at the time of being recruited into a preventive intervention program.

B. Attributable Risk

To engage in preventive interventions, one must identify the risk and/or protective factors that increase or decrease the probability of developing a particular disorder. An important concept from epidemiology is that of attributable risk. *Attributable risk* refers to the proportion of cases of a specific condition or disorder that are attributable to a specific factor. For instance, it is commonly known that tobacco smoking is related to lung cancer. However, lung cancer can also be caused by other factors. If we were to eradicate tobacco, a large proportion of lung cancer would be prevented, but not all cases. The proportion prevented would be the proportion of cases attributable to smoking, or the attributable risk.

Many factors have been linked to depression. Some of them are demographic factors that cannot be changed for the individual, such as sex, death of a parent during early childhood, or a family history of the disorder. Therefore it is important to focus on *modifiable* risk factors, especially those with a high level of attributable risk. From a preventive standpoint, one possible risk factor that is related to later episodes of major depression is the evidence of deficits in mood regulation. A potential strategy, therefore, is to identify individuals who have high symptom levels of depression, but who do not meet the criteria for a depressive disorder, and to teach such individuals methods to manage their moods. Such methods can come, for example, from cognitive–behavioral techniques that have been found to be useful in the treatment of depression. Some studies have already shown that depressive symptoms can be reduced in nonclinical populations that nevertheless show high depressive symptom levels when recruited. As of this writing, there have not been enough randomized controlled prevention trials to be able to say conclusively that new cases of major depression can be prevented. The development and evaluation of preventive interventions for depression and other mental disorders may be the next important stage in the development of mental health interventions.

IV. TREATMENT OF MAJOR DEPRESSION

Treatment interventions are divided into two sublevels: (1) case identification, to provide early treatment for cases of major depression that have not been identified previously; and (2) standard treatment, which accounts for the bulk of mental health intervention efforts.

The need for case identification efforts arises from the underdiagnosis of major depression and other depressive disorders in primary care clinics. Only 20% of individuals who meet criteria for major depression seek mental health services. However, more than 70% of those who meet criteria for major depression do seek health care, generally from a primary care physician. Yet, only about a third of individuals with major depression are so identified by their primary care providers. It is imperative, therefore, that primary care physicians and other health care providers learn to identify cases of depression so that individuals suffering from them may receive appropriate interventions.

Major depression is eminently treatable. Between 60% and 80% of individuals with major depression respond to either psychological or pharmacological treatments. Other less common types of treatment, such as light therapy and electroconvulsive therapy, have also been found effective for certain cases of major depression.

Treatments for depression vary in their theoretical assumptions and in the specific interventions used with patients. Certain common elements include an explicit helping relationship between the therapist and the patient, the identification of depression as a clinical disorder that requires treatment (as opposed to some type of "personal weakness"), an explanatory framework for the mechanisms that trigger and maintain the depression, and implicit or explicit recommendations for patient behaviors that are expected to bring about improvement.

Many types of psychological approaches are currently used in the treatment of depression. Those that have been most often subjected to randomized controlled outcome trials are the cognitive–behavioral therapies. Cognitive–behavioral therapies for depression are based on the hypothesis that mood is influenced by a person's cognitive and behavioral patterns. These patterns have been learned, usually in a social context, and can be modified. The purpose of therapy is to work with the patient to identify the cognitions (thoughts, assumptions, other mental processes) and behaviors (activity levels, interpersonal skills, and other physical or observable actions) that are most related to specific mood states. The goal of therapy is to reduce cognitions and behaviors that increase the probability of depressed states and augment those that decrease the probability of depression. [*See* BEHAVIOR THERAPY; COGNITIVE THERAPY.]

Another psychological approach to depression that has been repeatedly evaluated in randomized trials is interpersonal psychotherapy. This approach focuses on the influence that the interpersonal context has on triggering and maintaining depressive mood. The therapist reviews with the patient current and past interpersonal relationships as they relate to depressive symptoms. The focus of therapy usually centers on one or more of four major areas: grief, interpersonal disputes, role transitions, and interpersonal deficits.

Other psychological treatments have not been studied as extensively. However, brief approaches to therapy that specifically target depression have generally shown encouraging results.

Pharmacotherapy for depression has also been subjected to many randomized controlled trials. There are several types of antidepressants, all of which have approximately the same efficacy. Those developed most recently tend to have fewer side effects and lower lethality if used to attempt suicide. Pharmacotherapy is probably the most commonly used form of evidence-based treatment for depression in the United States, in part, because it is much more available than the psychotherapies. Antidepressants are prescribed at least as often by nonpsychiatric physicians as by psychiatrists. This has led to a strong (and controversial) emphasis on educating primary care providers to detect and treat depression in their setting before referring to mental health care providers. [*See* PSYCHOPHARMACOLOGY.]

Results of randomized trials do not always agree. Nevertheless, the preponderance of the evidence indicates that pharmacotherapy, cognitive–behavioral therapy, and interpersonal psychotherapy are all significantly effective in the treatment of major depression. The rate of improvement is generally faster for pharmacotherapy, but total improvement over a 20-week treatment is generally comparable across treatments, especially for mild and moderate cases of major depression. There appears to be some advantage to pharmacotherapy for more severe cases of depression, and clearly so for cases of depression with psychotic features in which antidepressants and antipsychotics may be prescribed simultaneously. A combination of psychotherapy and pharmacotherapy is often used in the treatment of depression. Most controlled studies have shown either additional improvement or no detectable difference in efficacy when both treatments are used. There appears to be no general disadvantage to the use of combined treatment. A major problem with treatment for depression is the high rate of relapse. This leads to a focus on maintenance strategies.

V. MAINTENANCE

The third large segment of mental health interventions identified by the Institute of Medicine is the area of *maintenance*. Even though the treatment of acute episodes of depression and other disorders may be quite effective, relapse or recurrence of such an episode can be not only as disruptive as the first experience of clinical depression, but, at times, even more demoralizing. The fear that this painful condition will recur can have a major impact on a person's outlook. Approximately 50% of persons who have had one major depressive episode have a second; 70% of those with two have a third; and 90% of those with three have a fourth. These figures suggest two important goals for the mental health field: preventing the first episode (as described earlier) and, if the first episode occurs, providing interventions that will maintain a healthy mood state, thus forestalling relapse and recurrence.

Current convention uses the terms relapse and recurrence in relatively well-defined ways. When treatment with antidepressants is effective, depressive symptoms diminish within a few weeks. In the 1980s, it was found that if antidepressant therapy was ended, a large proportion of patients began to exhibit symptoms again. The conclusion was that the processes underlying the mood dysregulation were still active, but that the medication was able to control the symptoms. Once medication ended, the symptoms reappeared. This reappearance was thought to be part of the same episode of depression. Now, the reappearance of symptoms within a year of the start of the episode is called relapse. Once the person has been free of clinical symptoms of depression for a year or more, the depressive episode is considered to be over. If symptoms reappear in the future, such an event is a recurrence.

Studies in which individuals who responded well to pharmacotherapy were followed for 1 or 2 years after treatment ended have found rates of relapse or recurrence as high as 70%. This has led to the recommendation that pharmacotherapy be continued for several months, and perhaps years, after the acute depressive episode has subsided. Some clinicians now state that for certain patients, lifetime maintenance pharmacotherapy is indicated.

Similar studies in which individuals who responded well to cognitive therapy have been followed have found much lower relapse rates of approximately 35% after 1 or 2 years. This has led to speculation that cognitive therapy may have an advantage in terms of reducing relapse or recurrence rates. More studies designed specifically to answer this question are needed.

What is clear at this time is that individuals who have had a depressive episode are at high risk for repeated episodes of clinical depression. These individuals should be taught to monitor their mood state and to obtain treatment as soon as possible after the onset of significant depressive symptoms in the future.

VI. HEALTHY MOOD MANAGEMENT: A DEVELOPMENTAL PERSPECTIVE

The development of effective mood management is an essential aspect of individual human growth. It is also a major factor in the health of a community. Among the major causes of death are several causes that appear to be influenced by mood problems. The top nine preventable causes of death, which account for about one half of all deaths in the United States, are tobacco, diet and exercise patterns, alcohol, microbial agents, toxic agents, firearms, sexual behavior, motor vehicles, and illicit use of drugs. Consider for a moment how many of these might be exacerbated by depressed mood.

The relationship between negative mood states and smoking and drinking has already been described. It is highly likely that illicit use of drugs follows a similar pattern. Diet and exercise certainly are affected by depressed mood. Deaths from firearms present an interesting illustration of how strong, and yet invisible to most of us, the impact of depression is on our society: few people are aware that for several decades over half the deaths from firearms in the United States have been suicides. Unprotected sexual behavior not only exposes individuals to sexually transmitted diseases, but also to unplanned pregnancies. And some proportion of motor vehicle accidents are related to alcohol and other substance abuse, or to reckless driving, which may be the result of desperate states of mind. The proportion of these factors that is attributable to depression is yet unknown, but is likely to be significant.

Many factors have been implicated in the development of deficits in emotion regulation. None appear to be necessary or sufficient to cause depression, nor are there known factors that offer complete protection from depression.

There appears to be a substantial genetic component in the more severe forms of depression, such as bipolar disorders and major depression. How this genetic influence is manifested physiologically is not yet known. Several biological abnormalities have been identified in subgroups of individuals exhibiting depression. However, most of them appear to occur during a depressed episode and to subside once a normal mood state is attained. None appear to be universally shared by clinically depressed individuals. Developmental influences also appear to be risk factors for depression, such as being born to a mother who is currently depressed, the loss of parents in childhood, and a high number of stressful life events. Social and environmental factors also have well-documented effects on depression. For example, poverty has been shown to account for approximately 10% of new cases of major depression.

The emotion regulation literature suggests that certain mechanisms can be used to affect whether a given emotion occurs or to modulate the intensity, duration, and tone of the emotion once it has been triggered. Factors that can come into play prior to the triggering of the emotion include changes in either the external or the internal environment, that is, either in the environment in which the individual is located (including the people in such an environment) or in the mind of the individual. Attention, memory, mental rehearsal, and the interpretation of the material brought into consciousness via these avenues, all can set the probabilities of certain emotions being triggered. Once an emotion is triggered, the responses of the individual to the emotion can maintain or diminish the intensity and duration of the emotion.

Developmental aspects of emotion regulation include the basic survival aspects of emotion expression in infants, including the instrumental functions of crying or smiling, cooing, and vocalizing; the development of language and its role in modulating emotional response when used by others and by the child; the differential reinforcement and punishment of specific emotions; acquiring expectations regarding which kinds of emotion regulation are possible by observing role models; and, as the individual moves into adolescence and adulthood, gaining greater ability to shape one's environment, choosing one's friends, activities, and school and work settings. Certain professional training includes fairly specific instructions regarding the types of emotional expression that are preferred, discouraged, or prohibited.

The development of healthy mood management or emotion regulation is a key prerequisite of mental health. As individuals develop, a large proportion attempt to modulate their mood by maladaptive methods, including the use of psychoactive substances. If these methods become part of the person's usual repertoire, they can have serious long-term consequences. The delineation of mood management strategies and their consequences deserves further study and dissemination.

Mood management skills are important in at least three broad contexts: work, relationships, and aloneness. The ability to maintain a healthy mood state in each of these situations appears to be necessary to good mental health. The theoretical factors that have been important in the development of treatment modalities can be integrated into a concept of mood management. Each addresses a different level of analysis: biological approaches focus on the neurochemical bases of emotion regulation, cognitive–behavioral approaches focus on psychological mediators of emotion regulation, and interpersonal approaches emphasize the influences of interpersonal relations on emotion regulation and dysregulation.

VII. CONCLUSION

Depression is an experience that has been shared by most human beings at one time or another. Thus, it can be thought of as a feeling state that is within the realm of normal functioning. If the frequency, intensity, and duration of this feeling increase, it can become a pathological process. After it crosses a certain threshold, criteria for which are now well-defined, it is diagnosed as a specific mental disorder. Mental health interventions that focus on this disorder include preventive, treatment, and maintenance interventions, of which treatment is the most developed and the most available. The public health impact of depression is considerable. Advances in the identification and dissemination of effective mood management strategies could have a major impact in the health of our societies.

BIBLIOGRAPHY

Akiskal, H. S., & McKinney, W. T. J. (1973). Depressive disorders: Toward a unified hypothesis. *Science, 182,* 20–29.

American Psychiatric Association. (1994). *Diagnostic and statistical manual of mental disorders* (4th ed.). Washington, DC: American Psychiatric Association.

Beck, A. T., Rush, A. J., Shaw, B. F., & Emery, G. (1979). *Cognitive therapy of depression.* New York: Guilford Press.

Beckham, E. D., & Leber, W. R. (Eds.). (1995). *Handbook of depression: Treatment, assessment, and research* (2nd ed.). New York: Guilford Press.

Bruce, M. L., Takeuchi, D. T., & Leaf, P. J. (1991). Poverty and psychiatric status: Longitudinal evidence from the New Haven Epidemiologic Catchment Area Study. *Archives of General Psychiatry, 48,* 470–474.

Depression Guideline Panel. (1993). *Depression in primary care: Vol. 1. Detection and diagnosis* (Clinical Practice Guideline No. 5 AHCPR Publication No. 93-0550). Rockville, MD: Department of Health and Human Services, Public Health Service, Agency for Health Care Policy and Research.

Depression Guideline Panel. (1993). *Depression in primary care: Vol. 2. Treatment of major depression* (Clinical Practice Guideline No. 5, AHCPR Publication No. 93-0551). Rockville, MD: Department of Health and Human Services, Public Health Service, Agency for Health Care Policy and Research.

Frank, E., Prien, R. F., Jarret, J. B., Keller, M. B., Kupfer, D. J., Lavori, P., Rush, A. J., & Weissman, M. M. (1991). Conceptualization and rationale for consensus definitions of terms in major depressive disorder: response, remission, recovery, relapse, and recurrence. *Archives of General Psychiatry, 48,* 851–855.

Gross, J. J., & Muñoz, R. F. (1995). Emotion regulation and mental health. *Clinical Psychology: Science and Practice, 2,* 151–164.

Lewinsohn, P. M., Hoberman, H., Teri, L., & Hautzinger, M. (1985). An integrative theory of depression. In S. Reiss & R. Bootzin (Eds.), *Theoretical issues in behavior therapy* (pp. 331–359). New York: Academic Press.

McGrath, E., Keita, G. P., Strickland, B. R., & Russo, N. F. (Eds.). (1990). *Women and depression: Risk factors and treatment issues.* Washington, DC: American Psychological Association.

Mrazek, P. J., & Haggerty, R. J. (Eds.). (1994). *Reducing risks for mental disorders: Frontiers for preventive intervention research.* Washington, DC: National Academy Press.

Muñoz, R. F., Hollon, S. D., McGrath, E., Rehm, L. P., & VandenBos, G. R. (1994). On the AHCPR Depression in Primary Care Guidelines: Further considerations for practitioners. *American Psychologist, 49,* 42–61.

Muñoz, R. F., & Ying, Y. (1993). *The prevention of depression: Research and practice.* Baltimore, MD: Johns Hopkins University Press.

Whybrow, P. C., Akiskal, H. S., & McKinney, W. T. (1984). *Mood disorders: Toward a new psychobiology.* New York: Plenum Press.

Domestic Violence Intervention

Sandra A. Graham-Bermann
University of Michigan

Domestic Violence Physical violence committed by one intimate partner against the other with the intention of causing physical pain or injury. Violence ranges from pushing, shoving, and slapping, to punching, hitting with an object, injuring, using a weapon, or threatening someone with a weapon. When such violence results in injury, women are likely to be the victims 95% of the time. Thus, domestic violence is a general term used to describe both woman-abuse and spouse-abuse. But, given the injury statistics, feminists argue that the term woman-abuse is a more accurate one, since it reflects the actual dynamics of domestic violence, and the term spouse abuse is not inclusive of the many abused women who may not be married to their abusive partners.

Emotional Maltreatment Psychological abuse of women includes repeated verbal assault, for example, threats, name calling, put downs, and other deprecating remarks, as well as tactics used by the batterer to control and constrict the woman's movement and behavior. Batterers use emotional maltreatment to wear down the woman and isolate her from others so as to subordinate and dominate her in the relationship. While domestic violence almost always includes the psychological intimidation and abuse of the partner, psychological abuse may or may not include physical assault.

Marital Conflict Verbal disagreements that range from subtle differences in opinion to heated arguments between married partners. There are several important differences between marital conflict and domestic violence. The first is that marital conflict is limited to verbal interaction, whereas domestic violence includes verbal, as well as mild and/or severe physical assault. Second, domestic violence is distinguished by the psychological maltreatment of the woman with the aim of controlling her actions and behaviors. Other important differences are that domestic violence spans the range of the intimate relationships and can include the actions of couples who are married, cohabiting, separated, or divorced.

Posttraumatic Stress Disorder (PTSD) A psychiatric diagnosis consisting of behaviors in evidence at least 3 months after witnessing or experiencing extremely distressing events. In this context, physical assault by an intimate partner may result in trauma reactions lasting beyond the violence events themselves. PTSD criteria include having a strong, negative reaction to the event, having nightmares and flashbacks of the event, avoiding people or places associated with the event, and physiological arousal in response to remembering the event. In order to qualify for the PTSD diagnosis, behavioral reactions must be tied to the specific traumatizing event and not reported as general stress symptoms. Delayed onset PTSD occurs when symptoms first manifest themselves at least

Copyright © 1998 by Academic Press.
All rights of reproduction in any form reserved.

6 months following the event. Both battered women and their children who witness the violence can have PTSD symptoms.

Primary, Secondary, and Tertiary Prevention Public health efforts that address identified problems on the societal level are called primary preventions. Thus, primary prevention against woman abuse would include programs and initiatives designed to change attitudes and behaviors that lead to and support violence against women. Secondary prevention refers to programs designed to help people considered to be at-risk for the identified problem. Secondary prevention against woman abuse would include programs to assist children of battered women, dating violence prevention programs, and educational efforts aimed at teaching social skills to children in the hopes of changing deleterious patterns of interacting with others. Tertiary prevention is reserved for those remedial efforts created to treat individuals after the abuse and/or harm has been perpetrated. Such interventions are usually referred to as treatment or therapy.

DOMESTIC VIOLENCE is now considered to be a serious public health problem, because one woman is battered every 15 seconds in the United States. The number of emergency room visits by battered women exceeds those caused by accidents and rape, and many battered women are killed by their abusers. Woman abuse refers to the physical and psychological maltreatment of a woman by a partner, usually in the context of an ongoing or recently terminated intimate relationship. Physical abuse to the woman is usually accompanied by acts designed to control her behavior and to intimidate her. These can include humiliating, shaming, threatening, coercing, isolating, and otherwise dominating the woman in order to establish her subordination within the relationship. For most batterers, the acts of physical assault are infrequent. However, verbal abuse, for example, threats to kill or to injure the woman, can have similar devastating effects, particularly for women who have been traumatized by previous assaults.

We know from national surveys that at least 3.3 million children live in homes where the mother is being abused. While children exposed to the battering of their mothers were once considered to be the "unintended victims" of domestic violence, more recent formulations have described woman abuse as also abusive to any child who watches these traumatic events. In addition, many children of battered women are themselves at-risk for abuse and serious injury during a battering incident. Domestic violence is a crime, a social problem, a public health epidemic, and a political issue in this country. Thus, efforts to intervene and to prevent domestic violence take many forms.

I. INTERVENTIONS FOR MEN WHO BATTER

A. Who Are the Batterers?

There is currently considerable debate in the research literature as to whether and how abuse is transmitted from one generation to the next. Retrospective studies have found high rates of transmission; upward of 60% of abusive parents or partner-abusers report having been abused themselves during their childhood. On the other hand, prospective studies have found rates between 18 and 40%. The distinction appears to be that a large majority of currently abusive parents or partners were abused as children, but a lower percentage of abused children grow up to be abusers. In addition, some initial research has indicated that boys who lived in families with violence (either spouse or child abuse) are more likely than are girls to be involved in violent dating relationships as adolescents. Other contextual variables may add to the risk, for example, living in a community with high rates of interpersonal violence, high levels of exposure to violence against women in movies and media, and low arrest and conviction rates of batterers. Although there are clearly other factors that influence whether or not an abused child will be involved in abusive relationships as an adult, the overall evidence shows that the childhood experience of abuse is an important risk factor for problems in relationships in adolescence and adulthood.

The results of studies of the typologies of batterers generally agree on at least three subtypes based on their violent behavior, the family history, as well as the personality characteristics and disorders of the batterer. First are the family-only batterers who show the least severe levels of emotional abuse and violence to their partner. This group of men is least likely to be violent outside the home, is less psychologically abusive, is more likely to report being satisfied in their marriages, and is less likely to have a history of being abused as children than other types of batterers. Substance abuse is associated with their violence only about half of the time. Within-family abusers do not appear to have clinical levels of depression or anger, but do appear to be jealous and to minimize their violent behavior. Approximately half of all batterers who enter treatment programs match the description of the family-only batterer.

The second categorical dimension is the pan-violent or antisocial batterer. Approximately one-fourth of batterers in treatment programs fit this description. Generally, pan-violent batterers have the highest rates of severe physical assault to their partners and are most likely to behave in violent ways in settings outside of the family. Not surprisingly, they have high rates of substance abuse, arrest, and involvement with the legal system. They are likely to have been severely abused as children and show only moderate levels of marital satisfaction, anger, and depression. Yet they are most likely to score high on antisocial personality disorder or psychopathy. That is, they are dominating and bullying, do not feel guilty about their abusive behavior, and lack empathy toward the victim.

The third type are dysphoric or have borderline personality disorders. This group is depressed, psychologically distressed, and emotionally volatile. They engage in moderate to severe levels of psychological and sexual abuse, as well as physical violence toward their partners. They are likely to be dependent on the woman and suspicious of her activities and motives. Intense jealousy characterizes these men. Approximately one-fourth of those who enter treatment are personality-disordered batterers.

Substance abuse may accompany battering, may precede battering, or may not be involved at all. We know that approximately half of all abuse incidents involve the use or abuse of drugs or alcohol but that the two are not inextricably linked.

B. Range of Programs and Underlying Theoretical Assumptions

The best intervention programs for batterers are those that take a comprehensive and coordinated approach to the problem. That is, communities that offer treatment programs that are tied to the police and judicial systems, as well as to programs that offer services to the victims of abuse, are better able to monitor the progress of the offender from initial arrest through several years of treatment than are services that focus on only one part of the problem. Some communities have antiviolence education campaigns, school-based antiviolence programs, mandatory arrest policies, and judges and probation officers who are sophisticated about the dynamics and patterns of abusers. Clearly, the strong and immediate response of professionals to domestic violence plays a part in reducing the chances that such violence in families will happen again. Psychoeducational intervention programs designed to stop the batterer's violent behavior take a number of forms. Many programs use a combination of strategies, but the unique properties of different types of programs will be explained. [*See* Community Mental Health.]

Programs that rely on a behavioral learning approach first identify factors that reinforce and maintain the abuser's behavior toward the woman. These behaviors typically include controlling her access to money and resources, monitoring her behavior when outside the home, restricting access to family and friends, verbal abuse aimed at undermining her sense of competence, and, of course, physical assault to reinforce the other forms of intimidation. Hence, in addition to the physical assault, the batterers' behaviors that serve to control and to limit the woman are the focus of treatment. Behavioral programs for batterers are typically group programs that use skills training to teach alternative behaviors. A prerequisite for most programs is to have the abuser take responsibility for his actions and to not blame the woman for his abusive behavior. By focusing on the behavior of the batterer, rather than on his explanations for events, behavioral programs seek to force recognition that the abuser is ultimately responsible for the violence.

Somewhat akin are programs that take a cognitive restructuring approach and recognize that cognitions or thinking processes play an important role in the development of abusive behavior. Many researchers have described cognitive-behavioral models designed to focus on skills training and attitude change. These programs are considered suitable for antisocial and generally violent batterers, in addition to the other batterer types. The assumptions of this model of treatment are that batterers who have been victimized during their childhoods, who hold rigid stereotypes about women, and who have poor social skills need direct teaching and education, rather than interventions that only require the ability to build trust and develop relationships with group leaders and other group members. Men who lacked adequate role models as children may not have learned appropriate interpersonal skills and may continue to rely on distorted cognitions and inappropriate problem-solving techniques in their relationships as adults. Without intervention, these men will continue destructive and hurtful patterns of interacting with the important people in their lives.

Cognitive-behavioral groups typically have 6 to 10 participants, and one or two leaders. They use a teaching and training format that may include homework and specific lessons each week. Cognitive-behavioral practices such as the rehearsal of new thoughts and behavior are standard fare. For example, participants learn to identify and to reinterpret their reactions to stressful events and to think differently about appropriate responses. There is a weekly emphasis on improving communication, building cognitive skills, and consciousness-raising about men's attitudes toward women's roles and violence against women.

Abusive and controlling behaviors toward a partner are reported each week in the group session. With the help of the group leaders, batterers can be confronted about their illogical thinking and reinforced when they take responsibility for their behavior and make a change toward more appropriate ways of relating to the women in their lives. Cognitive-behavioral groups typically discuss managing and expressing anger at women, they discuss alternative ways to express anger and other negative emotions, and they learn to respect the rights and wishes of others, including wives or partners and their children. Change is achieved through feedback, reinforcement from the group, as well as from social learning or modeling one's behavior on other members and leaders. [*See* BEHAVIOR THERAPY; COGNITIVE THERAPY.]

Another type of program employs relationship-based interventions and is considered to be most appropriate for batterers who experienced trauma during childhood. Psychodynamic theory is used to explain the ways in which the abuser's current behavior is the result of efforts to cope with past experiences of witnessing violence or being abused. It is thought that some men, in their efforts to overcome feeling inadequate and powerless in relationships as a child, have identified with the perpetrator, or currently try to gain control over traumatic memories by venting anger and behaving aggressively. The process-psychodynamic treatment model is focused on revisiting past relationships in order to work through and overcome the trauma in a supportive group setting. [*See* PSYCHOANALYSIS.]

These groups are not structured with a teaching agenda but rather they allow each participant the chance to explore the ways in which early abusive experiences have led to unhealthy patterns in relationships today. By uncovering past trauma and discussing it in a supportive group setting, the batterer can then realize the ways in which current violent behavior is an attempt to control past abuse and feelings of inadequacy related to the trauma. The goal is for men to be able to respect and to have empathy for others after having insights and empathy for themselves as children. The relationships of group members to the leaders and to one another are salient here and provide the support needed for this type of self-exploration. This is a relatively new approach to treating batterers and, thus far, it is not widely used.

C. Current Issues in Interventions for Men

1. Individual versus Group Therapy

A variety of treatment modalities exists for most types of psychological and behavioral problems, but group therapy is considered the treatment of choice for abusive men. Group sessions can range from 6 to 32 weeks in design. While individual therapy can focus on the behavioral, psychodynamic, or the cognitive methods described above, most experts in this field consider group therapy to be the most effective. There are several reasons. First, there are distinct benefits in discussing abusive behavior in front of other abusers. Many batterers are in denial about their own abusive behavior yet are able to identify violent behavior in other people. Thus, the group can be used to help break through an individual member's denial of his negative attitudes, or abuse toward his partner. Here the culture of violence is challenged by the group. Second, men can find comfort and support when they discover that others like them have had similarly difficult experiences during childhood, and/or suffer from the same feelings of frustration in dealing with the stress and the women in their lives. Group leaders also serve as living models of nonviolent men who are sensitive to their own and other peoples' needs.

2. Is Couples' Treatment Safe?

There is considerable debate in the field as to whether it is ever acceptable to treat a batterer and abused woman together as a couple. The underlying assumptions of couples' therapy are that both parties are able to participate fully in the treatment, that there are no power differentials supported by an external system, and that each person is free to discuss issues of importance to him- or herself and to the couple. However, when one partner is being abused and dominated by the other, these assumptions are often violated. That is, battered women may not be free to participate fully in the treatment, to disclose their opinions, or to report on the behavior of the abuser. Battered women know that there are serious and often severe consequences for revealing the abuse—they may be reprimanded, beaten, or even killed by their partner. We know from research studies that battered women who go to emergency rooms do not often report on the abuse when asked about it in the presence of the abuser. Similarly, battered women may not be free to discuss the most important and urgent issues in their lives (e.g., their victimization) in couples treatment.

Psychologists have argued that, by treating the couple, the focus of the problems may shift to the interactions between batterer and victim, thus deflect ing the batterer's responsibility for his abusive behavior onto features of the woman or of the couple. Obviously, many batterers would prefer to engage in couples' treatment where their actions would be considered as part of a system that includes the personality of the battered woman, her reactions to the violence, and her behavior that could be used to justify the abuse. Batterers regularly use denial and they blame the victim for her plight. The bottom line, however, is that the abuser alone is responsible for his violent behavior and until he receives non-couples' treatment to change his behavior, there is little that can be accomplished in the couples' treatment setting. Given the physical and emotional consequences to the woman, couples' treatment is considered by many to be completely safe only after the batterer has successfully completed an intervention program specifically designed to stop his violence.

Some therapists who endorse couples' treatment for domestic violence argue that not all physical abuse is severe or frequent, that not all violence is the sole responsibility of the abuser, and that battered women want to remain in their relationships, despite the risks to themselves. Yet many therapists may not be familiar with the dynamics of abusive relationships, may minimize the danger to the woman, and may see battering as an exaggerated form of marital conflict. Just knowing that the woman may be threatened with harm or may be harmed as a result of her participation in couples' treatment renders it particularly risky. Still, we know that when a woman is battered, the physical assault is but one of many forms of domination and control exerted by her partner. Nonetheless, once the batterer has completed a group intervention program, couples' treatment may be appropriate if the therapist has a firm grasp of the dynamics of domestic violence and is vigilant in monitoring the abuser's behavior. [*See* COUPLES THERAPY.]

D. Efficacy of Treatment

Studies of the effectiveness of treatment programs for men who batter show inconsistent results and have many problems. Even so, there is preliminary evidence that some forms of treatment work to reduce recidivism, or additional assaults, for some men when they stay in therapy. More recent studies have tried to sort out which qualities of particular programs are helpful, and for which men various types of programs are best suited.

1. Study Design and Criterion for Success

It is difficult to compare studies because they often measure different things. For example, some treatment programs are based on changing behavior, others on changing thinking, and still others rely on success in exploring childhood trauma. All programs for men work to stop the violence, to change attitudes about women, and in many, to increase the man's feelings of adequacy and reduce his level of anger. Success has traditionally been predicated on whether the program is effective in stopping the violence. Studies currently underway also include outcomes such as reducing the amount of sexual abuse and/or emotional maltreatment, eliminating the woman's fear, and reducing concomitant abuse of the children.

Given the above qualifiers, we can say that there are preliminary findings that some treatment is better than no treatment in reducing violence rates. In well-controlled studies, that is studies that use random assignment to treatment groups, outcomes varied not by the kind of treatment group but by the type of batterer in a particular group. In 1996, Saunders found that the cognitive-behavioral treatment was more effective for generally violent/antisocial batterers than for other types and that process-psychodynamic treatment was more successful for the dependent batterers than for other types. In each group less than half of the participants were violent 2 years following treatment. There is no evidence that programs that treat couples are effective in stopping the violence or are better than those that treat groups of men. Similarly, we have no evidence that individual treatment is more or less effective than group intervention programs.

2. Rates of Retention and Recidivism

A major problem with samples in research studies includes subject attrition, or dropping out of the research program before the end of the study. We do know that batterers who drop out of treatment are more likely to be young, to have substance abuse problems, and to have a longer history of abuse. Yet some offenders are so violent as to be considered untreatable and thus are not referred for intervention by courts, probation officers, or community agencies. They are seldom included in treatment outcome studies. In addition, women may not want to participate initially or to continue in research studies for a number of reasons, including deciding to return to the abuser, lack of interest, or out of fear for their safety.

3. Current Issues in Assessment

In doing program evaluation research it is essential to have more than one source of information about the abuser's behavior. Thus, multimethod studies that include police reports and arrest records, reports from the abusers and the women they assault, as well documentation of injuries from hospitals and doctors, are preferred. In addition, studies that have an extended posttreatment evaluation are more convincing as they give more evidence that the intervention has had a lasting effect. For example, some of the early outcome studies relied on only a 6-month period to test whether the batterer had changed his pattern of behavior. Some studies relied on the batterer's report of the amount of his violence. More recent studies have followed batterers for 2 to 4 years and beyond and have relied on reports from several sources. Finally, assessment of a range of batterer behaviors should be included in efforts to decide whether or not change has occurred. Studies can go beyond documenting rearrest (which essentially counts only about one-tenth of physical assaults), to include incidents of stalking, harassment, violating protection orders, as well as rates of psychological maltreatment of the woman.

II. INTERVENTIONS FOR BATTERED WOMEN

A. Impact of Battering on the Woman

Battered women are at high-risk for physical and psychological problems directly related to the violence and to the emotional abuse that they have endured. Battering by an intimate partner is considered to be the primary cause of injury to women ages 15 to 44. Some battered women may suffer contusions, bruises, or broken bones as a result of assault or they may be killed by their assailant. Although the vast majority of battered women do not seek treatment for their injuries, those who do use medical facilities do so for only the most severe injuries and often not after the first incident of abuse.

Many battered women are clinically depressed. They are more likely to have major depressive episodes than women with serious relationship problems that do not include violence. Depression and low self-esteem, in turn, influence the woman's coping, as she may become less active and more avoidant as she feels a loss of personal control. Recall that batterers strive to take control away from the woman so as to more easily dominate her. Several studies of battered women in shelters report that approximately 40 to 60% experience posttraumatic stress disorder related to the threats to their life, repeated physical assaults, and the extent and severity of abuse. However, with more time out of the abusive relationship, the rates of PTSD decrease, depression abates, and women can be helped to feel a sense of control over their lives once more.

B. Shelter-Based Programs

1. Goals and Range of Services

The battered women's movement started in the 1970s when the first shelters for women and children were created. Today there are more than 1300 shelters and thousands of service programs in the United States; most are overcrowded and have waiting lists. The immediate goal of most shelters is to provide safety to the woman. Referral for emergency medical care is often provided for those who arrive with injuries. Additional goals including providing legal advocacy for women, help in finding jobs, and social services. Many shelters offer support in the form of group programs and individual advocacy for women and some provide programs for their children. Ultimately, battered women need to find affordable shelter and ways to support themselves should they elect to leave the batterer for good.

2. Support Groups for Battered Women

The primary goals of most support groups are keeping the woman safe from harm and providing education about the dynamics of woman abuse. In addition, support groups are often the source of information about a range of topics from effective childcare methods to obtaining housing. The main topic of conversation in support groups is the abuse that the women have endured. For those who have left the abuser for the first time, or those who have never told anyone about their suffering, it is empowering and eye-opening to hear quite similar stories from other women with a range of educational, economic, and cultural backgrounds. Only women with shared experiences can resonate so strongly to one another's stories. Thus, the chief contribution of support groups within shelters is to provide a format for women to share and to explore what they have endured, and to then get help in becoming safe and avoiding the abuse. [*See* SUPPORT GROUPS.]

3. Shelter Parenting Groups

When battered women elect to come to a shelter, they are often escaping from a severe assault, leaving in the middle of the night, and taking their children and possessions with them to an unknown place. This stream of events often leaves the women and children confused, anxious, and eventually angry. Yet the women must assume complete control over their children, at a time when they may feel least up to the task. In addition, children who have been traumatized by violence are often agitated and aggressive, making the mother's job even harder. The problem is further compounded by having so many children in the same small space. Thus, support for the development of parenting skills is routinely provided in battered women's shelters. These groups focus on behavior management techniques, on identifying children's feelings, and on children's developmental needs.

4. Substance Abuse

There is currently a debate about whether some women are beaten because their own substance abuse renders them vulnerable to attack or whether they self-medicate in response to being abused over a period of years. These may be two distinct groups of women. Either way, many abused women suffer from addiction to drugs or alcohol. Recent studies have shown that a far greater percentage of substance-abusing battered women did not use or abuse substances before the start of the battering. Some women have reported that the batterer encouraged them to drink or to use drugs. Others have noted that the batterer forced them to use alcohol or drugs along with him. Nonetheless, many shelters address the issues of drug and alcohol dependency in their efforts to help battered women survive. These efforts can take the form of classes, support groups, or transportation to existing programs in the community.

5. Advocacy and Placement

Individual advocacy is an important part of most shelter programs as many battered women must decide whether to file charges, whether to stay out of the abusive relationship, whether to get a job, an apartment, or food stamps—all while recovering from the most traumatic events in their lives. Most battered women face a number of adjustments that require action immediately following assault. Recall, however, that, for some women, the healing process often brings with it renewed energy, less depression, and release from debilitating fears and nightmares associated with the abuse. Yet for others, the healing process takes more time. Many abused women are left with PTSD symptoms and a realistic fear of re-assault for years after separating from the batterer.

C. Coordinated Community Response

The battered women's movement has involved thousands of grass-roots workers and professionals, often battered women themselves, in efforts to combat violence against women. Most cities now have emergency hotlines, information directories, advocacy programs, and victim services. Many shelters and community groups work with law enforcement agencies, judges, and social service agencies to coordinate services from the time of the first emergency call to sentencing, treatment, and follow-up. In many states, volunteers and shelter workers have fought for legislation such as mandatory arrest laws and antistalking laws. The National Coalition Against Domestic Violence was established in 1978 to coordinate the efforts of workers from around the country and to disseminate information on various aspects of domestic violence.

1. Hospital/Emergency Room Interventions

Efforts are underway nationwide to train emergency room staff and medical students in the identification and treatment of violence against women. Currently, few medical schools spend more than a few minutes on evaluating and treating women for abuse injury. Studies of hospital clinics and emergency rooms reveal that many physicians do not recognize the signs of abuse and few ever ask the woman whether she is in a violent relationship or whether her injuries are the result of interpersonal conflict. When the batterer does accompany the woman to the ER oftentimes he may not be separated from the woman when she is questioned about her injuries. Clearly, policies aimed at educating emergency room personnel are needed to protect abused women and to facilitate the prosecution of the abuser. Just as in the case of rape, when a woman's claim of abuse is backed up by medical reports and photographs of her injuries, the case will be stronger in court. Many feminists argue that woman abuse will stop in this country only after men in positions of authority are willing to take a zero-tolerance stand against such violence. This will take primary prevention programs. Thus, coordinated efforts are underway in some communities to train police, physicians, prosecutors, and judges to reduce their tolerance for violence against women.

2. Community Support Groups for Women

Many communities offer free drop-in groups for battered women that have the same goals as those run within a shelter. These groups provide support on an as-needed basis and rely mostly on education, referral to services, and the chance to speak with other women about their experiences. The group leaders may be volunteers, formerly battered women and/or professionals, and the number of participants varies from week to week. Many women go to drop-in groups as a first step in getting help. Thus, they differ from shelter groups in that some women may still reside with their partner, while others may be in the process of leaving, may have already left, or may have returned. Once again, the important contribution of drop-in groups is the opportunity to listen to other women with shared experiences. Most often community drop-in groups are supported and run as part of the shelter program. Very few groups are provided by established clinical settings, such as mental health clinics, social service agencies, or private practice settings.

Some communities do provide longer term, or ongoing, clinical intervention groups for battered women. These are distinguished from drop-in groups by the stability of the group, for example, the same women return each week, and often by the presence of professionally trained group leaders such as social workers or psychologists. Ongoing groups take many forms and can last anywhere from several weeks to several years. Some programs are free, while others charge a nominal fee.

One program which adopts a feminist-ecological model in efforts to help women to overcome the effects of battering on their lives was created in 1985 by Ginette Larouche in Quebec, Canada. Feminists believe that woman abuse originates in a male-dominated society and that the responsibility for ending the violence rests with the community. The aims of the feminist model are to denounce woman abuse, to return responsibility for violence to the man, as opposed to the victim, and to focus on counterbalancing the negative consequences to the woman.

These groups take a social and psycho-educational approach that includes listening to the woman and providing active support, as well as clarification and education designed to explode myths perpetrated by the abuser. For example, many women come to believe that they are the cause of the violence against them, as batterers often cite small infractions by the woman as the reason for their violent behavior. Over time, some battered women come to believe the abuser and work diligently to avoid setting off a confrontation. These efforts are seldom successful and lead to low self-esteem, to self-blame, and to guilt, as well as to the risk of injury. Support groups provide battered women with information about their rights, available resources, and they empower women to endorse a broader range of gender roles. Along the way, it is hoped that tension is reduced, support is provided for reducing victim behaviors, and the woman's sense of autonomy is restored.

3. Individual Treatment

The exact number of battered women who receive individual therapy for their problems is unknown. Clearly, one difference in who obtains individual treatment is socioeconomic status. The ability to pay is associated with private therapy, although some community mental health centers accept low-fee clients that may include battered women. It is interesting to note that the socioeconomic status of women who are abused usually does not reflect the total household income. Many battered women are denied access to money and so must rely on public services. An additional constraint is that of using insurance to obtain treatment. Often insurance companies reimburse the account holder, who is not atypically the abuser. Efforts to keep treatment information confidential and away from the spouse might prove unsuccessful and thus are not worth the risk to some battered women.

Women enter individual therapy for a number of reasons, most often having to do with relationships and emotional disturbances such as depression. Battered women who are able to find a supportive therapist, one who understands the dynamics of woman abuse, can build the therapeutic, bridging relationship needed to explore their current lives.

D. What Works and Why

One of the most frequently heard complaints of care providers and shelter workers is that, despite their efforts, so many battered women elect to return to their abuser. Yet it is essential to note here that most battered women eventually DO leave their abusive partners for good. In one study, 67% eventually separated from or divorced an abusive partner and did not return.

Studies of the efficacy of treatment and intervention programs for battered women are few. The goals of treatment for women usually do not focus on stopping the violence but rather on the degree to which the woman is empowered, has increased her self-esteem, has reduced her depression, and has heightened her sense of autonomy. Overall results indicate that those women who receive treatment improve more than those who receive no treatment.

Studies of the correlates of violence and women's success at leaving the abuser show that both objective and subjective aspects of the woman's life are important to consider. Objectively, battered women cite fear, lack of money, unemployment, and other economic factors as reasons for returning to the abuser. Subjectively, the loss of friends, loss of intimacy with the batterer, loneliness, facing the anger of other relatives, or a misplaced sense of responsibility for the dysfunction in their relationships are the interpersonal reasons given by battered women for not leaving the abuser. However, we know that many battered women are at highest risk for injury or even death when the batterer becomes convinced that the relationship is over. Thus, treatment programs that address these concerns are most likely to lead to success.

How abuse is treated shows that, for many women, community resources are absent. Without help, many battered women cannot leave the abuser. For example, few men who abuse their wives are arrested and convicted of this crime. In most communities, if the batterer had assaulted someone outside the home, the chances that he would be arrested are much greater than if he elected to assault his partner. Many battered women do not have an extended family who will support them, they do not have police who will come to the home and arrest the perpetrator of violence, they do not have shelters with room for them, they do not have judges who will issue and then enforce restraining orders, and they do not have access to affordable housing, and to treatment for themselves or their children. Programs should evaluate and then address the woman's help-seeking history as part of the treatment she receives.

Just as there are different typologies of battering men, battered women's experiences vary as well. Researchers have shown that the varieties of abuse experienced by the woman are related to her ability to leave the abuser. One-third of the battered women most likely to leave and to stay out have partners who are unstable, explosive, and severely abusive. About one-fifth are rarely physically abused, but experience severe emotional abuse. These women are most likely to have a stable relationship with the abuser and are most likely to stay. Another one-fifth have extensive and chronic abuse but may leave and return several times before being able to successfully live apart from the abuser. Approximately 10% leave only when the abuser starts to abuse the children as well. Those who are least likely to leave, who repeatedly go back to the perpetrator despite severe physical violence, are most likely to have a family history of violence, to have been abused themselves as children, and to think that violence is inescapable and expected. Programs to help battered women could take these typologies into account and tailor their services to the needs of the individual woman. In the future, outcome studies may include the entire community as the sample, to see whether education efforts have had an impact on attitude change, whether there have been fewer repeat offenders, whether arrest rates have increased, and whether the number of women who are abused by a partner each year has decreased.

III. PREVENTIVE INTERVENTIONS FOR CHILDREN EXPOSED TO DOMESTIC VIOLENCE

A. Children's Reactions to Witnessing Domestic Violence

Children whose mothers have been physically and emotionally abused are considered victims of family violence. We know from research studies that individual children respond differently to the violence, from those who evidence major psychological disorders and posttraumatic stress symptoms, to those who appear resilient and unaffected by the trauma. Approximately 40 to 60% of children who witness the abuse of their mothers are above the clinical cutoff level on measures of mood and behaviors. That is, they are in need of clinical treatment for their anxiety, depression, and aggressive behavior. In one study, more than half of the children who witnessed domestic violence had symptoms of posttraumatic stress, and 13% qualified for a full Posttraumatic Stress Disorder (PTSD) diagnosis—the diagnosis first given to returning combat veterans who showed extreme stress reactions to the atrocities witnessed during war.

Most children who observe violence in the family are worried and concerned about the behavior of their father and the welfare of their mother relative to children who have not observed such violence. Many of these children feel anxious because they harbor a terrible family secret—one that they often are unable to share with friends. In this instance, they may avoid or withdraw from social contacts. Other children may behave aggressively with peers and find themselves rejected by others, socially neglected, or avoided. Without some intervention, these lessons and reactions can interfere with a child's social and emotional development. Yet there is often little opportunity for children to discuss their perceptions, worries, and fears, or to get new information.

B. Theoretical Assumptions of Programs for Children

Social learning theory tells us that children learn about violence and aggressive tactics as a result of being exposed to the abuse of their mothers. In the process children develop attitudes about violence, and learn lessons about power in relationships. Children are highly likely to believe that at least some of the blame for the parents' conflicts resides within themselves. In some families, the children are directly blamed for the fighting in the family. As children get older, they are much more capable of seeing alternative explanations as causes for the events happening around them. However, children raised in violent families may either attempt to reject the aggressive behavior of the adults in their family, or they may attempt to wholly incorporate this aggressive behavior. Both approaches are problematic. For most children, these conflictual role models hamper the child's efforts to move forward with a clear sense of competence.

Children's reaction to the violence is mediated by their level of cognitive development. Preschool-age children are considered to be egocentric. That is, they understand the world in terms of themselves. Thus, younger children are more likely to blame themselves for their parents' problems and/or to believe many of the threats made by the batterer. They are often frightened yet unable to discuss what is happening. Most children aged 6 to 12 understand that one person may have different feelings than another in response to different situations or events. In terms of understanding domestic violence, the school-age child is able to imagine various causes for the violence. In particular, the child can see the causes of domestic violence as beyond those immediately connected with her- or himself. The child also is able to play out or imagine other possibilities or outcomes to domestic conflict.

C. Programs for Preschoolers

While many communities have programs designed to aid and support battered women and to treat the batterers, the development of children's programs lags far behind. In many communities there are simply no services available for children of abused women. When services do exist, they often take the form of drop-in groups in shelters. Programs designed for younger children most often have the goals of providing support and building self-esteem. For reasons stated above, younger children are less cognitively mature, and hence, less able to consider and to process the distressing events in their family. Yet they are no less affected by these events. We know from the few research studies on preschool-age children of battered women that they are more likely to have difficulty modulating negative emotions and solving problems in social situations than children who have not been exposed to such abuse. Therefore, programs that emphasize the role-modeling of appropriate social interaction may be very helpful to these children.

It is generally believed that the best way to help young children is to help their mothers. Thus, programs that focus on honing and developing better parenting skills, in addition to keeping the mother safe, indirectly serve to help the young child. Programs that involve both the mother and the child may be the most successful of all, as they focus on interaction and provide an opportunity to enhance and to support parenting efforts. However, many battered women need to have their own support before they can attend to the needs of their youngest children. In this case, child care and groups for preschool children are necessary. Also, many of the youngest children of battered women are often cared for by their older siblings. Efforts to include relief and skill building for these older children may be additional and appropriate ways to provide for the preschool-age child's needs.

D. Programs for Children Ages 6 to 12

The strategy most widely recommended for working with children of abused mothers is the small group format. These groups can be either ongoing, with the same children meeting over a set period of time, or drop-in, where the participants vary from week to week. Drop-in groups are typically found in shelters whereas ongoing groups for children are best suited for children in the community. Children who come to shelters following the abuse of their mothers are in need of an accepting environment, and of the self-esteem-enhancing activities usually provided by drop-in groups. It is a time when children need to recover and receive support in mastering their anxiety, but not to uncover their deepest fears and worries about the violence in their lives.

Before children can be expected to discuss the trauma in their lives, it is necessary to build trusting relationships. When these relationships are strong, they facilitate disclosure and the child's acceptance of the group leader's support. Thus, ongoing groups that build relationships both with the group leader and with the other group members are considered the most appropriate intervention strategy either before or after the child's stay in a shelter. Efforts by group leaders and therapists to disconfirm negative stereotypes and distorted expectations about family and gender roles focus on experiential exercises, such as those described below for the children in one intervention group program. Strategies such as role playing or puppet play are expected to show greater changes in the children's understanding of the experience of domestic violence over strategies using direct teaching, dialogue, or discussion alone.

"The Kids' Club: A Preventive Intervention Group Program for Children of Battered Women" is a time limited, 10-week clinical program designed by Sandra Graham-Bermann in 1992. This intervention is directed at three levels. The goal at the cognitive level is to improve the child's knowledge base about family violence and conflict resolution. By expressing and identifying feelings, fears and worries associated with fighting in the family, children learn that others their age have similar, negative reactions to the violence. Discussions of safety planning teach children different ways of responding to violence. The goal at the social level is to build skills and to change behavior in interaction with others. Here, discussions of gender roles and practicing alternative problem-solving strategies provide a platform for discussing social behavior and expectations. At the relationship level the focus is on building trust and gaining support from both the group and the group leaders. Relationships with peers in the group are equally important in that there is a special quality of relief and comfort in being with other children who share the "secret" of domestic violence in their own families. This atmosphere allows children to feel less stigmatized and less alone in their distress, to exchange information and impressions, and to validate their feelings of outrage and sadness.

Children between the ages of 6 and 12 are accepted into two groups based on their age. They may or may not be living with the batterer. Each group is led by two therapists who receive weekly supervision of their work. Here, group leaders are master's-level or doctoral-level clinical psychologists and social workers. The curriculum helps children to discuss a specific aspect of domestic violence and how it affects their lives each week, although there is no pressure for children to participate or to disclose anything about themselves or their families. In fact, all activities are designed to use displacement. For example, group leaders seek the child's thoughts, referring to children as "experts on what most kids really think," thus making it both safe and compelling for the child to give his or her advice.

As a result of participating in the group, it is hoped that children learn that the violence between parents is not their fault, that they have a right to feel angry at the perpetrators of the violence, and even at their mothers, and that they can employ a broader range of conflict resolution skills, along with the understanding that physical aggression is not an acceptable way of coping with family stress and conflict.

E. Parenting Support and Education Programs

One program designed specifically to address the needs of battered women through empowering them as parents was designed in 1994 by Graham-Bermann and Levendosky. Many battered women do not identify their own needs and are reluctant to seek help for themselves, but are often quite worried about their children. On the other hand, many battered women cite the children's needs as a primary reason for staying with the abuser. Specifically, the women want to have a family, think it is important for children to have a father, and worry about whether they could manage raising children alone. When society reinforces the importance of having a man as the head of the family, many battered women feel caught in the bind of whether an abusive father is better than no father at all. Further, it is often difficult for women as mothers to claim power and to take control of their families. Battered women often struggle with asserting themselves as mothers and in handling aggression by their children.

The parenting support program provides basic education about domestic violence, advocacy for women to obtain services in the community, and a support group where the woman can share and process issues related to both the violence and to parenting children under these most difficult family circumstances. Two trained clinicians (social workers or clinical psychologists) serve as leaders for each group of approximately five to eight women. It is essential that the group leaders receive weekly supervision for their work, in order to reduce the potential for secondary traumatization from the many vivid and horrific stories that are heard each week.

The groups begin with each woman telling her story, including her present circumstances and concerns. A list of worries about children and concerns about parenting is kept. Each session emphasizes both the emotional and physical abuse as well as child-rearing issues. Along the way, these parenting topics are addressed—discipline and controlling negative behavior in children, mothers' worries and fears about their children, the impact of woman abuse on the child, understanding children's developmental needs, having fun with children, helping children to identify emotions, and communication in the mother–child relationship. Group leaders make referrals as needed to shelters, lawyers, doctors, and other advocates and community agencies that provide support for battered women.

This program is designed to serve only as a starting point for battered women to think about issues associated with domestic violence and raising healthy children. The aim is not to cover all that can be learned about any subject in a few hours' time, but to provide an opportunity for the women to discover their shared concerns and to learn new strategies for dealing with the very real problems presented by their children. In this way it is hoped that battered women may experience a sense of empowerment as they become more effective mothers to their children.

F. Assessment of Intervention Efficacy

While the best programs are firmly grounded in theory and take into account the results of previous research on children exposed to domestic violence, we know little about whether these programs are effective and for which children they are most effective. Some of the risk variables that should be considered are the duration of the abuse, the number of abusive partners, other stressful family and neighborhood events, the child's role in family violence, and the presence of physical abuse to the child. Protective factors may include the amount of support available to the child and the mother, as well as the response of the community to the violence. The timing of the assessment, relative to the violence events, should also be considered, as many children exposed to domestic violence do not show evidence of dysfunction at the time of assessment. These children may be either resilient or unaffected by the events, or more likely, they may show symptoms later. Finally, children whose mothers join support groups for abused women, or who remove themselves from a violent situation through separation and divorce, may be expected to fare better in treatment programs than those in families with ongoing abuse.

Some fathers successfully complete programs designed to address domestic aggression. Studies have shown a concomitant decrease in child abuse by some graduates of domestic aggression treatment programs. Thus, some children have seen a resolution to the battering, and have witnessed a parent acting in the child's interest. Other children from woman-abusing families have extensive contact with positive male adult figures, such as grandparents or teachers, who may serve as alternative role models. Efforts to test the efficacy of intervention programs for children are underway in several states, with projects funded by the National Injury Prevention Center, Centers for Disease Control in Atlanta, Georgia.

IV. PREVENTIVE INTERVENTIONS FOR ADOLESCENTS EXPOSED TO DOMESTIC VIOLENCE

A. Developmental Strengths and Needs of Adolescents

Teenagers are in an important transitional period in terms of gaining their independence and establishing their identities apart from the family, and in solidifying social relationships with friends. In addition, patterns of relating to others are formed with intimate partners during adolescence. For teens whose mothers are abused, these tasks can be complicated by the deleterious models of male and female adult behavior that they have witnessed and, perhaps, incorporated and taken as their own. Further, teenagers who have witnessed domestic violence are more likely to be depressed, to behave in antisocial ways, and to be physically aggressive and anxious than are teens from nonviolent families. In addition to the psychological scars, teenagers may be recovering from physical abuse and injury, as they are more likely to intervene in parents' fights than are younger children.

The cognitive skills of teenagers vastly exceed those of younger children. At this point, most adolescents can consider many causes for events, can think abstractly, and can entertain a range of possible outcomes to events. They are able to take a longer time perspective and to envision their futures more clearly than are younger children. At the same time, biological changes require the management and regulation of more intense emotions, such as anger and love, as well as sexual urges. Programs designed to address their needs must take into account their longer histories of coping with domestic violence, as well as the developmental tasks of establishing themselves as competent, well liked, and independent from their families.

Research studies tell us that the long-term effects of witnessing domestic violence differ for boys and for girls, with many boys at-risk for repeating violence in relationships with others outside the home. Males who have grown up around men who use power and control tactics need to learn other ways of communicating and they to develop skill in nonviolent conflict resolution. Females who have witnessed their mothers as victims of violence, or have been abused themselves, may need to develop a better understanding of themselves as competent, they may need to learn more about self-protection and about intolerance for various forms of abuse and harassment. While complicated by many developmental changes, adolescence is considered a good time to intervene, as children are forming their own intimate relationships and are beginning to put into practice the models that they have learned.

B. Domestic Violence Intervention Programs for Teenagers

The program "Promoting Healthy, Nonviolent Relationships: A Group Approach with Adolescents for the Prevention of Woman Abuse and Interpersonal Violence" was created by David Wolfe in 1994. It was based on his extensive clinical work and research with children living in abusive homes. The three main elements of the program are information dissemination, skills development, and social action learning. The program is unique as it capitalizes on adolescents' interest in forming and maintaining healthy relationships with members of the opposite sex. It takes a positive view of adolescents' development rather than the "youth as problem" approach that characterizes many other intervention programs designed for this age group. Finally, the program includes the adolescents themselves in finding solutions to the broader problem of woman abuse in their community.

One-third of the program is focused on understanding gender stereotypes, attitudes toward women, and violence in intimate relationships. These concepts are placed in the context of the broader society as each adolescent seeks to expose myths and to learn the ways in which aggression against women is promulgated in the media and in the culture. Group facilitators work with questionnaires, active exercises, video presentations, and group discussion to explode myths and to get at the facts. Discussion of dating violence is included.

The second section focuses on skills development and requires change at the level of the individual. Here each participant works to improve the ways in which he or she interacts with members of the opposite sex. Males learn about noncoercive communication and listening skills, while females learn personal safety skills. Assertiveness training is geared toward empowering youth to take responsibility for their interpersonal signals and actions.

The social action part of the program actively engages group members in working together to identify and to challenge some aspect of violence in their own community. First, there is a series of exercises aimed at teaching group members about resources available to teenagers, men, and women in their community. Next, group members develop a social action or a fundraising activity in which they all participate. Examples include setting up a display about stopping sexual assault in a shopping mall and selling t-shirts to raise funds for a local battered women's shelter. In this way teenagers put their skills to use on the broader community level. Along the way they learn to respect one another and themselves, to think differently about sex roles and family roles, and to develop healthier relationships as they work together to stop violence against women.

V. PREVENTIVE INTERVENTIONS IN COMMUNITY SETTINGS

There is considerable debate in the field as to whether it is better to move intervention efforts into established institutional settings—places that have traditionally not been responsive to abused women—or to focus on community-based services. However, help is needed throughout each community. A similar debate occurs over whether volunteers or professionals are best equipped to bring the most help to battered women and their children. Yet, these labels can be misleading when they dichotomize roles. For example, they do not recognize the number of professionals who are battered women, the number of volunteers who are professionals, and the professional training of shelter workers. Further, many theorists and researchers have taken an ecological perspective and they have conceptualized the problem and hence the solutions to woman abuse on a number of levels. On the societal level primary prevention has focused on national policy to bring attention to the problem and to obtain needed funds. On the community level both professional and volunteer workers share secondary prevention initiatives to provide services and to work on prevention with children. Some of these efforts are described below.

Social skills building and violence prevention programs are now offered in many schools. They are designed to offer education to all children but are considered to be particularly useful to children exposed to violence in the home. Typically, these programs include identifying feelings associated with violence, teaching and modeling alternative problem-solving skills, and demonstrating intolerance for violence at home, at school, and in the community. By addressing the problems early on, rather than waiting until after violent patterns have been established, it is hoped that all children can be empowered to respond to violence, and that those who have witnessed violence at home can get help. Concomitantly, some schools have trained teachers and counselors how to respond to children exposed to domestic violence and how to make referrals to provide for their needs.

Police departments in some communities provide training for dealing with domestic violence, for when and how to make arrests of batterers, for identifying battered women, and for providing for the needs of both women and children in the family following a domestic assault. These training programs include educating officers about the impact of domestic violence on women and children, and teaching them how to handle the often confusing presentation of abused women when asked to file complaints about the assailant, how to inform women of their rights to protection, and how to obtain services for victims of such abuse. Some police departments have developed domestic violence units and have hired social workers and psychologists specifically trained to work with women and children before and during the court process.

In some communities police department and battered women's shelters work hand in hand to track abusers, to identify women at risk for repeated abuse, and to monitor compliance with the conditions of an abuser's probation. Such efforts are sorely needed, as studies of both the training of police officers and the attitudes they hold toward domestic violence cases show that many officers avoid these calls or handle them quickly because they feel uncomfortable dealing with these issues. However, the legal understanding of domestic violence has come a long way from early identification of this as a "family problem" to our current understanding of the social, emotional, and economic costs to individual women, to children, and to the larger community.

Similarly, the legal community has expanded its understanding of domestic violence and what is needed to provide protection to women and children. Hence, many states have enacted mandatory arrest laws and antistalking ordinances with strict penalties and sentencing guidelines. There is currently some debate as to whether mandatory arrest reduces the occurrence of domestic violence or whether it puts the woman at greater risk for abuse. In addition, the cost of arresting all batterers has been a significant burden for some communities. However, research has shown that younger abusers and those with an active criminal history were more likely to abuse after a restraining order was issued than were older and less violent men. In the future, researchers should be able to provide more sophisticated answers to these questions as they move away from gross generalizations of whether mandatory arrest works to deciding for whom it works best. Then, policies and laws can be tailored to the needs of individual perpetrators and victims to provide the most effective, safest, and economical response to domestic violence.

Innovative educational initiatives sponsored by some communities include postering in subways and on buses and using billboards and newspaper advertisements in efforts to stop violence against women. Other cities have started campaigns with easily identifiable slogans and logos, such as "zero tolerance for violence against women." In some areas businesses and other volunteer groups have worked with local shelters to sponsor communitywide events in support of stopping the violence. These efforts reflect the growing knowledge that societal attitudes that condone violence against women need to change. Challenging the culture of violence in communities is another way to protect women and to inoculate children against commiting or tolerating violence in their lives.

VI. CONCLUSIONS

Domestic violence is a serious public health problem in America with far-reaching consequences for women and children. Efforts to stop the violence have taken many forms and include diverse settings such as community shelters, schools, courts, hospitals and clinics, and research institutions.

While treatment outcome research is in its infancy, there is some preliminary evidence that certain kinds of interventions work better for particular batterer types than for others, that some offenders may not be helped by traditional interventions, and that even brief intervention programs are better than no treatment at all. Group treatment is generally preferred to individual or couples' treatment. Those batterers who drop out of treatment, and are therefore hardest to treat, are likely to be young substance abusers with a long history of violence.

Interventions for women generally take the form of shelter programs and group treatment programs. However, few communities offer interventions designed specifically to meet the needs of children exposed to domestic violence. While most battered women eventually do leave their abusive partners, those who have access to social and financial support, and who feel protected in the community and by the police, are more likely to leave.

Current efforts can be seen in communities that take an ecological or multilayered approach to the problem. That is, they offer coordinated responses to domestic violence in terms of primary, secondary, and tertiary prevention. Educational programs aimed at reducing the culture of violence against women and school-based programs that teach nonviolent problem solving and social skills are primary preventions.

Dating violence programs for teenagers and psychoeducational intervention programs for younger children exposed to domestic violence are examples of innovative secondary preventions. It is hoped that in the future communities that take the initiative in preempting and combating violence against women will need fewer treatment programs and police units to respond to domestic violence after it occurs.

BIBLIOGRAPHY

Buzawa, E. S., & Buzawa, C. G. (1996). *Domestic violence: The criminal justice response* (2nd Ed.). Thousand Oaks, CA: Sage Publications, Inc.

Edelson, J. L., & Eisikovits, Z. C. (Eds.) (1996). *Future interventions with battered women and their families.* Thousand Oaks, CA: Sage Publications, Inc.

Edelson, J. L., & Tolman, R. M. (1992). *Intervention for men who batter: An ecological approach.* Newbury Park, CA: Sage Publications, Inc.

Graham-Bermann, S. A. (1992). *The kids' club: A preventive intervention program for children of battered women.* Ann Arbor: University of Michigan, Department of Psychology.

Graham-Bermann, S. A., & Levendosky, A. A. (1994). *The moms' group: A parenting support and intervention program for battered women who are mothers.* Ann Arbor: University of Michigan.

Larouche, G. (1985). *A guide to intervention with battered women.* Montreal: Corporation professionnelle des travailleurs sociaux du Quebec.

Saunders, D. (1996). Cognitive-behavioral and process-psychodynamic treatments for men who batter: Interaction of abuser traits and treatment models. *Violence and Victims,* 11(4), 393–414

DSM-IV

John J. B. Allen
University of Arizona

Comorbidity The co-occurrence of two or more mental disorders in the same individual.
Diagnosis The determination of the nature of a disease. Although in most branches of medicine this implies that the cause of the disorder has been identified, this is often not the case with psychiatric diagnosis using the *DSM-IV*, which involves assigning a diagnostic label on the basis of the observed and/or reported behaviors and symptoms.
Etiology The cause of a disorder.
Heterogeneity The situation where individuals who share the diagnosis of a particular disorder do not share all symptoms in common. A heterogeneous disorder is one where people with the disorder can present with a variety of different symptoms.
Mental Disorder The *DSM* defines mental disorder as a pattern of behavior, or psychological features, occurring in an individual that are currently associated with any of the following: a subjective sense of distress; impairment in important areas of function, such as work, school, relationships; or a significantly increased risk of posing a danger to oneself or others, or of losing an important freedom.
Prognosis Estimating the likely course and outcome for those with a mental disorder.
Reliability Consistency of diagnosis. If diagnoses can be assigned reliably, an individual will be assigned the same diagnosis across differing circumstances (e.g., different diagnosticians).
Validity The extent to which a diagnosis is meaningful. A valid diagnosis allows that individuals with the diagnosis can be distinguished from individuals with other diagnoses and from individuals with no diagnosis. Valid diagnoses should also provide useful information about the etiology, treatment, or prognosis of the mental disorder.

DSM-IV is the abbreviation for the *Diagnostic and Statistical Manual of Mental Disorders,* 4th Edition. The *DSM-IV* details the diagnostic criteria for nearly 300 mental disorders, and nearly 100 other psychological conditions that might be the focus of professional attention, thereby providing a standardized system of classification that is intended to be used internationally. The *DSM-IV* also provides systems for noting medical conditions and stressors that may be related to the psychological conditions, and for noting how the individual's functioning (for example, job performance or ability to care for one's self) may be affected.

I. THE PURPOSE OF DIAGNOSIS

Diagnosis of psychological symptoms using the *DSM-IV* entails classifying observable symptoms, or reports

Copyright © 1998 by Academic Press.
All rights of reproduction in any form reserved.

of such symptoms, into discrete categories termed mental disorders. A mental disorder (defined above) represents a pattern of behavior or psychological features that in some way causes the person distress or impairment. Moreover, a mental disorder is conceptualized in the *DSM-IV* as a problem or dysfunction that resides within an individual, rather than a problem that results from a conflict between that individual and society. This caveat is important because it is supposed to prevent the misuse of diagnostic labels for the purpose of social control, applying them to individuals whose values or beliefs differ from those of the majority.

Assigning a diagnosis using the *DSM-IV* does not necessarily suggest that the etiology (cause) of the symptoms is known, but only than an individual's symptoms meet the criteria for the particular mental disorder. For example, two individuals might meet the criteria for a diagnosis of Major Depressive Disorder, but might develop these symptoms after a very different set of circumstances; one person might experience these symptoms only after a series of troubling setbacks (e.g., financial, legal, and relationship problems) while another might experience these symptoms after an apparently unstressful period. Although one might imagine that the etiology of the depression differs for these two individuals, they would both receive the same diagnosis using the *DSM*.

Assigning a diagnostic label may have profound implications for the person receiving the diagnosis. On the one hand, diagnostic labels may allow individuals to receive the treatment they are seeking. On the other hand, such labels may have a stigmatizing effect for the person diagnosed. Consider, for example, how you might think about yourself, and how others might begin to think about you and to treat you, if they learned you had received a diagnosis of a severe psychosis—schizophrenia. Diagnostic labels convey a wealth of information, some of it intended, some of it not. Because assigning a diagnostic label may have profound effects on how people may view the person who receives the label, the diagnosis of mental disorders should be taken seriously, and should have the potential for some clear benefits for those diagnosed.

What, then, is the purpose of diagnosing mental disorders? First, diagnosis should help us identify a homogeneous group of individuals. For example, many different disorders may entail delusions—beliefs that most persons in an individual's culture would regard as false, such as the belief that one can read verbatim another's thoughts. Yet despite similarity in this particular symptom, individuals with delusions may differ in important ways. Delusions are associated in some cases with the ingestion of psychoactive substances (e.g., amphetamines), in others with a disturbance in mood (e.g., mania or depression), and in others with hallucinations and disorganization of thought (e.g., schizophrenia). These different diagnoses, while sharing a symptom in common, may differ in other important ways. By identifying patterns of symptoms that tend to occur together, important differences between individuals with a common symptom may be identified, such as the cause of the disorder, the most effective treatments, or the prognosis for the future.

Second, diagnosis should help in the planning of treatment. For example, the delusional behavior that can be seen in both mania and schizophrenia will typically be treated by different drugs. Similarly, knowing that the delusional behavior results from use of psychoactive substances suggests a different intervention; i.e., stopping use of the substance causing the symptom.

Third, diagnosis can facilitate communication among professionals. A diagnostic label provides a succinct means of conveying information. For example, if, after an assessment interview, a mental health professional determines that an individual needs to be referred to another mental health professional or facility, the diagnostic label can summarize much of the information. Of course the diagnosis does not summarize all relevant information, but can reduce the amount of description required to round out the assessment picture. Another instance in which diagnostic labels facilitate communication is the case of communication between mental health professionals and insurance providers. Given particular diagnoses, insurance providers will authorize reimbursement for particular treatments, without the need to review the entire assessment interview.

II. A BRIEF HISTORY OF THE DEVELOPMENT OF THE *DSM-IV* AND ITS PREDECESSORS

Over the last several thousand years, many systems have existed for diagnosing mental disorders. The *DSM* series is relatively recent, with the first edition of the *Diagnostic and Statistical Manual* (now referred to as *DSM-I*) appearing in 1952. The manual has been revised several times since, with the *DSM-II* appearing in 1968, the *DSM-III* appearing in 1979, a minor revision—the *DSM-III-R*—appearing in 1987, and the current version of the manual—the *DSM-IV*—appearing in 1994. In contrast to the *DSM* series, most earlier systems detailed only a handful of diagnostic categories.

Several categorization systems existed for use in the United States prior to the development of the *DSM*. These systems included: simple systems with between one and seven diagnostic categories to aid in collecting census data concerning mental illness during the nineteenth century; a system for statistically tallying information on patients in mental hospitals in the early twentieth century; a system developed by the U.S. Army, and modified by the Veteran's Administration, for use with servicemen; and several editions of a system developed by the World Health Organization (WHO). Since the latter part of the nineteenth century, the WHO had ben publishing the *International Classification of Disease* (*ICD*), a comprehensive listing of medical conditions. With the sixth edition (*ICD-6*), mental disorders were included for the first time. In each revision of the *DSM* series, an attempt was made to coordinate the system with the corresponding revision of the *ICD* system. Each of the disorders listed in the *DSM-IV* has a corresponding code in the most recent versions of the *ICD*, namely the *ICD-9-CM* and *ICD-10*.

The *DSM-I* was the product of The American Psychiatric Association Committee on Nomenclature and Statistics, and contained 106 mental disorders, with an emphasis on being clinically useful. *DSM-II* added 76 new disorders and, unlike its predecessor, encouraged rather than discouraged assigning multiple diagnoses to each patient. Both *DSM-I* and *DSM-II* were similar in format, providing a description of the disorder, but lacking detailed criteria by which to diagnose the disorder. *DSM-III* represented a major change, with each disorder possessing tangible, operational criteria. This change was inspired by research that showed that clinicians using the previous *DSM* versions failed to agree on a diagnosis for a surprisingly large percentage of the patients. Although inconsistency in information provided by the patients, and inconsistencies in the type of information gathered by clinicians could explain some of the disagreement, a vast majority of the problem lay with the diagnostic criteria themselves. The descriptions were overly broad, were often vague, sometimes included reference to unobservable processes, and often overlapped with descriptions of other diagnostic categories. The operational criteria of the *DSM-III* referred to observable or reportable symptoms, with specific numeric criteria for frequency and duration of symptoms. The *DSM-III* for the first time included a *multiaxial* system of diagnosis (see below), a feature that has been retained in subsequent revisions.

In contrast to earlier systems, which contained only a few broad and severe diagnostic categories that were likely to be relevant to governmental and institutional interests, the *DSM* series was designed to be of use to the clinical psychiatrist; *DSM* therefore focused on a broader range of symptoms, including less severe forms of disturbance that might be treated outside of institutional settings. The origins of this trend began a decade prior to the publication of the *DSM-I*, as military and Veterans Administration psychiatrists found a need for additional diagnostic categories to cover the psychiatric conditions resulting from the stress of combat. These conditions were less severe and less chronic than the few severe categories that existed prior to World War II. Moreover, these conditions could be treated in an outpatient setting rather than through institutionalization.

As a diagnostic system was developed to delineate these broader, less severe, diagnostic categories, it became impossible to unequivocally link each diagnostic category to a specific etiology. The *DSM* series, therefore, established diagnostic categories on the basis of the pattern of symptoms and their appearance over time, remaining largely agnostic with respect to etiology (with some clear exceptions). This *descriptive categorical approach* defines discrete categories of mental illness, based primarily on observable symptoms. In contrast to an etiologically based system, where each diagnostic category is included because a cause has been scientifically established, the decision to include a diagnostic category in the descriptive system must be based on informed judgments of experts as to whether the symptoms co-occur in such a manner to merit the inclusion of a discrete category defining those symptoms. Although such judgments will ideally be influenced by scientific research, some subjectivity is inevitable.

The development of *DSM-IV*, in particular, involved many individuals chosen for their expertise in a variety of areas. A 27-member *DSM-IV* Task Force worked with 13 Work Groups, each comprised of up to a dozen members. Additionally, each task force relied on the advice of committees of up to 100 people. Members of these committees represented many different specializations and professions, with medical doctors having the largest representation. Over the course of 6 years, a three-step process was followed to increase the likelihood that changes would be based on the basis of research findings, rather than the whim of committee members. This three-step process involved literature reviews, reanalysis of previously collected data sets, and field trials to assess the reliability of several alternative criterion sets. New diagnostic categories were included when the Task Force considered that sufficient evidence existed to justify the addition of a new category in terms of antecedent indicators (e.g., family history or precipitating situations), concurrent indicators (e.g., physiological and psychological symptoms that co-occur), and predictive indicators (e.g., response to treatment, prognosis). Conversely, in a few instances, a category from the *DSM-III-R* was removed when insufficient evidence existed to merit retaining it.

The *DSM-IV,* therefore, ideally represents the informed scientific judgment of many experts in the mental health field. On the other hand, these judgments are inevitably shaped and limited by the current scientific knowledge base, the previous diagnostic systems that form the basis for scientific research, the particular composition of the Task Force and Work Groups, and the idiosyncratic preferences of these various committee members. The *DSM-IV,* therefore, may best be viewed as one more chapter of a work in progress.

III. ORGANIZATION AND CONTENTS OF THE *DSM-IV*

The *DSM-IV* details a *multiaxial* system of diagnosis, meaning that individuals are assessed in multiple areas, or along multiple dimensions or *axes.* Axis I contains 15 major classes of mental disorders. Axis II contains personality and developmental disorders. Axis III contains medical conditions. Axis IV provides for the notation of psychological, social, and environmental stressors that may affect diagnosis. Axis V provides for a measure of the individual's function in areas such as work, social activities, and self-care. The multiaxial system is designed to encourage a comprehensive evaluation of biological, social, and psychological factors relevant to each person's presenting symptoms. The multiaxial system also provides a means for detailing differences between those with identical diagnoses. With respect to the example provided at the beginning of the chapter—two depressed individuals who developed symptoms after different life events—Axis IV would provide a way of summarizing that one individual developed depression only after a series of troubling setbacks while another developed depression in the absence of such events.

A. Axis I: Clinical Disorders and Other Conditions That May Be a Focus of Clinical Attention

Almost all mental disorders or conditions that may be a focus of clinical attention appear on Axis I, with a few exceptions that appear on Axis II. Axis I organizes mental disorders into 15 major groups of disorders, as presented in Table I. Most of the groups in Table I were created based on the similarity of symptoms of disorders within that group, although in some cases disorders are grouped together because of the typical age at which symptoms first appear (Disorders Usually First Diagnosed in Infancy, Childhood or Adolescence), or because of common etiology (Mental Disorders due to a General Medical Condition, Substance-Related Disorders, Adjustment Disorders). In many cases, an individual may receive more than one Axis I diagnosis, although some diagnoses by definition will preclude another diagnosis.

Each disorder on Axis I includes a set of diagnostic criteria, which are typically a combination of *monothetic* (i.e., all conditions of the criterion must be met) and *polythetic* (i.e., only some from among a larger set of conditions must be met) criteria. For example, to diagnosis Attention Deficit/Hyperactivity disorder, an individual must meet the following criteria: (a) either 6 or more symptoms (from among 9) of inattention, *or* 6 or more symptoms (from among 9) of hyperactivity-impulsivity (*polythetic*); (b) some symptoms are present and causing impairment before age 7 (*monothetic*); (c) impairment is seen in at least two settings, such as school and home (*monothetic*); (d) the symptoms clearly cause impairment in func-

Table I Examples of Disorders in Each of the 15 Major Groups Listed on Axis I of *DSM-IV*

Group	Examples of Disorders
Disorders Usually First Diagnosed in Infancy, Childhood, or Adolescence	Attention Deficit/Hyperactivity Disorder, Autistic Disorder
Delirium, Dementia, and Amnestic and Other Cognitive Disorders	Dementia of the Alzheimer's Type, Vascular Dementia
Mental Disorders Due to a General Medical Condition	Mood Disorder Due to a General Medical Condition (e.g., stroke, hypothyroidism)
Substance-Related Disorders	Alcohol Abuse, Nicotine Dependence, Caffeine Intoxication, Cocaine Withdrawal
Schizophrenia and Other Psychotic Disorders	Schizophrenia, Delusional Disorder, Schizoaffective Disorder
Mood Disorders	Major Depressive Disorder, Bipolar I Disorder (aka Manic Depression), Dysthymic Disorder
Anxiety Disorders	Agoraphobia, Social Phobia, Panic Disorder, Obsessive-Compulsive Disorder, Posttraumatic Stress Disorder
Somatoform Disorders	Somatization Disorder, Hypochondriasis
Factitious Disorders	Factitious Disorder
Dissociative Disorders	Dissociative Identity Disorder (*formerly* Multiple Personality Disorder), Dissociative Amnesia
Sexual and Gender Identity Disorders	Sexual Dysfunctions (e.g., Male Erectile Disorder), Paraphilias (e.g., Exhibitionism, Pedophilia), Gender Identity Disorder
Eating Disorders	Anorexia Nervosa, Bulimia Nervosa
Sleep Disorders	Primary Insomnia, Narcolepsy, Sleep Terror Disorder
Impulse-Control Disorders Not Elsewhere Classified	Kleptomania, Pyromania, Pathological Gambling

tioning (*monothetic*); and (e) the symptoms are not better accounted for by another mental or physical disorder (*monothetic*). Polythetic criterion sets have advantages and disadvantages. The primary advantage is that polythetic sets reduce the number of diagnostic categories required, since people with highly similar but nonidentical symptoms can receive the same diagnosis. If, by contrast, each and every criterion were required, such highly similar people would require different diagnoses. The primary disadvantage to polythetic criterion sets is symptom heterogeneity, where people with the same diagnosis may be quite different in terms of their symptoms. In fact, in the case of some disorders, it is possible that two individuals with the same diagnosis may not share a single symptom in common.

There are also disorders that appear on Axis I that do not have such clearly defined criterion sets. There are over 40 disorders that include "NOS" in their name, an abbreviation for Not Otherwise Specified. These disorders are diagnosed if the symptoms resemble those of another diagnosis but fail to meet the full criteria required for diagnosis. For example, Anxiety Disorder NOS is a diagnosis for cases in which there is "prominent anxiety or phobic avoidance that do not meet the criteria for any specific Anxiety Disorder" (p. 444) or meet criteria for Adjustment Disorder.

Also found for each disorder (other than NOS disorders) listed on Axis I are other sections providing more detailed information that may be of use to clinicians. The *Diagnostic Features* section provides an overview of the essential features of the disorder, along with examples and definitions of criteria and terms that are part of the criterion set for that disorder. The *Subtypes and/or Specifiers* section delineates subtypes of the disorder (e.g., Catatonic Subtype of Schizophrenia) or specifiers of the disorder (e.g., Postpartum Onset for Major Depressive Disorder), where applicable. The *Recording Procedures* section includes information to assist in reporting the correct name of the disorder and the associated five-digit code that corresponds to the disorder. These five-digit codes correspond to the codes listed in the *International Classification of Disease* (9th edition, with clinical modification), the diagnostic system of the

World Health Organization that includes both medical and mental disorders.

The *Associated Features and Disorders* section describes symptoms that, while not necessary for the diagnosis of the disorder, are often seen in persons with the disorder. This section also includes a listing of other mental disorders that are commonly comorbid (likely to co-occur) with the disorder, and includes a listing of laboratory findings, clinical findings from examination, and medical conditions that may be associated with the disorder. The *Specific Age, Culture, or Gender Features* section details information concerning how the symptoms of a disorder may differ as a function of these demographic variables, including how symptoms may present differently in children and the elderly, how particular symptoms of the disorder may present differently in different cultures, and the proportion of women and men among those with the disorder. The *Prevalence* section provides information estimating how common the disorder is thought to be. These estimates are taken from large-scale epidemiological studies when possible, and include estimates of point prevalence (prevalence at any point in time) as well as lifetime prevalence (the proportion of people that in their lifetimes will experience the disorder). The *Course* section details information concerning onset and progression of symptoms, as well as the prognosis for remission and for relapse. In this section are included the typical age (or ages) of onset, factors that may predispose one to develop the disorder, and information concerning whether symptoms may worsen or improve with age. Also included in this section are estimates of whether a disorder is likely to involve one episode, multiple episodes with symptom-free periods between episodes, or chronic unremitting symptoms. The *Familial Pattern* section summarizes evidence concerning whether the disorder and related disorders are more common in the first-degree biological relatives of those with the disorder than members of the general population. This section also summarizes the results of twin or adoption studies, when available. Finally, the *Differential Diagnosis* section provides information to assist the diagnostician in distinguishing the disorder from other disorders that may appear similar or that may share symptoms in common. This section highlights the differences between disorders that could possibly be confused (e.g., Major Depressive Disorder versus Adjustment Disorder with Depressed Mood or, in the elderly, Dementia).

B. Axis II: Personality Disorders and Mental Retardation

On Axis II are listed Personality Disorders and Mental Retardation. These disorders, by definition, are present for a substantial period of time (i.e., years). Although Axis I disorders may also be present for similar lengths of time, enduring symptoms are fundamentally part of these Axis II disorders. Also listed on Axis II are other traits or prominent features of a person's personality that a clinician deems maladaptive (e.g., frequent use of denial, excessive impulsivity).

In addition to the Personality Disorders, Mental Retardation appears on Axis II and is defined by (a) significantly below average intellectual abilities; (b) significant problems with adaptive functioning, defined as serious problems in carrying out duties expected for the person's age (e.g., self-care, interpersonal skills, work); and (c) an onset of these symptoms before the age of 18. Mental Retardation is placed on Axis II because of its pervasive and persistent effects on a person's function. It is worth noting that in the previous version of the *DSM* (*DSM-III-R*), other developmental disorders such as Autism and learning disorders were also listed on Axis II; these disorders, however, are listed on Axis I in *DSM-IV*.

As the term Personality Disorder implies, people with these disorders have characterological features that create difficulties. *DSM-IV* defines a Personality Disorder as follows:

> A Personality Disorder is an enduring pattern of inner experience and behavior that deviates markedly from the expectations of the individual's culture, is pervasive and inflexible, has an onset in adolescence or early adulthood, is stable over time, and leads to distress or impairment (p. 629).

Upon a casual reading of the criteria for the various personality disorders, one may see many descriptions that may seem applicable to oneself or others at times. Symptoms of various personality disorders include, as examples, emotional lability, feelings of emptiness, bearing grudges, lacking close friends, suspiciousness, impulsivity, suggestibility, feeling envious, concern with criticism or rejection, difficulty in making everyday decisions, and perfectionism. In fact, many writers have criticized the *DSM* series' Personality Disorders for pathologizing anyone who simply may be different, or difficult. A Personality Disorder, however, can (in theory) be distinguished from what might be considered normal variation in personality because a Personality Disorder is *persistent, pervasive,* and *pathological.*

By persistent, it is meant that the pattern of behavior in Personality Disorders is consistent over time. Whereas people without personality disorders may from time to time, after a bad day or following certain triggering events, display some of the features of certain personality disorders (e.g., difficulty controlling anger), such persons do not do so often or with any consistency.

By pervasive, it is meant that the behavior in Personality Disorders is seen across many different situations in the person's life. Whereas people without personality disorders may demonstrate some features of certain personality disorders in restricted situations (e.g., one is extremely suspicious of a difficult coworker; e.g., one doubts the fidelity of a spouse or sexual partner after a previously difficult and unfaithful relationship), such persons do not do so across situations (e.g., with coworkers, with spouse or partner, and with neighbors).

By pathological, it is meant that the severity of the symptom in Personality Disorders exceeds that which would be considered acceptable or normal by most people. Hot tempers, while not well-liked, are not necessarily pathological, but repeatedly getting into physical fights could be considered excessive. Daydreaming of a life more fantastic than one's own may be an occasional brief escape, but losing hours lost in fantasy could be considered excessive. Impulsive spontaneity can be fun, but impulsivity that results in overextended spending sprees, sexual indiscretions, or reckless driving could be considered excessive. Feeling empty and lonely are a part of the human condition, but suicide attempts that result from these feelings could be considered excessive. In each of these examples, what makes the behavior pathological in Personality Disorders involves the intensity of the subjective feeling, an impairment in judgment, and the degree to which the subjective feeling is translated into unacceptable or problematic behavior.

The personality disorders are organized by their apparent similarity into three clusters. Cluster A, the odd and eccentric cluster, includes the Paranoid, Schizoid, and Schizotypal Personality Disorders. Cluster B, the dramatic, emotional, and erratic cluster, includes the Antisocial, Borderline, Histrionic, and Narcissistic Personality Disorders. Finally, Cluster C, the anxious and fearful cluster, includes the Avoidant, Dependent, and Obsessive-Compulsive Personality Disorders. In addition to general criteria for Personality Disorders, each disorder has its own polythetic criterion where an individual must have some minimum number (ranging from 3 to 5 for various disorders) from among a larger number (ranging from 7 to 9 across disorders) of symptoms.

C. Axis III: General Medical Conditions

On Axis III are listed general medical conditions that may be relevant to the disorder(s) listed on Axes I and II. The presence of Axis III should not be taken to suggest a mind–brain dualism, with Axes I and II representing problems of the mind in the absence of a physiological basis. On the contrary, mental experience is rooted in the function of the brain. Axis III is included in the *DSM* to encourage a comprehensive evaluation and a consideration of the various ways in which a general medical condition may be related to mental disorders.

There are several ways in which medical conditions may be related to mental disorders. First, the medical condition may be the direct cause of the mental condition. For example, hypothyroidism (Axis III) can lead to a syndrome of depressed mood known as Mood Disorder due to Hypothyroidism (Axis I). Similarly, Alzheimer's Disease (Axis III) produces Dementia of the Alzheimer's type (Axis I), and systemic infections (Axis III) can produce a Delirium (Axis I).

The second manner in which a general medical condition may be relevant to a mental disorder is that the medical condition may be related to the development of the mental disorder, but not through direct physiological means. For example, an Axis I disorder such as Major Depression or Adjustment Disorder with Depressed Mood might follow in reaction to learning of one is diagnosed with a malignant melanoma (Axis III).

Finally, an Axis III medical condition, while not related to the appearance of the symptoms of a mental disorder, might be relevant in the treatment of a disorder. For example, certain antidepressant medications might be ill-advised in the presence of certain cardiovascular conditions. Alternatively, someone with a severe psychosis (Axis I) might have a medical condition (Axis III) that needs careful monitoring or treatment (e.g., diabetes), and might be unable to adhere to the treatment without assistance.

D. Axis IV: Psychosocial and Environmental Problems

Axis IV is included for detailing psychological, social, and environmental problems that may be relevant to the presenting mental disorder. Such problems may have influenced the development of the disorder, may have developed as a consequence of the disorder, may be relevant to the selection of an appropriate treatment, or may influence the prognosis for recovery. Although both positive (e.g., job promotion) and negative (e.g., job loss) life events can be perceived as stressful, typically only the negative events are detailed on Axis IV unless the positive event is clearly related to the mental disorder. Moreover, only events during the last year are typically noted, unless remote events still appear to be a significant influence on the mental disorder. Examples of problems that could be listed on Axis IV include death of a loved one, divorce, problems with school, unemployment or other job problems, homelessness or a difficult living situation, financial troubles, lack of insurance, legal troubles, or experiencing a natural disaster.

A careful assessment of the problems listed on Axis IV may suggest that, in some cases, the most appropriate intervention will not focus on the individual (as is the case with psychological counseling or the prescription of psychotropic medication), but rather on the broader social environment in which the individual must exist. In such cases, the primary intervention could involve not only mental health professionals (e.g., providing family therapy), but teachers, landlords, lawyers, insurance companies, and so on. On the other hand, some mental disorders may arise in the relative absence of psychosocial and environmental problems and suggest that the treatment might most fruitfully focus on the individual.

E. Axis V: Global Assessment of Functioning

Axis V provides a scale for the assessment of a person's overall level of functioning. Ratings reflect a continuum of mental health to mental illness and range from 100 (exemplary) to 1 (inordinately poor). Taken into account in making the rating are the person's psychological, social, and occupational functioning. Limitations due to purely physical limitations (e.g., spinal cord injury) are not considered when making the rating. The severity of psychological symptoms and the potential for suicide or violence are important determinants of the person's functioning rating. Global functioning is typically rated for the period surrounding the current evaluation, although it may be useful to rate, in addition, previous time periods to provide an indication of how well or poorly the individual may function at other times.

At the top end of the scale (81–100) are people who are models of mental health. These scores are reserved for those fortunate individuals who not only are without impairment, but exhibit many of the traits considered to be mentally healthy (superior functioning, wide range of interests, social effectiveness, warmth, and integrity). Just below this range (71–80) are individuals with no significant symptoms or impairment, but who lack the positive mental health features. Below this range are scores that will likely characterize a majority of individuals in need of psychological or psychiatric treatment. Those in the upper range (31–70) will most likely be capable of receiving outpatient treatment, whereas those in the lower range (1–40) will most likely require inpatient treatment.

F. Appendices to the *DSM-IV*

Included in the *DSM-IV* are 10 appendices. The appendices include a guide to facilitate differential diagnosis, a glossary, alphabetical and numerical listings of the diagnoses described in the manual, a summary of changes between the *DSM-IV* and the previous version of the *DSM*, comparisons of *DSM-IV* codes to the codes in two editions of the International Classification of Diseases, and a listing of contributors.

Worth special mention are two other appendices, *Criteria Sets and Axes Provided for Further Study*, and an *Outline for Cultural Formulation and Glossary of Culture-Bound Syndromes*. The first of these lists entries that were considered for inclusion in the *DSM-IV*, but were not included due to insufficient evidence. The disorders or axes are listed in the appendix to encourage research that will provide sufficient evidence to include or exclude these entries from future editions of the *DSM*. The appendix encourages researchers to study refinements in these sets of criteria. Examples of entries in this appendix include Caffeine Withdrawal, alternative descriptions of Schizophrenia and other disorders related to Schizophrenia, other variants of depressive disorders, Premenstrual Dysphoric Disorder, Mixed Anxiety-Depressive Disorder, a series of Medication-Induced Movement Disorders, and Passive Aggressive Personality Disorder (which appeared as an Axis II disorder in the previous edition of the *DSM*). The proposed Axes include a scale to measure strategies for coping with emotional states, termed the Defensive Functioning Scale, and two scales modeled after Axis V to measure functioning in specific areas (relationships, and social/occupational).

The appendix covering cultural variations in the presentation of mental disorders provides information that might be of assistance in evaluating individuals from cultures other than one's own. One could mistakenly label as mental illness behaviors that appear abnormal from one's own culture, but that would not be regarded as aberrant by members of the culture from which the individual originates. For example, hearing voices is typically considered a psychotic symptom by members of the mental health community, although within some religious groups the experience is supported and interpreted as an experience that is to be heeded or revered. When diagnosing, one needs to take into account how such symptoms would be viewed by fellow members of an individual's culture, which may be include religious, ethnic, racial, and geographic influences.

IV. EVALUATION OF DIAGNOSTIC SYSTEMS: RELIABILITY AND VALIDITY

A discussion of the validity of a diagnostic system must first assume that diagnoses can be assigned reliably. Reliability of diagnosis simply means that the same diagnoses will be assigned to individuals across different circumstances. Such different circumstances might involve the passage of time (in the case of test-retest reliability) or different diagnosticians (in the case of inter-rater reliability). Because symptoms of mental illness often wax and wane, test-retest reliability may not be the most appropriate means of assessing the reliability of diagnosis, since we might expect diagnoses to change over time. The standard method of assessing the reliability of the diagnosis of mental illness, therefore, is inter-rater reliability, or the extent to which two (or more) independent raters agree on the presence or on the absence of a mental illness.

A. Calculation of Inter-Rater Reliability

In assessing inter-rater reliability, one could simply calculate the overall proportion of agreement between two independent raters. This approach, however, fails to account for the proportion of time that two raters would agree merely by chance. For example, imagine that two raters agree on the presence or absence of depression 70% of the time. Although this might appear promising, one needs to compute the likelihood that they would agree by chance alone. To illustrate, imagine that these two diagnosticians each "diagnose" 100 individuals for depression with the flip of a coin. Each diagnostician therefore labels 50 individuals depressed, and 50 nondepressed. Of the 50 individuals labeled depressed by the first diagnostician, half (25) will also be diagnosed as depressed by the second diagnostician (since the second diagnostician is independently "diagnosing" by a coin flip). Similarly, among the 50 individuals labeled nondepressed by the first diagnostician, 25 will be similarly labeled by the second diagnostician. Therefore, by chance alone, these two diagnosticians would agree for 50 (25 + 25) of the 100 individuals.

Of course diagnosticians do not diagnose by coin flips, but the calculation of chance agreement follows in a similar fashion. Assume that in a particular clinic, based on the observation of symptoms, each diagnostician identifies half of the patients as depressed. Also assume, for the moment, that the diagnosticians' ratings agree only for reasons of chance. The raters would agree that 25 of the patients merit a diagnosis of depression, and would agree that 25 do not, yielding an overall agreement of 50/100 cases, or 50%. The actual agreement of 70%, while higher than that expected by chance, is not as promising as it initially appeared.

To account for chance agreement, a corrected estimate of agreement, termed *Kappa,* is often calculated:

$$\kappa = \frac{p_o - p_c}{1 - p_c}$$

Kappa reflects the extent to which the observed proportion of agreement (p_o; e.g., 70%) exceeds the proportion of agreement expected by chance (p_c; e.g., 50%), expressed as a proportion of the difference between perfect agreement (1.0) and chance agreement (e.g., 50%). Stated differently, Kappa reflects the improvement beyond chance actually obtained by the diagnosticians, expressed as a proportion of the maximum possible improvement beyond chance. Kappa therefore ranges from 0 (chance agreement) to 1.0 (perfect agreement). A Kappa of .50, for example, would indicate that the agreement of the diagnosticians fell midway between chance and perfect agreement. In the hypothetical example above, where 70% agreement was obtained, but 50% was expected by chance:

$$\kappa = \frac{p_o - p_c}{1 - p_c} = \frac{.70 - .50}{1 - .50} = \frac{.20}{.50} = .40$$

For *DSM-III* diagnoses, Kappas range from near 0 to near 1. Reliability data, while provided as an appendix in *DSM-III,* have been conspicuously absent from *DSM-III-R* and *DSM-IV* manuals. The reliability data from the *DSM-IV* field trials is promised to appear in Volume V of the *DSM-IV Sourcebook,* a compendium of the literature reviews and empirical research on which *DSM-IV* is based. Two years after the publication of the *DSM-IV,* however, only Volumes I and II of the *Sourcebook* have appeared in print. It is reasonable to assume that Kappas will again span a broad range, but on average be slightly higher than those associated with earlier versions of the *DSM.*

While Kappa provides a simple metric for summarizing agreement beyond chance, Kappa is not a panacea. Kappa is influenced by base rates of diagnosis, and Kappa provides no direct evidence of validity. The base-rate problem results when diagnoses are assigned very frequently or virtually never. In such cases, even small increases beyond chance can result in an appreciable value of Kappa. This can be problematic since the rate of many mental disorders in the general population is rather low. Imagine that two diagnosticians agree on only 4% more cases than would be expected by chance for a disorder that affects 5% of the population. If each of these diagnosticians label 5% of the sample with the diagnosis, they will agree that 90.25% (.95 * .95) of the people do not have the disorder, and will agree that fewer than 1% (.05 * .05 = .25%) of the people have the disorder. In other words, by chance alone, they would agree 90.5% of the time. If their actual agreement exceeds this by 4% (94.5%), Kappa would be .42. As can be seen from the preceding examples, it required agreement that was 20% higher than that expected by chance to achieve a Kappa in the range of .4 when the baserate of diagnosis was in the range of 50%, but it only required agreement that exceeded chance by 4% to achieve a similar Kappa when the base rate was quite low. The interpretation of Kappa is not absolute, as Kappa is considerably influenced by the base rate of diagnosis.

A second form of the base-rate problem stems from the fact that the base rate of disorders may vary dramatically by setting. For example, while schizophrenia is quite rare in the general population, it is considerably more prevalent among patients in a psychiatric hospital. Because the value of Kappa is influenced by the baserate of the diagnosis, Kappa can vary by setting even when raters apply criteria consistently across these settings.

The second caveat to consider is that Kappa provides no direct evidence of the validity of diagnosis. High values of Kappa merely indicate agreement. In fact, independent of any correspondence to the actual symptoms, perfect agreement ($\kappa = 1.0$) would be obtained if both diagnosticians agreed that every individual had the diagnosis in question. Therefore, while high values of Kappa may be necessary to ensure validity, they are by no means sufficient. Moreover, it is possible to alter diagnostic criteria to improve inter-rater agreement as indexed by Kappa, but to sacrifice validity in the process. For example, by making the criteria for a disorder increasingly tangible, one might increase agreement at the expense of making the criteria so narrow that many individuals no longer meet the criteria, despite having symptoms that many people would consider to be essential features of the disorder.

A final caution to keep in mind when considering the reliability of diagnosis, whether it be measured by Kappa or some other index, is that two raters can disagree for a variety of reasons, only some of which may reflect a poor system of diagnostic classification. For example, the particular method used to assess the symptoms (e.g., a standardized interview versus an unstructured interview) can determine what symptoms are elicited. Moreover, poor training of the diagnosticians can also lead to poor reliability. Research studies of mental illness, therefore, typically employ highly trained diagnosticians who use a standard structured interview to inquire about each of the symptoms of the disorder under study.

Reliability, therefore, should not be the sole standard by which the adequacy of diagnostic criteria are judged. Although this sounds obvious, there is a tendency for researchers to use high reliability as evidence of the adequacy of diagnostic criteria; this may be tempting since a single number can provide a summary of reliability whereas establishing validity is considerably more complicated.

B. Validity

When considering whether a set of diagnostic criteria have validity, one is asking whether assigning the diagnostic label provides valuable information—beyond the specific symptoms that begot the diagnosis—about a person with a particular diagnosis. There may be many such *external indicators* of validity, but three of the most important would include etiology, treatment, and prognosis. Additionally, and perhaps most primary, a valid system of diagnosis should allow one to clearly make distinctions between one disorder and another, and between a disorder and the absence of a disorder. Individuals who share a diagnosis should be similar to one another (in terms of symptoms, etiology, response to treatment, or prognosis) and should be clearly different than individuals with other diagnoses or individuals with no diagnosis. If such a clear delineation is not possible, then there is insufficient evidence to justify the existence of the diagnostic category. The *DSM-IV* in particular has been criticized for inadequately distinguishing between mental disorders and normal variations in behavior. For example, although significant depressive symptoms that follow the death of a loved one are considered a normal reaction (for a period, incidentally, of up to 2 months), depressive symptoms following other major losses or setbacks (e.g., divorce, diagnosis with a terminal illness) are considered evidence of the mental disorder Major Depression.

In terms of etiology, a valid system would ensure that people with the same diagnostic label would share a common etiology. In some instances in the *DSM-IV,* this is clearly the case (e.g., Alcohol Withdrawal Delirium, also known as "delirium tremens"); in other instances, it is likely that people with the same diagnosis may have different etiological influences (e.g., Major Depressive Disorder).

In terms of treatment, a valid system should suggest particular treatments that are likely to be effective for a particular disorder. Alternatively, since no treatments are 100% effective, a valid system should inform us of the likelihood that different treatments may be effective for the disorder. For example, given an episode of Major Depression that has lasted less than 2 years, there is a 50 to 70% chance that an individual will experience remission using one of several antidepressant medications, or by receiving one of two varieties of psychotherapy.

In terms of prognosis, a valid system should provide an indication of what is likely to happen in the future given that a person has a particular diagnosis. For example, given that a person has experienced one episode of Major Depression, there is approximately a 50% chance that the person will experience another at some point in life. Given that one has a personality disorder diagnosis, it is likely that the pattern of behavior will continue for quite some time, if not indefinitely.

V. CHALLENGES TO VALIDITY AND FUTURE DIRECTIONS IN DIAGNOSIS

The *DSM-IV,* like its predecessors, has adopted a *descriptive categorical approach* to diagnosis, which assumes that there exist *discrete categories* of mental illness that can be defined—for most diagnoses—primarily on the basis of observable symptoms. Discrete categories of illness dichotomize individuals into those who do, and those who do not, have the illness; borderline cases are categorized into one or the other category (or given one of the may NOS diagnoses). When the etiology of an illness is known, the categorical approach is defensible and is likely to provide useful information. For example, people either do or do not have a history of a stroke. Within the category of those with strokes, there are certainly gradations in severity, but there is a clear delineation between those who have, and those who have not, experienced a stroke. In the case of most mental disorders, by contrast, there are not such obvious distinctions between the presence and the absence of the condition. For example, *DSM-IV* requires that five of nine symptoms be present in order to make the diagnosis of a Major

Depressive Episode. Certainly people who meet four of the nine symptoms are not free of depression, yet they would not be categorized as having a Major Depressive Episode.

Strictly speaking, a categorical approach assumes that there exist necessary and sufficient features for categorical membership. Although the *DSM-IV* adopts a categorical approach, there are many instances of disorders that do not have necessary or sufficient criteria. Consider for example, the case of Obsessive-Compulsive Personality Disorder, for which an individual must meet at least four of eight possible criteria to receive the diagnosis. None of the individual criteria are necessary and, moreover, two individuals could both meet criteria and share not a single one of the criteria in common. In other words, there can exist considerable heterogeneity in symptoms among those who share a common diagnosis.

Strictly speaking, a categorical approach also assumes that categories are either nested, or mutually exclusive. For example, a square is a special (nested) case of a rectangle, but is mutually exclusive with the category of circle. For diagnoses of mental illness, by contrast, there exists considerable overlap (comorbidity) of diagnoses. A recent large-scale community study found that, across the life span, about one-sixth of the population had three (or more) diagnoses, and that this group accounted for over half all diagnoses. Such high comorbidity certainly raises questions as to whether the categorical approach to diagnosis is justified. When comorbidity of diagnoses is observed, it is unclear whether the different disorders reflect different manifestations of the same underlying cause, whether one disorder served to facilitate the development of another, or whether the disorders resulted from different underlying causes and merely co-occurred by chance. Comorbidity can also present an enigma in terms of treatment, as it can be unclear which disorder to treat, or how to coordinate treatments for different disorders.

A modification to the classical categorical approach is the *prototype* approach, in which exemplars (also known as prototypes) of a given diagnosis become the standard for comparison. Each individual is compared to the diagnostic prototypes, and assigned the diagnosis associated with the best-fitting prototype. Such a system has several advantages. Such a system eliminates the problem of borderline cases, since such cases will receive a diagnosis if they are more similar to the diagnostic prototype than to any other prototype. Such a system also virtually eliminates the need for the NOS categories, which in the *DSM* seem to have become the "wastebasket" for many borderline or unusual cases. On the other hand, a prototype system has its drawbacks. Prototypes stem from the perceptions of the diagnosticians, and therefore may fail to reflect important features of a disorder that are not easily observable (e.g., lab findings). Moreover, the use of prototypes may make the identification of new disorders more difficult, and instead simply reify the implicit theories that people have about forms of mental illness. Finally, to distinguish mental health from mental illness, one would presumably require a prototype of mental health. Although it could be difficult to define a single prototype for each diagnostic category, it might be even more challenging to define the prototype(s) for mental health.

Other modifications to the categorical approach of the *DSM-IV* have been proposed, including eliminating categories entirely. The dimensional approach involves assessing individuals along a set of relevant dimensions. Under such a system, an individual would receive a quantitative rating along each dimension in the diagnostic system. Although the conceptual simplicity of a category may be lost using such a system, such a system could possibly convey more information about each individual, would eliminate the problem of classifying borderline cases, and would have no problems of comorbidity. On the other hand, many diagnosticians prefer the yes-or-no simplicity of categorical diagnosis, and may be likely to establish idiosyncratic cutpoints on the dimensions, such that those individuals scoring above a certain value would be considered to have a particular categorical diagnosis. Additionally, it is no trivial matter to determine the relevant set of dimensions to use in such a system.

In the final analysis, there may exist some types of problems for which a categorical system is well-suited, and others where a dimensional approach may hold greater utility. The *DSM-IV* is already an amalgam of different approaches to categorization, with some diagnoses clearly defined by etiology, and others defined solely by the presence of particular symptoms. This may reflect the nature of different forms of mental illness. Some forms may have a single causal factor that is more potent than all other contributing factors, and have a homogeneous set of symptoms that appear.

Others, by contrast, may have multiple determinants, and may present with a heterogeneous set of symptoms that differ for each individual.

The *DSM-IV* is the current version of the most widely-used diagnostic system for mental disorders. If history provides an accurate indication, many other revisions—some major, and some minor—are likely to follow, with considerable controversy and debate surrounding each.

BIBLIOGRAPHY

American Psychiatric Association (1987). *Diagnostic and statistical manual of mental disorders* (3rd ed., revised). Washington, DC: American Psychiatric Association.

American Psychiatric Association (1994). *Diagnostic and statistical manual of mental disorders* (4th ed.). Washington, DC: American Psychiatric Association.

Cantor, N., Smith, E. E., deSales French, R., & Mezzich, J. (1980). Psychiatric diagnosis as prototype categorization. *Journal of Abnormal Psychology, 89,* 181–193.

Clark, L. A., Watson, D., & Reynolds, S. (1995). Diagnosis and classification of psychopathology: Challenges to the current system and future directions. *Annual Review of Psychology, 46,* 121–153.

Kessler, R. C., McGonagle, K. A., Shanyang, Z., Nelson, C. B., Hughes, M., Eshlemen, S., Wittchen, H., Kendler, K. (1994). Lifetime and 12-month prevalence of *DSM-III*-R Psychiatric Disorders in the United States: Results from the National Comorbidity Study. *Archives of General Psychiatry, 51,* 8–19.

Kirk, S. A., & Kutchins, H. (1992). The selling of DSM: The rhetoric of science in psychiatry. New York: Walter de Gruyter, Inc.

Robins, L. N., & Barrett, J. E. (1989). The validity of psychiatric diagnosis. New York: Raven Press Ltd.

Rosenhan, D. L. (1973). On being sane in insane places. *Science, 179,* 250–258.

Wakefield, J. C. (1996). DSM-IV: Are we making progress? *Contemporary Psychology, 41,* 646–652.

Family Therapy

Philip Barker
University of Calgary and Alberta Children's Hospital

Circular Causation A causal chain in which there is a series of events, each influencing another, the process continuing in a circular manner.
Disengagement The opposite of enmeshment (see below).
Enmeshment The close emotional involvement of two or more people.
Family Structure The ways in which the different family members, or groups of members, are allied, and the nature and strengths of the alliances.
Family System The parts of a family and the ways in which they interact to make up a functioning entity that is more than the sum of the parts.
Linear Causation One event causes another but the second event does not affect the first event.
Strategic Therapy A therapeutic method that uses a carefully planned, usually indirect, approach to promoting changes in families.

FAMILY THERAPY is a treatment approach that takes the family unit as its focus. Family therapists understand the emotional and behavioral problems of individuals as often being related to problems in the family systems of which they are part. They believe that by working to promote change in the family, the symptoms and problems of the family's members will be resolved, or at least ameliorated. Sometimes, but less often, it is the family as a group that presents with problems. An important feature of the family therapy approach is an emphasis on the concept of *circular,* rather than *linear* causation. Family therapists are reluctant to regard events or behaviors in families as due to single, isolated causes, but tend to see them as parts of, usually complex, chains of events.

I. THE DEVELOPMENT OF FAMILY THERAPY

The family therapy approach to the treatment of mental health problems was developed during the years that followed the Second World War. Psychotherapists of various mental health disciplines, together with researchers from other disciplines, began to look at their patients' families as possibly contributing to the disorders they were treating. The idea that families might have a part in the genesis of psychiatric disorders was not new. Freud and others from the early days of psychoanalysis had postulated that the early childhood family relationships of their patients had caused the neurosis with which these patients presented. In those early days, however, the response was to separate the patients from their families for treatment. This was accomplished either by seeing patients for treatment on their own while having minimal or no contact with their families; or by admitting them to psychiatric hospitals or other institutions where they could be cared for and treated away from the supposed adverse influences of their families. What *was* new was the idea that it was possible to work with families, in the here and now, to change their

Copyright © 1998 by Academic Press.
All rights of reproduction in any form reserved.

ways of functioning; and that this might be a quicker and more effective approach than individual psychotherapy with individual patients.

One of the first to point out the importance of the family was Christian Midelfort whose book, *The Family in Psychotherapy,* was published in 1957. Despite its promising title, however, this was not truly a book about family therapy. More important was Nathan Ackerman's *The Psychodynamics of Family Life,* published the following year. Like many of the pioneers of family therapy, Ackerman came from a background of psychoanalytic training, and his first book reflects this. But he pointed out that while psychiatrists had become adept in the retrospective study of mental illness and in the careful examination of family histories, they had not yet cultivated an equivalent skill in the study of current family processes. Ackerman went on to suggest that, by acquiring skills in working with whole family groups, we would add a new dimension to our understanding of mental illness as an ongoing process—and one that changes with time and the conditions of group adaptation.

By 1966 Ackerman's thinking had developed further and his second book, *Treating the Troubled Family,* was probably the first true single-author family therapy book published. By the mid-1960s many groups, several of which had commenced their studies and treatment of families in the 1950s, were publishing their findings. Among the other early pioneers in family therapy were Murray Bowen, Don Jackson, John Elderkin Bell, Don Jackson, Jay Haley, John Weakland, Virginia Satir, Lyman Wynn, Salvador Minuchin and Ivan Boszormenyi-Nagy. Each therapist, or group of therapists, developed a particular approach and theoretical framework. While these often differed substantially, they had in common their focus on the family group and how it functioned. The enthusiasm of some of these pioneers was unbounded, and extreme claims for the effectiveness, or at least the potential, for family therapy were sometimes made. All, or almost all, psychiatric problems came to be seen by some as residing, not in individuals, but in the processes of interaction going on in the person's family or other social group or groups.

Over the years, most of these extreme views have become modified. Family therapy has come to be regarded as a useful therapeutic option and the treatment of choice in many cases. But it is not a cure-all and it may need to be used along with other treatments. The almost religious zeal of some of the early pioneers has been toned down by the harsh reality of clinical experience and the results of research. Many of the pioneers paid particular attention to patients with schizophrenia, the origins of which, they believed, lay in the family. However the failure of family therapy to prove effective as a primary treatment, combined with increasing knowledge of the neurochemical and biological correlates of the condition and the greater effectiveness of pharmacological treatments, has resulted in a shift of focus toward other disorders. Nevertheless, more recent research has shown that family factors are by no means irrelevant in schizophrenia, and may determine whether relapse occurs after patients return home following treatment in hospital.

II. THEORETICAL CONCEPTS

A. Systems Theory

A way of thinking about families that was seized on early in the development of family therapy was that of *general systems theory.* This theory, originally developed in the 1950s, is concerned with how parts are organized into wholes. Although it was not designed with families in mind, systems theory was found to fit in well with the thinking of many of the early family therapists. The idea that families are open systems has continued to be central to the work of virtually all family therapists. The task of the systems-based therapist thus becomes that of first determining how the family system is functioning, and then facilitating any changes that appear to be required in the way it functions. The systems-oriented therapist expects that once the needed changes in family functioning have been achieved, the symptoms of the member(s) who have been experiencing difficulties will be resolved, or at least ameliorated.

What exactly are the basic principles of systems theory that family therapists have found useful? In summary, they are that:

- Families, and other social groups, are systems that have properties that are more than the sum of the properties of their parts.

- Certain general rules govern the functioning of such systems.
- Every system has a boundary. The boundaries of family systems are permeable in varying degrees, so that some families are more readily, and to a greater extent, influenced by what is going on around them than are others.
- Family systems typically reach relatively steady states; that is, each family settles down to function in its own characteristic way, although change can occur; indeed growth and evolution are usual as the composition of the family changes, its members age, and changes occur in the wider systems of which it is a part.
- The amount and quality of the communications between the parts of the system, are important features.
- The concept of *circular causality* is preferred to that of *linear causality*.
- Family systems, like other systems, appear to be purposeful. They serve such purposes as the rearing of children; the provision of mutual comfort and a context for the expression of the marital partners' sexuality; and the promotion of the economic security of the family group.
- Systems are made up of *subsystems* and are parts of larger *suprasystems*.

Many individuals and families come to therapists asking to be told the "cause" of the problem that is concerning them. They tend to see causality in linear terms. An example of linear causality is the action of a man who puts up his umbrella when it starts to rain. The cause is clear—it is raining—and so is the result—up goes the umbrella. It is not usually believed that putting up the umbrella affects the weather. But in families things are seldom, if ever, that simple. If person A tells person B to do something, and B does it, this in turn will affect the behavior of A, who may, for example, be more likely to ask B to do the same task again when the need arises. There may also be similar, or perhaps opposite, effects on the behavior of other family members.

Let us consider a family in which there is a boy who is anxious about going to school. When it is time to leave for school, the boy cries, clings to his mother, and refuses to leave the house. The mother turns for help to her husband. He fails to give her support and even blames her for not being firm enough with the boy. Instead he speaks angrily to his son. This increases the boy's anxiety and his tears flow even more freely. This leads to the mother becoming yet more worried and upset; she comforts the boy and then turns with even greater force to her husband who gets even more angry with the boy, and perhaps with the mother also. So whose problem is it? Is it the mother's anxiety about her son that results in her being unable to support her son calmly in the task of separating from her to go to school? Or is the basic problem that of a boy who is (for whatever reasons) emotionally immature and constitutionally prone to react anxiously in situations perceived as threatening? Or is the real problem a dysfunctional parental or marital relationship? Or maybe the cause of it all is an angry, dominating, verbally abusive father? And so on. In other words, who or what is causing the problem? Considering this scenario, some might try to answer these questions in a straightforward way. The family therapist interested in circular causality, however, would not consider it useful to do so. All the problems implied in the questions might indeed exist but none is "the cause." They are all simply—or perhaps not so simply—part of a circular process. To put it another way, they all reflect characteristics of the way the family systems works.

B. Learning Theory

Many other theoretical concepts are used by family therapists. Therapy, whether or not it is addressed to the family system, may be looked on as a teaching and learning process. When we are treating families there is nearly always a need for the family to learn such things as new ways of relating to each other; new approaches on the part of the parents to rearing their children; new ways of allocating the tasks the family members must, between them, ensure are done; perhaps a new type of marital relationship.

While few family therapists would regard themselves simply as teachers, and family therapy is much more than telling people what they should do, learning must happen during the treatment if change is to occur. Learning is conceptualized to occur in several ways:

a. In *respondent conditioning,* a behavior is learned when a rewarding stimulus is paired with a desired behavior. Pavlov's much quoted dogs learned to associate the ringing of a bell with the presentation of food. After a while they salivated in response to the ringing of the bell, without the presentation of any food.

b. In *operant conditioning* the circumstances following a behavior are altered either to reinforce the behavior or to extinguish it. In other words it consists of the systematic, and, ideally, carefully planned, application of positive and negative responses (or, in everyday language, rewards and punishments).

c. *Modeling* is the process by which people acquire behaviors by imitating others. It need not be, and usually is not, a conscious process. Therapists can, and regularly do, model behaviors during their sessions with their clients. The respectful way the therapist addresses family members; how the therapist talks or plays with a child; or how the therapist reacts to things family members do or say—all these and many other behaviors carry messages.

d. *Learning by cognition* occurs when a person thinks something through and comes to a conclusion as a result. In lay terms, it is the process of "figuring things out."

All of these learning processes may occur during family therapy. The therapist must devise ways of tapping into the potential all people have to learn new behaviors, concepts, and ways of viewing things.

C. Communications Theory

The processes of communication within families are of great interest to family therapists. In many families with problems, communication is deficient in some way. It may be insufficient, unclear, indirect or contradictory, or the information communicated may be just incorrect. Also important is the process of communication between therapist and family. Much attention has therefore been given to communication theory by family therapists.

Therapists are concerned with *syntax,* the grammatical rules of a language; *semantics,* the meaning of words and how they are put together to convey meaning, including the clarity of language and how it is used in particular situations; and *pragmatics,* the study of the behavioral effects of communication. These latter effects are related as much to the nonverbal communications that go along with the words spoken, as to the words themselves. Indeed sometimes the nonverbal is the essence of the communication—a laugh, perhaps.

Many other aspects of communication have been studied by family therapists. Communications can define relationships; how we talk to our bosses may be very different than how we talk to our employees, our children, or our spouses. Also it is impossible, if one is in the presence of another person, not to communicate. Simply remaining silent, or looking away or busying oneself with someone or something else can carry powerful messages.

Family therapists are interested in whether communications between family members are *symmetrical* or *complementary.* In symmetrical communication the participants are on an equal footing. Complementary interaction occurs when the participants are not on an equal footing; examples would be many (but not necessarily all) doctor–patient, penitent–confessor, teacher–student, and master–servant interactions.

Two other types of communication merit mention here. One is the paradoxical statement. A simple example is the sentence, "I am lying." Another would be, "I will call you when you least expect me to." Related to this is the much written about "double-bind." This is a rather more sophisticated way of giving contradictory messages simultaneously. The double-bind occurs when there are two people in an intense relationship. Two injunctions are given that are incompatible, but the person concerned feels a strong need to obey them both. The subject cannot discuss the conflict (in other words metacommunication—that is, communication about the communication—is not possible), and cannot escape from the situation. Cinderella was placed in a double-bind when her stepmother told her that of course she could go to the ball at the palace, but she must finish the work allocated to her before she could get ready. This was impossible in the time available and only the intervention of her fairy godmother and the latter's magic spell enabled Cinderella to attend.

The double-bind has been frequently observed in the families of patients with schizophrenia, and in the early days of family therapy it was thought by some that it played a part in the causation of the condition. The idea was that, after repeated "double-bind" experiences over a long period of time, a person might be driven to forsake reality for a psychotic world. In due course, however, it was discovered that the double-bind was common in many other families and it is no longer generally considered to be an important etiological factor in schizophrenia. Much the same applies to the concept of "communication deviance," a form of aberrant communication described during the early studies of schizophrenic patients. More recently, evidence has emerged that "expressed emotion" is important. While a high level of expressed emotion in the family is not thought to be a *cause* of schizophrenia, it does seem that it may lead to relapse after treatment away from the family has been successful in producing a remission.

D. Family Structure

The concept of *family structure,* either overtly expressed or implied, is common to many schools of family therapy. It was well described by Salvador Minuchin in his 1974 book, *Families and Family Therapy.* It is related to systems theory concepts in that the perceived "structure" in a family system consists of the various subsystems in the family and the nature—that is strength and permeability—of the boundaries between them.

A typical, well-functioning family might have quite a simple structure: a parental subsystem and a child subsystem. In two-parent families some would distinguish the parent subsystem from the marital subsystem, since the way a couple relate as a marital pair is often distinct from how they function as parental couple. There might be expected to be a well-defined, but not overly rigid and impermeable boundary between the parental and the child subsystems.

The nature of the boundaries that exist between the subsystems in families is of great interest to the structural family therapist. Related to this are the concepts of *enmeshment* and *disengagement.* Enmeshment is said to exist when the boundaries between family members or subsystems are weak and readily permeable; it implies an overclose involvement of those concerned. When families members are enmeshed, their behaviors and, often, emotional states have marked effects on each other. In contrast to this, if members are disengaged, the behavior of one member will have little effect on those with whom the member is disengaged.

In a less well-functioning family one might find a different subsystem pattern. For example, there might be a subsystem consisting of the mother in an enmeshed relationship with one or two children, and another comprising the father. The boundary between the two subsystems might be robust, with little interaction or communication of feeling between them.

Many other family structures may be encountered; indeed the possibilities are limitless. In larger families there may be more than one child subsystem; for example, an older child subsystem and a younger child one, or male and female subsystems. And the structural problems may not be confined to the nuclear family. The extended family—grandparents, uncles, aunts, and other relatives—may be involved. So may friends, school staff and others, depending on the boundary between the family and its suprasystems.

E. Family Development

Families are not static entities. They change and develop. Among the considerations the therapist working with a family must take into account and is where the family is in its life cycle, for families have life cycles, just as individuals do. Moreover, many family problems prove to be associated with difficulties in proceeding from one stage of the life cycle to the next.

The family life cycle has been described and subdivided in a variety of ways. In summary, however, it is generally as follows. The starting point is arbitrary:

- The single adult person.
- Two single adults get together as a couple. Traditionally they get married, but in many societies nowadays a formal marriage ceremony is not required. This may be termed the childless couple stage.
- The couple have a child, often going on to have several more. We now have the couple with young children.
- The oldest child starts school. The family enters the stage of the couple with school-age children.
- The oldest child enters adolescence.
- The first child (it need not be the oldest) leaves home. This is the family launching its children into the wider world.
- The last child leaves home. This is the start of the "empty nest" stage.
- Retirement, aging, and grandparenthood.

The above is necessarily an oversimplification. Clearly, a family can be, and indeed will often be, in several stages at the same time. Some children may be in school while others have not started; some will have reached adolescence and others will not have. The parents may even have retired before all the children have left home. An additional complication is that many families do not follow the above course. We see, for example, family groups that have only contained one parent from the start; others disrupted by divorce or the death of one parent; blended families of various types; homosexual couples, with or without children; families in which it is the grandparents who are caring for the children.

What the family therapist must do, with every family that presents, is determine where the family is in its life cycle, and whether it is encountering any difficulty in moving from one stage to the next. It is often found that a family has functioned well at one stage, perhaps before the arrival of children, but does less well at the next, for example, when a third member, in that case a newborn child, is added. But any transition can present a challenge, as can single parenthood, blended family situations, and other special circumstances—for example, the incarceration of a family member.

The family therapist's work becomes even more complex when families have become split up because of separation or divorce, an increasingly common scenario in many contemporary societies. The children's time may be divided between the separated parents, whose conflicts and disagreements may persist despite the separation or divorce. Emotional problems, conflicts of loyalties, financial hardship and disputes, and custody and access issues may be sources of stress to all concerned. Often the children suffer most, and they sometimes come to play the role of pawns in ongoing "battles" between their parents. One or both parents may be in new relationships, which can complicate matters further.

In these situations the therapist may come to play the role of mediator, maintaining a neutral stance and being careful not to become overidentified with the point of view of any party. At the same time the well-being of all concerned, especially the children (who tend to be most at risk), must be the primary concern of the therapist. In these often unfortunate, even tragic, situations therapists may need to cast their nets wide and involve more than just the specific family grouping that has initially sought help—regardless of who is paying.

III. SCHOOLS OF FAMILY THERAPY

Many different approaches have been, and continue to be, used by therapists in their efforts to promote change in families. As the field developed, most of the pioneers became identified with particular methods, and so "schools" of family therapy came to be identified. Nevertheless, there was, from the start, much overlap between the methods of different therapists and schools. It can also be difficult to know how far the success of a particular approach is due, on the one hand, to the theoretical underpinnings and the methods used and, on the other hand, to the personality and charisma of the therapist. Many of the pioneers were powerful personalities, with well-developed interpersonal skills and great powers of persuasion. Even today, the ability of therapists to establish rapport with the families they treat, and to be convincing in the interventions they offer, is probably at least as important as their theoretical persuasion or the school of therapy to which they subscribe. Subject to the above provisos, here are brief descriptions of some of the main schools of family therapy.

A. Structural Family Therapy

We have seen how this approach looks at the subsystem pattern within the family and the nature and strength of the boundaries between the subsystems. Structural therapists first assess the existing family structure and how this may be related to the problems the family is experiencing; and then they set out to assist the family in making the changes that seem to be needed. The following are considered:

- The arrangements, or unwritten "rules," that govern the interactions between family members.
- The flexibility of the family's way of functioning, and how easily it can change.
- The family's "resonance." This is the extent to which family members are enmeshed or disengaged.
- The family's life context, that is, the relevant suprasystems.
- The family's developmental stage.
- How the symptoms of the family member(s) who are presented for treatment fit into the family's transactional patterns.

B. Approaches Using Communications Theory

Here the emphasis is on the patterns and styles of communication in the family. It was observed, from the earliest days of the family therapy movement, that families with symptomatic members often had major communication problems. These may involve:

- The cognitive understanding of what the members are saying to each other. What one member intends to convey to another is not correctly understood.
- The communication of feeling. It is often important, if a family is to function well without any members developing symptoms, for the members to be able to communicate effectively to each other how they feel.
- Communication and power. Jay Haley has eloquently pointed out that when one person communicates with another, that person is maneuvering to define a relationship. This probably does not apply to every communication. Some are simply intended to provide needed information, such as what time it is. Yet if one person has persistently to ask another one—the same other one—for the time this may say something about the relationship between the two.

Distinguishing one school of family therapy as particularly concerned with communication should not be taken to mean that therapists of other schools are not interested in family communication. It is merely a matter of emphasis. Indeed, Haley, who has been described as being of the "communication and power" school, also emphasizes the importance of establishing appropriate hierarchical arrangements within families—a concept that has much in common with structural therapy.

C. Behavioral Family Therapy

Therapists who take a behavioral approach lean heavily on learning theory. They understand the dysfunctional or deviant behaviors occurring in the families they treat as learned responses that can be replaced by more functional behaviors and ways of reacting by the use of behavioral techniques such as those outlined above. A prominent practitioner of and researcher in behavioral interventions with families is Gerald Patterson. Like most behaviorists he tends to be precise in his definition of problem behaviors, carrying out a careful analysis of what is happening—especially what appears to be maintaining the undesired behaviors—before devising interventions in the family system designed to produce behavioral change. [*See* BEHAVIOR THERAPY.]

D. Extended Family Systems Therapy

The extended family systems approach is sometimes referred to as the "three generational approach." Therapists of this school pay particular attention to the extended families of their patients. They are impressed by the way behaviors and ways of relating seem to be handed down from one generation to the next. They emphasize the role of the families of origin of the family members in influencing current family functioning; and they play close attention to the ongoing relationships the families they treat have with their extended families. Many of their therapeutic interventions take into account, or actually involve, the extended family.

Murray Bowen has often been included among the ranks of the "extended family systems" school, and rightly so, but his own theory differs from that of most others. He has maintained that many family problems arise because the family members have not differentiated themselves psychologically from their families of origin, a problem he saw himself having before he made a "voyage of discovery" to his family of origin. He also described the "undifferentiated ego mass," later preferring the term "nuclear family emotional system." A major aim of the therapist using Bowen's theory is to assist family members in differentiating themselves from the "undifferentiated ego mass." This, he asserts, enables them to function independently and autonomously, for example, as members of their own newly created families.

Whether there is a true *school* of extended family therapy may be questioned. Indeed it is probable that none of the schools we are discussing here exists in pure form. What we are describing are the points, the aspects of therapy, to which each school pays particular attention.

E. Experiential Family Therapy

Therapists who come under the "experiential" rubric tend to eschew theory. Instead, they join the family system and allow themselves to become involved in the intense interactions between the family members. Carl Whitaker and Walter Kempler are the best-known proponents of this approach. They do not offer us a consistent theory, but rather trust their instincts, or what Whitaker called, "The accumulated and organized residue of experience, plus the freedom to allow the relationship to happen, to be who you are with the minimum of anticipatory set and maximum responsiveness to authenticity and to our own growth impulses." This school of therapy is probably best experienced; if you cannot do that, the next best thing is to read the writings of Whitaker, Kempler, and their ilk.

F. Psychodynamic Family Therapy

In a sense, this is a contradiction in terms, since family therapy is concerned with family systems, and not primarily with the psychopathology of family members. But many of the figures who played major roles in the early development of family therapy came to it from a psychoanalytic background. As far as there is such a thing as psychodynamic family therapy, it seems to be therapy that aims to help family members gain insight into themselves and how they react with each other. [*See* PSYCHOANALYSIS.]

Psychoanalytic thinking informed the early work of Nathan Ackerman, as well as that of Virginia Satir. However, Satir was a therapist of many parts who seemed to draw her ideas from a wide variety of sources.

G. Strategic Family Therapy

The "strategic" school of therapy is less well defined than some of the other schools. Cloe Madanes, in her 1981 book, *Strategic Family Therapy,* suggested that it is the "responsibility of the therapist to plan a strategy to solve the client's problems." She saw strategic therapy stemming from the work of Milton Erickson, who often used indirect means of promoting change in his patients. These means are discussed below in the section "Indirect Interventions and Injunctions." A problem with the term "strategic therapy," however, is that presumably every effective therapist uses strategies of some sort in attempting to assist families make the changes they seek. It is thus somewhat imprecise.

This brief overview comes nowhere near to covering all the schools of, or approaches to, family therapy. It is presented to make the point that there are many possible approaches to the task of helping families change.

IV. ASSESSING FAMILIES

Regardless of their theoretical orientation, all therapists must first come to an understanding of the changes in the family system that need to be made to resolve the problems that therapy is to address. This involves some sort of assessment, although how detailed it is varies from therapist to therapist. The experiential therapists probably emphasize assessment least. Therapists of most other schools have systematic ways of assessing families along a variety of parameters. As an example, we will consider the Process Model of Family Functioning, which resembles and was in part derived from McMaster Model of Family Functioning. This considers six aspects of family functioning:

A. Task Accomplishment

Task accomplishment is similar to the "problem solving" of the McMaster model. It involves:

- Identifying the tasks to be accomplished;
- Exploring what approaches might be used and selecting one;
- Taking action;
- Observing the results of the action and making any necessary adjustments.

Both models consider three categories of tasks: *basic, developmental,* and *crisis.* Basic tasks are such things as the provision of food, clothing, and shelter. Developmental tasks are those required as the family moves from one developmental stage to the next. Crisis tasks are those presented by such events as the death or serious illness of a family member, job loss, natural disaster, or migration from one culture or another.

B. Role Performance

In a well-functioning family each member has a role, or habitual pattern of behavior. Together, these ensure that everything that needs to be done is done, and each family member's role is an appropriate one. In dysfunctional families it may be found that members, often those with symptoms, have assumed "idiosyncratic" roles, such as family scapegoat, "parental" child, sick member, or disturbed or "crazy" member.

C. Communication, Including Affective Expression

We have seen how important communication is in families, and what some of the main communication problems tend to be. In many families, problems in communication are among the main issues that need to be addressed in therapy.

D. Affective Involvement

This is the degree and quality of family members' interest in and concern for one another. The following types of involvement have been distinguished:

- Lack of involvement. The family members occupy the same house but behave rather like strangers.
- Interest or involvement devoid of feelings.
- Narcissistic involvement. In this case, one family member is involved with another to bolster his or own feelings of self-worth, not because of any real concern for the other person.
- Empathic involvement. Here there is real caring and concern for the needs of the other person. This results in responses which meet the needs of that person.
- Overinvolvement, or enmeshment. This was described above.

E. Control ("Behavior Control" in the McMaster model)

This is a measure of he influence the family members have on the behavior of other family members.

F. Values and Norms

This dimension appears only in the Process Model.

The above is but one of many schemata that are used by therapists of differing schools to understand the families that seek their help. It is quoted to give a flavor of the types of information that interest family therapists.

V. HELPING FAMILIES CHANGE

Promoting change is, of course, the essence of family therapy. To achieve this the therapist must have a coherent theory of change. This can be based on any of the theoretical schemes outlined above, or on others that exist. The therapist's theory of change is then the basis for the interventions he or she employs. The actual techniques used vary widely, but certain stages are required:

a. The establishment of rapport. As rapport develops, the participants become intensively involved with each other; trust also develops. The process has been given other names; some therapists refer to it as "joining" the family or "building working alliances." The process may occur quickly or it may take an entire session, even several. It involves both verbal and nonverbal techniques. Time spent establishing rapport is, however, seldom wasted. Lack of sufficient rapport is a major cause of failure in family therapy—and indeed in most endeavors that involve relationships with others.

b. Intervening in the family system. Having joined with the family, there are many ways the therapist may intervene in its transactional patterns. They may be divided into direct and indirect interventions.

A. Direct Interventions or Injunctions

Since family therapy aims to help families find new ways of functioning, a simple and straightforward approach is to offer the family suggestions, designed to help them make the changes that the assessment has shown to be needed in their way of functioning. The suggestions might be concerned with how family members could behave differently toward each other, or communicate more effectively, or alter their respective roles in the family—or whatever appears to be needed. They will also be related to the therapist's theory of change.

Direct injunctions should be more than the giving of common-sense advice, because they must be based on a careful assessment of the changes the family needs to make. Families presenting for therapy, while aware that they have problems, or that family members have symptoms, often do not know what changes are needed to achieve the objectives they desire. Indeed, when asked what they are seeking from therapy, many family members reply by saying that they want answers to "why" questions such as: "Why is my child stealing?" "Why won't my teenager daughter eat properly?" "Why have my husband and I drifted so far apart?"

"Why" questions are not unreasonable, but giving definitive answers to them is often difficult and frequently impossible. Who really knows the true motivation of anyone doing anything? It is generally better to focus on the changes that are desired by the participants, and how these may be achieved, than to spend time discussing the possible reasons why problems exist. The family members may be asked to describe, preferably in some detail, how things will be when treatment has come to a successful conclusion. (It is better to talk about *when,* not *if,* treatment has been successful; this is the process of "programming for success.") The desired state is sometimes referred to as the "outcome frame."

Once the outcome frame has been established the therapist, using the information that has been obtained during the assessment of the family, can then devise some interventions. Direct ones should probably be the first to be used, unless the history shows that they have been given a fair trial previously and have proved unsuccessful. Examples of direct interventions are:

- Rehearsing the family in communication techniques; these might aim to promote the direct, clear, and sufficient communication of information, opinions, and feelings between family members;
- Discussing the roles the various family members have been playing, and how these might be altered if it appears that alterations would be helpful;
- Proposing behavioral interventions to deal with undesired behaviors, or promote desired behaviors, on the part of the children;
- Suggesting, or modeling, more respectful ways for the family members to interact with each other;
- Helping family members to affirm and support each other, instead of the mutual criticism that is often encountered in families with problems.

Behavioral family therapy tends to use predominantly direct methods. The contingencies that appear to be controlling the behaviors that need to be changed are addressed directly.

Therapists of most schools are open to addressing dysfunctional patterns of interaction directly, and in some families this approach proves effective, especially when it is used in the context of a high degree of rapport. Unfortunately, especially in the more severely dysfunctional families, direct injunctions may be rejected or are not given an adequate trial even if lip service is paid to implementing them.

B. Indirect Interventions or Injunctions

The changes that may result from direct interventions, as outlined in the section above, tend to be what are often referred to as "first order change." This implies that although the behaviors of one or more family members have changed, there have not been the more fundamental changes in the family that may be needed and are implied by the term "second order change." Direct interventions may leave the functioning of the family system fundamentally unchanged, even though communication may be clearer, roles better defined, and so on.

The terms "strategic" and "systemic" are used for treatment approaches that aim to bring about more radical changes. These may involve alterations of perspective among the family members, so that some aspects of the way the family functions come to be viewed and understood in new ways. This is the process of "reframing"—the giving of different meaning to behavior, feelings or relationships. In "developmental reframing," for example, the antisocial behavior of an adolescent may be reframed as "immature," rather than "bad." "He's not really a bad kid, he's just having trouble growing up." Getting a family, including the young person who is displaying the troublesome behavior, to see the problem behaviors in this light represents second order change. The very process of developmental reframing may affect the young person's behavior. It may not be so acceptable to see oneself as immature, as opposed to being the strong, rebellious young person who does his or her own thing.

Many indirect interventions have been described. Here are brief descriptions of some of them:

- Reframing and positive connotation. Reframing—the giving of a different meaning to a behavior, or a pattern of behaviors—is the basic aim of most, if not all, indirect interventions. We have encountered one form—developmental reframing. Positive connotation is but a form of reframing, although it is an important one. For example, a parent's abusive behavior toward a child may be reframed (positively connoted) as a laudable attempt to correct the child's behavior. Therapy then can address the question of how the parent can develop better methods of achieving that goal. There are indeed few behaviors that cannot be positively connoted; what is required in doing so is the separation of the behavior from the motive behind it.

- Communication by metaphor. Metaphor is a long-established way of conveying messages indirectly and in a nonthreatening way. Situations may be reframed, new perspectives offered, and solutions to problems suggested without the issues being raised directly. Stories, anecdotes, other relationships, rituals, tasks, objects, and artistic productions may all carry meaning metaphorically.
- Paradoxical directives and related devices. When direct interventions have failed, it may be effective to suggest that, as "everything" has been tried, it may be better to leave things as they are. This effectively turns responsibility for change over to the family. Moreover, if they have, unconsciously, been trying to "defeat" the therapist, the only way they can now do so is by making the changes the therapist is advising against. Related to this are the declaring of therapeutic impotence and prescribing interminable therapy.
- Prescribing rituals and tasks. As we have seen, these may have metaphorical meaning, but they can also be used to interrupt repetitive, dysfunctional patterns of behavior. Examples are the "odd-days-even-days" routine, whereby parents take turns putting their children to bed; or the "same-sex parenting" plan, whereby the father is given responsibility for the boys in the family and the mother for the girls,
- Using humor. Helping family members to laugh at what they have been doing can, in the right situation, and in the context of profound *rapport,* be an effective change-promoting technique.
- Presenting alternative solutions or courses of action. This can be done by having the therapist admit to being uncertain about what is the best course of action and offering two or more; by having a "Greek chorus" observing though the one-way observation screen (a device widely used in family therapy) and sending in varying messages, or disagreeing with the therapist's ideas; or by staging a debate in the therapy room, the observers coming in to discuss possible solutions. Such strategies have several potential advantages. They make the point that there are choices to be made and that there is not necessarily only one possible solution to a problem; they invite families to take some responsibility for making changes; and they operate from the "one-down" position, that is, the therapist(s) are not presented as all-knowing experts seeking to impose their solutions on the family.
- Externalizing the problem. This is a process whereby a symptom is labeled or personified. "'Uncertainty' has taken over your life." "How can you win the battle with 'Mr. Anger'?" The family, or an individual, is then invited to consider ways of defeating or otherwise dealing with the externalized object.

The above are but examples of what are often called strategic therapy techniques. Others have been described and only the creativity of the therapist limits the possibilities. Such techniques are not used only in family therapy; they have application in individual therapy as well as in other fields of endeavor such as teaching and selling.

BIBLIOGRAPHY

Barker, P. (1992). *Basic family therapy* (3rd ed.). Oxford: Blackwell.

Barker, P. (1996). *Psychotherapeutic metaphors: A guide to theory and practice.* New York: Brunner/Mazel.

Duvall, E. M., & Miller, B. C. (1984). *Marriage and family development* (6th. ed.). New York: Harper & Row.

Epstein, N. B., Bishop, D. S., & Levin, S. (1978). The McMaster model of family functioning. *Journal of Marriage and Family Counselling, 4,* 19–31.

Imber-Black, E. (Ed.). (1993). *Secrets in families and family therapy.* New York: Norton.

Madanes, C. (1981). *Strategic family therapy.* San Francisco: Jossey-Bass.

Minuchin, S. (1974). *Families and family therapy.* Cambridge, MA: Harvard University Press.

Nichols, W. C. (1996). *Treating people in families: An integrative framework.* New York: Guilford.

Palazzoli, M. S., Boscolo, L., Cecchin, G., & Prata, G. (1978). *Paradox and counterparadox.* New York: Jason Aronson.

Steinhauer, P. D., Santa-Barbara, J., & Skinner, H. (1984). The process model of family functioning. *Canadian Journal of Psychiatry, 29,* 77–88.

Whitaker, C. A. (1976). The hindrance of theory in clinical work. In P. Guerin, (Ed.), *Family therapy: Theory and practice.* New York: Gardner.

Hypnosis and the Psychological Unconscious

John F. Kihlstrom
University of California, Berkeley

Automatic Processes Perceptual–cognitive processes that are initiated involuntarily, executed outside phenomenal awareness, and consume no attentional resources.
Data-Driven Processes Perceptual–cognitive processes that are based on the perceptual structure of a stimulus.
Episodic Memory Memory for personal experiences, each associated with a unique spatiotemporal context (see contrasting *Semantic Memory*).
Explicit Memory Conscious recollection, as manifested in a person's ability to recall or recognize some past event (see contrasting *Implicit Memory*).
Factor Analysis A statistical technique that provides a concise summary of the correlations among a large number of variables.
Hypnotizability Individual differences in response to hypnosis, as measured by standardized psychological tests such as the Stanford Hypnotic Susceptibility Scales.
Implicit Memory Any effect on task performance that is attributable to a past event, independent of conscious recollection of that event (see contrasting *Explicit Memory*).
Preattentive Processing The perceptual–cognitive processing that occurs before attention has been paid to a stimulus.
Priming The facilitation of perceptual–cognitive processing of a stimulus (known as a target) by presentation of a prior stimulus (known as a prime). In repetition priming, prime and target are identical (e.g., water–water); in semantic priming, prime and target are related in terms of meaning (e.g., ocean–water).
Semantic Memory Context-free memory for factual information (see contrasting *Episodic Memory*).

HYPNOSIS is a social interaction in which one person (the subject) responds to suggestions given by another person (the hypnotist) for imaginative experiences involving alterations in perception, memory, and the voluntary control of action. In the classic case, these responses are associated with a degree of subjective conviction bordering on delusion and an experience of involuntariness bordering on compulsion. The psychological unconscious refers to the proposition that mental states—cognitions, emotions, and motives—can influence ongoing experience, thought, and action outside of phenomenal awareness and voluntary control.

Copyright © 1998 by Academic Press.
All rights of reproduction in any form reserved.

I. HISTORY OF HYPNOSIS

The origins of hypnosis extend back to the ancient temples of Aesculapius, the Greek god of medicine, where advice and reassurance uttered by priests to sleeping patients was interpreted by the patients as the gods speaking to them in their dreams. Its more recent history, however, begins with Franz Anton Mesmer (1734–1815), who theorized that disease was caused by imbalances of a physical force, called animal magnetism, affecting various parts of the body. Accordingly, Mesmer thought that cures could be achieved by redistributing this magnetic fluid—a procedure that typically resulted in pseudoepileptic seizures known as "crises." In 1784, a French royal commission chaired by Benjamin Franklin and including Lavoisier and Guillotin among its members concluded that the effects of mesmerism, while genuine in many cases, were achieved by means of imagination and not any physical force. In the course of their proceedings, the commissioners conducted what may well be the first controlled psychological experiments.

Mesmer's theory was discredited, but his practices lived on. A major transition occurred when one of Mesmer's followers, the Marquis de Puysegur, magnetized Victor Race, a young shepherd on his estate. Instead of undergoing a magnetic crisis, Victor fell into a somnambulistic state in which he was responsive to instructions, and from which he awoke with an amnesia for what he had done. Later in the nineteenth century, John Elliotson and James Esdaile, among others, reported the successful use of mesmeric somnambulism as an anesthetic for surgery (although ether and chloroform soon proved to be more reliably effective). James Braid, another British physician, speculated that somnambulism was caused by the paralysis of nerve centers induced by ocular fixation; in order to eliminate the taint of mesmerism, he renamed the state "neurhypnotism" (nervous sleep), a term later shortened to hypnosis. Later, Braid concluded that hypnosis resulted from the subject's concentration on a single thought (monoideism) rather than from physiological fatigue.

Interest in hypnosis was revived in France in the late 1880s by Jean Martin Charcot, who thought hypnosis was a form of hysteria. Charcot believed that both hypnosis and hysteria reflected a disorder of the central nervous system. In opposition to Charcot's neurological theories, A. A. Liebeault and Hippolyte Bernheim, two other French physicians, emphasized the role of suggestibility in producing hypnotic effects. Pierre Janet and Sigmund Freud also studied with Charcot, and Freud began to develop his psychogenic theories of mental illness after observing the suggestibility of hysterical patients when they were hypnotized.

In America, William James and other early psychologists became interested in hypnosis because it seemed to involve alterations in conscious awareness. The first systematic experimental work on hypnosis was reported by P. C. Young in a doctoral dissertation completed at Harvard in 1923, and by Clark Hull in an extensive series of experiments initiated at the University of Wisconsin in the 1920s and continued at Yale into the 1930s. Also at Wisconsin during Hull's time was Milton Erickson, whose provocative clinical and experimental studies stimulated interest in hypnosis among psychotherapists (Hull knew Erickson at Wisconsin, but the immediate source of Hull's interest in hypnosis was Joseph Jastrow, who was Hull's mentor). In England, Hans Eysenck studied hypnosis and suggestibility as part of his classic explorations of personality structure.

After World War II, interest in hypnosis rose rapidly. Ernest Hilgard, together with Josephine Hilgard and Andre Weitzenhoffer, established a laboratory for hypnosis research at Stanford University. Hilgard's status as one of the world's most distinguished psychologists helped establish hypnosis as a legitimate subject of scientific inquiry. Also important in this revival were Theodore Sarbin, Martin Orne, Theodore Barber, and Erika Fromm. Hypnosis is now a thriving topic for both scientific inquiry and clinical application, and is represented by such professional organizations as the Society for Clinical and Experimental Hypnosis, the American Society of Clinical Hypnosis, and other affiliates of the International Society of Hypnosis. The *International Journal of Clinical and Experimental Hypnosis*, the *American Journal of Clinical Hypnosis*, the *Australian Journal of Clinical and Experimental Hypnosis*, and *Contemporary Hypnosis* (formerly the *British Journal of Experimental and Clinical Hypnosis*) are among the leading journals publishing hypnosis research.

II. INDIVIDUAL DIFFERENCES

The Abbe Faria, another follower of Mesmer, recognized individual differences in response to animal magnetism as early as 1819, and there are large individual differences in response to hypnosis as well. Hypnosis has little to do with the hypnotist's technique and very much to do with the subject's capacity, or talent, for experiencing hypnosis. Hypnotizability is measured by standardized psychological tests such as the Stanford Hypnotic Susceptibility Scale or the Harvard Group Scale of Hypnotic Susceptibility. These instruments are work samples, analogous to other performance tests. They begin with a hypnotic induction in which the subjects are asked to focus their eyes on a fixation point, relax, and concentrate on the voice of the hypnotist (although suggestions for relaxation are generally part of the hypnotic induction procedure, people can respond positively to hypnotic suggestions while engaged in vigorous physical activity). The hypnotist then gives suggestions for further relaxation, focused attention, and eye closure. After the subjects close their eyes, they receive further suggestions for various imaginative experiences. For example, they may be told to extend their arms and imagine a heavy object pushing their hands and arms down, or that a voice is asking them questions over a loudspeaker, or that when they open their eyes they will not be able to see an object placed in front of them. Posthypnotic suggestions may also be given for responses to be executed after hypnosis has been terminated, including posthypnotic amnesia, the inability to remember events and experiences which transpired during hypnosis. Response to each of these suggestions is scored in terms of objective behavioral criteria—do the subjects' arms drop a specified distance over a period of time, do they answer questions realistically, do they deny seeing the object, and so on.

Hypnotizability, so measured, yields a roughly normal (i.e., bell-shaped) distribution of scores. Most people are at least moderately responsive to hypnotic suggestions, while relatively few people are refractory to hypnosis and relatively few (so-called hypnotic virtuosos) fall within the highest level of responsiveness. Cross-sectional studies of different age groups show a developmental curve, with very young children relatively unresponsive to hypnosis and hypnotizability reaching a peak at about the onset of adolescence; scores drop off among middle-aged and elderly individuals. Hypnotizability assessed in college students remains about as stable as IQ over a period of 25 years.

Although hypnotizability is generally assessed in terms of a single-sum score, factor-analytic studies reveal a degree of multidimensionality. Hypnotic suggestions can be classified roughly as ideomotor (involving the facilitation of motor responses), challenge (involving the inhibition of motor responses), and cognitive (involving alterations in perception and memory). These factors are themselves intercorrelated, so that a general dimension of hypnotizability emerges at a higher level, much like Thurstone's solution to the structure of intelligence in terms of primary mental abilities and a superordinate general intelligence.

Even though hypnosis is a product of suggestion, it is a mistake to identify hypnotizability with suggestibility. In fact, suggestibility itself is also factorially complex. Eysenck distinguished among primary (e.g., direct suggestions for the facilitation and inhibition of motor activity), secondary (implied suggestions for sensory–perceptual changes), and tertiary (e.g., attitude changes resulting from persuasive communications) forms of suggestibility; a further form of suggestibility is the placebo response. Hypnotizability is correlated only with primary suggestibility, and this is carried mostly by the relation between primary suggestibility and the ideomotor and challenge components of hypnotizability.

There is some controversy over whether hypnotizability can be modified. Some clinical practitioners, influenced by the theories of Milton Erickson, believe that virtually everyone can be hypnotized, if only the hypnotist takes the right approach, but there is little evidence favoring this point of view. Similarly, some researchers believe that hypnotizability can be enhanced by developing positive attitudes, motivations, and expectancies concerning hypnosis, but there is also evidence that such enhancements are heavily laced with compliance. As with any other skilled performance, hypnotic response is probably a matter of both aptitude and attitude: negative attitudes, motivations, and expectancies can interfere with performance, but positive ones are not by themselves sufficient to create hypnotic virtuosity.

The role of individual differences makes it clear that

in an important sense, all hypnosis is self-hypnosis. The hypnotist does not hypnotize the subject. Rather, the hypnotist serves as a sort of coach, or tutor, whose job is to help the subject become hypnotized. Although it takes considerable training and expertise to use hypnosis appropriately in clinical practice, it takes very little skill to be a hypnotist. Beyond the hypnotist's ability to develop rapport with the subject, the most important factor determining hypnotic response is the hypnotizability of the individual subject.

III. CORRELATES

Hypnotizability is not substantially correlated with most other individual differences in ability or personality, such as intelligence or adjustment. Interestingly, it does not appear to be correlated with individual differences in conformity, persuasibility, or response to other forms of social influence. However, in the early 1960s, Ronald Shor, Arvid Ås, and others found that hypnotizability was correlated with subjects' tendency to have hypnosis-like experiences outside of formal hypnotic settings, and an extensive interview study by Josephine Hilgard showed that hypnotizable subjects displayed a high level of imaginative involvement in domains such as reading and drama. In 1974, Auke Tellegen and Gilbert Atkinson developed a scale of absorption to measure the disposition to have subjective experiences characterized by the full engagement of attention (narrowed or expanded) and blurred boundaries between self and object. Absorption is the most reliable correlate of hypnotizability (by contrast, vividness of mental imagery is essentially uncorrelated with hypnosis), although the statistical relation is too weak to permit confident prediction of an individual's actual response to hypnotic suggestion. So far as the measurement of hypnotizability is concerned, there is no substitute for performance-based measures such as the Stanford and Harvard scales.

Absorption seems to be a heretofore unappreciated aspect of individual differences. The scales of the Minnesota Multiphasic Personality Inventory, California Psychological Inventory, and other such instruments do not contain items related to absorption, which may explain their failure to correlate with hypnotizability. However, absorption is not wholly unrelated to other individual differences in personality. Recent multivariate research has settled on five major dimensions—the Big Five—which provide a convenient summary of personality structure: neuroticism (emotional stability), extraversion, agreeableness, conscientiousness, and a fifth factor often called openness to experience. Absorption is correlated with openness.

Actually, the definition of the fifth factor as openness is somewhat controversial, with some theorists arguing for alternative interpretations in terms of intellectance (i.e., the appearance of being intelligent) or culturedness. Openness itself proves to be heterogeneous: some facets (richness of fantasy life, aesthetic sensitivity, and awareness of inner feelings) resemble absorption, while others (need for variety in actions, interest in ideas, and liberal value systems) relate to sociopolitical liberalism. In fact, hypnotizability is correlated with the absorption component of openness, but not with liberalism or intellectance. This pattern of differential correlates indicates that intellectance, absorption, and liberalism are different dimensions of personality and should not be lumped together. In stimulating the discovery of absorption, and in clarifying the nature of the fifth factor in the Big Five structure, research on individual differences in hypnotizability has contributed to understanding in the broader domain of personality.

Researchers have been interested in biological correlates of hypnotizability as well as in those which can be measured by paper-and-pencil tests. Although hypnosis is commonly induced with suggestions for relaxation and even sleep, the brain activity in hypnosis more closely resembles that of a person who is awake. The discovery of hemispheric specialization, with the left hemisphere geared to analytic and the right hemisphere to nonanalytic tasks, led to the speculation that hypnotic response is somehow mediated by right-hemisphere activity. Studies that used both behavioral and electrophysiological paradigms have been interpreted as indicating increased activation of the right hemisphere among highly hypnotizable individuals, but positive results have proved difficult to replicate and interpretation of these findings remains controversial.

It should be noted that hypnosis is mediated by verbal suggestions, which must be interpreted by the subject in the course of responding. Thus, the role of the left hemisphere should not be minimized. One interesting proposal is that hypnotizable individuals show greater flexibility in deploying the left and right hemispheres in a task-appropriate manner, especially when they are actually hypnotized. Because involuntariness is so central to the experience of hypnosis, it has also been suggested that the frontal lobes (which organize intentional action) may play a special role. A better understanding of the neural substrates of hypnosis awaits studies of neurological patients with focalized brain lesions, as well as brain-imaging studies (e.g., positron-emission tomography, magnetic resonance imaging) of normal subjects. [*See* Brain Scanning/Neuroimaging.]

IV. EXPERIMENTAL STUDIES

Right from the beginning of the modern era, a great deal of research effort has been devoted to claims that hypnotic suggestions enable individuals to transcend their normal voluntary capacities—to be stronger, see better, learn faster, and remember more. However, research has largely failed to find evidence that hypnosis can enhance human performance. Many early studies, which seemed to yield positive results for hypnosis, possessed serious methodological flaws, such as the failure to collect adequate baseline information. In general, it appears that hypnotic suggestions for increased muscular strength, endurance, sensory acuity, or learning do not exceed what can be accomplished by motivated subjects outside hypnosis.

A special case of performance enhancement has to do with hypnotic suggestions for improvements in memory—what is known as hypnotic hypermnesia. Hypermnesia suggestions are sometimes used in forensic situations, with forgetful witnesses and victims, or in therapeutic situations to help patients remember traumatic personal experiences. Although field studies have sometimes claimed that hypnosis can powerfully enhance memory, these anecdotal reports have not been duplicated under laboratory conditions.

A 1994 report by the Committee on Techniques for the Enhancement of Human Performance, a unit of the U.S. National Research Council, concluded that gains in recall produced by hypnotic suggestion were rarely dramatic and were matched by gains observed even when subjects are not hypnotized (in fact, there is some evidence that hypnotic suggestion can interfere with normal hypermnesic processes). To make things worse, any increases obtained in valid recollection are met or exceeded by increases in false recollections. Moreover, hypnotized subjects (especially those who are highly hypnotizable) may be vulnerable to distortions in memory produced by leading questions and other subtle and suggestive influences.

Similar conclusions apply to hypnotic age regression, in which subjects receive suggestions that they are returning to a previous period in their lives (this is also a technique used clinically to foster the retrieval of forgotten memories of child abuse). Although age-regressed subjects may experience themselves as children, and may behave in a childlike manner, there is no evidence that they actually undergo either abolition of characteristically adult modes of mental functioning or reinstatement of childlike modes of mental functioning. Nor do age-regressed subjects experience the revivification of forgotten memories of childhood.

One phenomenon that has received a great deal of attention is hypnotic analgesia—in large part because of the obvious clinical uses to which it can be put. A comparative study of experimental pain found that among hypnotizable subjects, hypnotic analgesia was superior to morphine, diazepam, aspirin, acupuncture, and biofeedback. Hypnotic analgesia relieves both sensory pain and suffering. It is not mediated by relaxation, and the fact that it is not reversed by narcotic antagonists would seem to rule out a role for endogenous opiates. There is a placebo component to all active analgesic agents, and hypnosis is no exception; however, hypnotizable subjects receive benefits from hypnotic suggestion that outweigh what they or their insusceptible counterparts achieve from plausible placebos.

Psychological explanations of hypnotic analgesia come in two primary forms. On the one hand, it is argued that hypnotized subjects use such techniques as self-distraction, stress-inoculation, cognitive reinterpretation, and tension management. While there is no doubt that cognitive strategies can reduce pain, their success, unlike the success of hypnotic suggestions, is not correlated with hypnotizability and thus is unlikely to be responsible for the effects observed in hypnotizable subjects. Rather, hypnotic analgesia seems to be associated with a division of consciousness which prevents the perception of pain from being represented in conscious awareness, without altering the physiological effects of the pain stimulus.

A great deal of research has also been devoted to the posthypnotic amnesia frequently displayed by hypnotizable subjects. This form of forgetting does not occur spontaneously and may be reversed by administration of a prearranged signal without the reinduction of hypnosis, so it does not represent a form of state-dependent learning. However, the reversibility of amnesia does indicate that its mechanisms may be located at the retrieval stage of memory processing, rather than at the encoding or storage stages. Posthypnotic amnesia does not prevent words studied during hypnosis from being used as free associates or category instances, indicating that posthypnotic amnesia is a disruption of episodic, but not semantic, memory. Moreover, the production of studied items as instances and associates is actually facilitated, resulting in priming effects. Similarly, posthypnotic amnesia does not affect retroactive inhibition or savings in relearning. Skills acquired during hypnosis are preserved afterward, even though the subject cannot remember the acquisition trials. This assortment of findings indicates that although posthypnotic amnesia disrupts explicit expressions of episodic memory (such as recall), it spares implicit expressions.

Other phenomena of hypnosis can also be understood in terms of the explicit–implicit distinction. For example, hypnotizable subjects given suggestions for deafness deny hearing anything; yet they show speech dysfluencies under conditions of delayed auditory feedback. And when given suggestions for blindness, they deny seeing anything, yet show priming effects from stimuli presented in their visual fields. With the analogy between explicit and implicit memory, we may say that hypnotic suggestions for blindness, deafness, and the like impair explicit perception while sparing implicit perception.

V. CLINICAL APPLICATIONS

Hypnosis has been used in clinics for both medical and psychotherapeutic purposes. By far the most successful and best documented of these has been hypnotic analgesia for the relief of pain. Clinical studies indicate that hypnosis can effectively relieve pain in patients suffering pain from burns, cancer and leukemia (e.g., bone marrow aspirations), childbirth, and dental procedures. In such circumstances, as many as one half of an unselected patient population can obtain significant, if not total, pain relief from hypnosis. Hypnosis may be especially useful in cases of chronic pain, where chemical analgesics such as morphine pose risks of tolerance and addiction. Hypnosis has also been used, somewhat heroically perhaps, as the sole analgesic agent in abdominal, breast, cardiac, and genitourinary surgery, and in orthopedic situations, although it seems unlikely that more than about 10% of patients can tolerate major medical procedures with hypnosis alone.

Hypnotic suggestion can have psychosomatic effects, a matter that should be of some interest to psychophysiologists and psychoneuroimmunologists. For example, several well controlled laboratory and clinical studies have shown that hypnotic suggestion can affect allergic responses, asthma, and the remission of warts. A famous case study convincingly documented the positive effects of hypnotic suggestion on an intractable case of congenital ichthyosiform erythroderma, a particularly aggressive skin disorder. Such successes have led some practitioners to offer hypnosis in the treatment of cancer. While there is some evidence that hypnosis can have effects on immunological processes, more research in this area is needed, and hypnosis should never be substituted for conventional medical treatments in such cases.

Hypnosis has also been used in psychotherapy, whether psychodynamic or cognitive–behavioral in orientation. In the former case, hypnosis is used to promote relaxation, enhance imagery, and generally loosen the flow of free associations (some psychodynamic theorists consider hypnosis to be a form of adaptive regression or regression in the service of the ego). However, there is little evidence from controlled outcome studies that hypnoanalysis or hypnotherapy are more effective than nonhypnotic forms of the same treatment. By contrast, a 1995 meta-analysis by Kirsch and colleagues showed a significant advantage when hypnosis is used adjunctively in cognitive–behavioral therapy for a number of problems. In an era of managed mental health care, it will be increasingly incumbent on practitioners who use hypnosis to document, quantitatively, the clinical benefits of doing so. [*See* Behavior Therapy; Cognitive Therapy; Psychoanalysis.]

Hypnosis is sometimes used therapeutically to recover forgotten incidents, as for example in cases of child sexual abuse. Although the literature contains a number of dramatic reports of the successful use of this technique, most of these reports are anecdotal and fail to obtain independent corroboration of the memories that emerge. Given what we know about the unreliability of hypnotic hypermnesia, and the risk of increased responsiveness to leading questions and other sources of bias and distortion, such clinical practices are not recommended. Similar considerations obtain in forensic situations. In fact, many legal jurisdictions severely limit the introduction of memories recovered through hypnosis out of a concern that such evidence might be tainted. The Federal Bureau of Investigation has published a set of guidelines for those who wish to use hypnosis forensically, and similar precautions should be used in the clinic. [*See* CHILD SEXUAL ABUSE.]

Returning to strictly therapeutic situations, an important but unresolved issue is the role played by individual differences in the clinical effectiveness of hypnosis. As in the laboratory, so in the clinic: a genuine effect of hypnosis should be correlated with hypnotizability. It is possible that many clinical benefits of hypnosis are mediated by placebo-like motivational and expectational processes—that is, with the "ceremony" surrounding hypnosis, rather than with hypnosis per se. An analogy is to hypnotic analgesia, which appears to have a placebo component available to insusceptible and hypnotizable individuals alike, and a dissociative component available only to those who are highly hypnotizable. Unfortunately, clinical practitioners are often reluctant to assess hypnotizability in their patients and clients out of a concern that low scores might reduce motivation for treatment. This danger is probably exaggerated. On the contrary, assessment of hypnotizability by clinicians contemplating the therapeutic use of hypnosis would seem to be no different, in principle, than an assessment of allergic responses before prescribing an antibiotic. In both cases, the legitimate goal is to determine what treatment is appropriate for what patient.

It should be noted that clinicians sometimes use hypnosis in nonhypnotic ways—practices which tend to support the hypothesis that whatever effects they achieve through hypnosis are related to its placebo component. There is nothing particularly hypnotic, for example, about having a patient in a smoking-cessation treatment rehearse therapeutic injunctions not to smoke and other coping strategies while hypnotized. It is likely that more successful use of hypnosis as an adjunct to the cognitive–behavioral treatment of smoking, excessive weight, and similar habit disorders would be to use hypnotic suggestions to control the patient's awareness of cravings for nicotine, sweets, and the like. Given the ability of hypnotic suggestions to control conscious perception and memory, such strategies might well have therapeutic advantage—but only, of course, for those patients who are hypnotizable enough to respond positively to such suggestions.

VI. THEORIES

The dual nature of hypnosis, in which alterations in consciousness occur in an interpersonal context, has meant that theoretical attempts to understand the phenomenon have been entangled in dichotomies. This has been the case since Mesmer, who thought his effects were due to a magnetic fluid, while the French royal commission attributed them to imagination. Charcot thought hypnotizability was a matter of neurology, while Liebeault and Bernheim emphasized suggestion. Sometimes these dichotomies are manifested within a single individual: Braid began with ideas about the paralysis of nerve centers and ended up emphasizing attention, imagination, expectation, and personality.

In the modern era these dichotomies are still visible, if somewhat obscured by theoretical nuance. Thus, the traditional (if perhaps somewhat tacit) view that hypnosis involves a "special" or "altered" state of consciousness is opposed by a variety of social–psychological or cognitive–behavioral views which assert that hypnotic behavior is a result of processes that are in every sense ordinary. However, there is considerable heterogeneity of viewpoint within each camp, which is sometimes ignored by the other side (a common feature of intergroup relations, according to social psychologists). Among those who are sometimes labeled as state theorists (including the present writer) are cognitive psychologists who think that hypnosis involves dissociative processes, psychoanalysts who invoke adaptive regression in the service of the ego, and neuroscientists who emphasize the inhibition of cortical structures. Among the critics of the state view are some who claim that hypnotic effects can be produced in the absence of a hypnotic induction, so long as subjects are appropriately motivated and instructed. There are others who emphasize the importance of prescriptive social roles played out by both hypnotist and subject, the self-fulfilling effects of expectancies, and the role of attributional processes and self-deception. While some social–psychological and cognitive–behavioral theorists have spent a great deal of time debunking exaggerated or erroneous claims about hypnosis, this has been no less true for some state theorists.

Although it is sometimes popular to portray this theoretical dispute as a kind of enduring debate, there is as much controversy within each camp as there is between camps, and in the final analysis most hypnosis research is designed more to illuminate the nature of specific hypnotic phenomena such as analgesia or amnesia than to provide evidence for any overarching theory of hypnosis. Nevertheless, scientists are trained to test hypotheses derived from theories, and, if possible, to test single hypotheses that will decide between competing theories, so that any empirical evidence obtained tends to be construed as evidence for one view or another.

In the early 1960s, J. P. Sutcliffe published a pair of seminal papers that contrasted a credulous view of hypnosis, which holds that the mental states instigated by suggestion are identical to those that would be produced by the actual stimulus state of affairs implied in the suggestions, with a skeptical view, which holds that the hypnotic subject is acting *as if* the world were as suggested. This is, of course, a version of the familiar dichotomy, but Sutcliffe also offered a third view: that hypnosis involves a quasi-delusional alteration in self-awareness—a delusion that is constructed out of the interaction between the hypnotist's suggestions and the subject's interpretation of those suggestions. Hypnosis is simultaneously a state of (sometimes) profound cognitive change, involving basic mechanisms of perception, memory, and thought, and a social interaction, in which hypnotist and subject come together for a specific purpose within a wider sociocultural context. A truly adequate, comprehensive theory of hypnosis will seek understanding in both cognitive and interpersonal terms. We do not yet have such a theory.

VII. PSYCHOLOGICAL UNCONSCIOUS

The psychological unconscious refers to the idea that mental states—cognitions, emotions, and motives—can influence ongoing experience, thought, and action outside of phenomenal awareness and voluntary control. Although the discovery of the unconscious is commonly attributed to Sigmund Freud, in fact, interest in unconscious mental states and processes goes back to the eighteenth century philosopher Leibnitz, who argued for the importance to perception of subliminal stimuli, and the nineteenth century psychophysicist Helmholtz, who argued that conscious perception results from unconscious inferences about environmental stimuli. Within contemporary cognitive psychology and cognitive science, interest in the psychological unconscious is almost entirely divorced from Freud and psychoanalysis.

In early cognitive psychology, the psychological unconscious was conceived as part wastebasket and part file cabinet. On the one hand, it was the repository for unattended inputs or for those contents of the sensory registers and short-term memory (STM) that had been rendered unavailable by virtue of decay or displacement. On the other hand, the unconscious was identified with the latent contents of long-term memory (LTM), which are brought into awareness when they are copied from LTM to STM. Later, acceptance of the distinction between automatic and effortful processes led to the idea that unconscious mental processes were executed automatically, without drawing on attentional resources. The upshot has been the identification of the unconscious with the unattended, and the rise of the notion that unconscious processing is limited to perceptual and other low-level, presemantic analyses.

More recently, unconscious processing has frequently been identified with the distinction between automatic and controlled mental processes. In some respects, the models for automatic processes are innate reflexes, taxes, instincts, and learned stimulus–response connections formed through classical and instrumental conditioning. Automatic processes are initiated independent of conscious intentions, are executed outside of awareness, and cannot be terminated until they have run to completion. Moreover, it appears that their execution consumes no attentional resources, so that they do not interfere with other ongoing perceptual–cognitive activities. Automatic processes are unconscious in the strict sense of the term: they are never directly available to conscious awareness and are known only by inference.

The automatic–controlled distinction refers to perceptual–cognitive processes engaged in the course of perceiving, remembering, and thinking. The implication is that percepts, memories, and thoughts themselves are available to conscious awareness. Logically, however, availability is no guarantee of accessibility, raising the possibility that mental contents as well as mental processes might be unconscious. In fact, a wealth of experimental evidence, involving both brain-damaged patients and normal subjects, supports a distinction between explicit and implicit memory. Amnesic patients or normal subjects who show preserved priming in the absence (or independent) of recall or recognition, constitute evidence for unconscious memory.

The explicit–implicit distinction can be extended to other psychological domains as well. In perception, for example, there is considerable evidence that stimuli which are subliminal, masked, or unattended can have effects on cognition and behavior even though the stimuli themselves are not consciously perceived. In cases of "blindsight," patients who have suffered damage to the striate cortex of the occipital lobe are able to respond appropriately to visual stimuli even though they are unable to see them. These experimental outcomes illustrate a distinction between explicit and implicit perception, analogous to the explicit–implicit distinction in memory. Explicit perception refers to the conscious perception of current events, as exemplified by the ability to locate and identify objects. By contrast, implicit perception refers to any effect of a current event on ongoing experience, thought, or action in the absence (or independent) of conscious perception, as exemplified by subliminal perception or blindsight.

The explicit–implicit distinction may also be relevant to discussions of thinking and problem solving. For example, intuitions about the solution to a problem, in the absence of conscious awareness of the solution itself, may be an example of implicit thought; incubation may reflect increases in activation associated with an implicit thought; and insight may occur once an implicit thought crosses the threshold required for conscious awareness.

It should be noted that the explicit–implicit distinction may be relevant to emotion and motivation as well as cognition. Many theorists distinguish among three components of an emotional response: subjective (or cognitive), referring to the person's conscious feeling state; behavioral, referring to overt motor activities associated with the emotion; and physiological, referring to associated covert somatic changes. Researchers have observed that these three components are not always positively intercorrelated, a situation known as desynchrony. A particular form of desynchrony, in which the subjective component of emotion is absent while the behavioral and physiological components persist, is tantamount to a dissociation between explicit and implicit emotion.

Implicit perception, memory, and thought serve as examples of preconscious cognition, in which the percepts and memories lie on the fringes of consciousness. Were the encodings deeper, or the retention interval shorter, or the retrieval cues richer, implicit memories might be consciously accessible. So, too, for implicit percepts: we would be conscious of them if only the stimuli contributing to implicit perception effects were of greater intensity or duration, or unmasked, or presented within the focus of attention. In general, the processing of preconscious percepts and memories is analytically limited. For example, the repetition priming effects obtained in the typical study of implicit memory are mediated by traces that represent the perceptual structure, but not the meaning, of the event in question. Semantic priming effects have been obtained in subliminal perception, but they are very weak and short-lived. Apparently, the conditions under which preconscious processing occurs do not permit very much to be done, cognitively, with these percepts and memories.

Hypnosis is relevant to the psychological unconscious because the phenomena of hypnosis appear to expand the boundaries of unconscious processing beyond the automatic and the preconscious. For example, the priming effects which are preserved in posthypnotic amnesia reflect semantic processing: the items in question were deeply processed at the time of encoding. Finally, the impairment in explicit memory is reversible: posthypnotic amnesia is the only memory disorder studied under laboratory conditions where implicit memories can be restored to explicit recollection. Taken together, then, these properties of priming in posthypnotic amnesia reflect the unconscious influence of semantic representations formed as a result of extensive attentional activity at the time of encoding. The priming itself may be an automatic influence, but it is not the sort that is produced by automatic processes mediated by a perceptual representation system or by presemantic or data-driven processing.

A second example is provided by posthypnotic suggestion, which appears to have a quasi-compulsive quality to it, especially when—as so often happens—the subject is unaware (by virtue of posthypnotic amnesia) that he or she is responding to the experimenter's cue. Thus it appears to be an automatic response to stimulation, but careful examination indicates that responding to the posthypnotic cue consumes attentional resources and interferes with other ongoing activities. Even though the posthypnotic suggestion is executed outside of the subject's awareness, and is experienced as involuntary, it is not automatic in the technical sense of being attention-free.

The identification of the psychological unconscious with automatic processing and with preconscious percepts and memories is popular, but if the phenomena of hypnosis are to be taken seriously, it is also misleading. Studies of hypnotic phenomena indicate that deep, semantic processing can occur without concurrent or retrospective awareness of what has been processed, and behavior executed outside of awareness can nonetheless consume attentional resources. The major contribution of hypnosis to our understanding of the psychological unconscious is the realization that there is more to consciousness than attention. At the very least, the phenomena of hypnosis seem to require another category, besides automatic processes and preconscious contents, in the taxonomy of unconscious mental life: subconscious contents. Subconscious percepts are in no sense subliminal or unattended; subconscious memories are in no sense weakly encoded. Yet neither are accessible to conscious awareness.

VIII. DISSOCIATION AND SUBCONSCIOUS PROCESSING

Hilgard and others have suggested that the phenomena of hypnosis and similar phenomena observed in other altered states indicate that consciousness can be divided, so that attentive, semantic processing can proceed outside phenomenal awareness. Hilgard's neodissociation theory of divided consciousness characterizes the mind as a set of modules that monitor and control mental functions in different domains. In the normal case, these modules are organized to be able to communicate with each other and with a central cognitive structure—what Hilgard calls the executive ego—which serves as the end point for all conscious inputs and the point of origin for all conscious outputs. This executive ego provides the cognitive basis for the phenomenal experiences of awareness and intentionality.

However, neodissociation theory also asserts that certain conditions, one of which is hypnosis, can alter the integration of the various cognitive structures. If the lines of communication between two subordinate structures are cut, they may perform input–output functions in the absence of any coordination between them. If the communication between a subordinate structure and the executive ego is disrupted, the domain-specific module will perform its function in the absence of the phenomenal experience of awareness and intentionality. In descriptive terms, both cases constitute states of dissociation.

Neodissociation theory holds that responses to suggestions are executed by the subordinate cognitive substructures, alone or in combination, independent of involvement of the executive ego. In the case of posthypnotic amnesia, for example, the events and experiences of hypnosis are processed by modules dedicated to learning and memory; when the suggestion for posthypnotic amnesia is given, the normal communicative link between these modules and the executive control structure is disrupted. Thus, when the executive control structure tries to gain access to these memories in order to respond to an explicit memory test, it cannot do so. However, implicit memory functions such as priming, which do not require conscious access mediated by the executive control structure, are unimpaired. Similarly, posthypnotic suggestions are executed by the relevant substructures without involvement of the executive. Because the executive has no awareness of this activity, the behavior in question is experienced as automatic, even though it may be quite complex and cognitively demanding. Although some critics have interpreted dissociation theory as implying that dissociated activities should not interfere with other ongoing functions, it should be apparent that such a system of dissociated control may well make considerable demands on cognitive resources, resulting in decrements in the performance of simultaneous tasks.

How this dissociation occurs is not well understood. However, the neodissociation theory of divided consciousness, proposed in the context of hypnosis, has stimulated a revival of interest in various forms of dissociation observed clinically, such as psychogenic amnesia, fugue, and multiple personality (dissociative identity disorder). In addition to these clinical syndromes, which fall under the diagnostic rubric of "dissociative disorders," it has been noted that the various "conversion disorders," such as functional blindness, deafness, and paralysis, are essentially dissociative in nature. In each case, some aspect of perception or memory is split off from awareness. Research on the mechanisms of dissociation is at an early stage, but it is already clear that the phenomena of hypnosis, and the clinical syndromes which they resemble, expand the domain of the psychological unconscious and constitute major challenges to our understanding of the nature of conscious and unconscious mental life.

ACKNOWLEDGMENT

Preparation of this article was supported by Grant #MH-35856 from the National Institute of Mental Health.

BIBLIOGRAPHY

Bowers, K. S. (1976). *Hypnosis for the seriously curious.* Monterey, CA: Brooks/Cole.

Fromm, E., & Nash, M. R. (Eds.). (1992). *Contemporary hypnosis research.* New York: Guilford.

Gauld, A. (1992). *A history of hypnotism.* Cambridge, UK: Cambridge University Press.

Hilgard, E. R. (1965). *Hypnotic susceptibility.* New York: Harcourt, Brace, and World.

Hilgard, E. R. (1977). *Divided consciousness: Multiple controls in human thought and action.* New York: Wiley-Interscience.

Hilgard, E. R., & Hilgard, J. R. (1975). *Hypnosis in the relief of pain.* Los Altos, CA: Kaufman.

Lynn, S. J., & Rhue, J. W. (Eds.). (1991). *Theories of hypnosis: Current models and perspectives.* New York: Guilford.

Olness, K., & Gardner, G. G. (1988). *Hypnosis and hypnotherapy with children* (2nd ed.). Philadelphia: Grune & Stratton.

Rhue, J. W., Lynn, S. J., & Kirsch, I. (Eds.) (1993). *Handbook of clinical hypnosis.* Washington, DC: American Psychological Association.

Sheehan, P. W., & Perry, C. W. (1976). *Methodologies of hypnosis: A critical appraisal of contemporary paradigms of hypnosis.* Hillsdale, NJ: Erlbaum.

Spanos, N. P., & Chaves, J. F. (Eds.) (1989). *Hypnosis: The cognitive–behavioral perspective.* Buffalo, NY: Prometheus Books.

Spiegel, H., & Spiegel, D. (1978). *Trance and treatment: Clinical uses of hypnosis.* Washington, DC: American Psychiatric Press.

Meditation and the Relaxation Response

Richard Friedman, Patricia Myers, and Herbert Benson

Harvard Medical School

Fight-or-Flight Response Physiological arousal of the sympathetic nervous system which prepares an organism to either fight or run away from a perceived threat.
Central Nervous System Neural activity that occurs within the brain and the spinal cord.
Meditation Any activity that focuses conscious attention.
Peripheral Nervous System Neural activity that occurs outside the brain and spinal cord including the sympathetic branch of the autonomic nervous system.
Relaxation Response An integrated physiological response that is the opposite of the fight-or-flight response—i.e., it reduces physiological arousal. The relaxation response is elicited by two simple steps: (1) focusing attention on a word, sound, prayer, phrase, image, or physical activity, and (2) passively ignoring distracting thoughts and returning to the repetition.
Sympathetic Nervous System A branch of the human body's autonomic nervous system. In response to stress, sympathetic nervous system activity automatically increases resulting in the fight-or-flight response. During meditation or other mental focusing techniques, sympathetic nervous system activity is decreased, resulting in the relaxation response.

Over the past several decades, hundreds of scientific studies have documented the deleterious effects of psychological stress on the psychological, behavioral, and physiological functioning of humans. Upon exposure to psychological stress a series of central and peripheral nervous system changes occurs that compromise our ability to think effectively and behave appropriately. psychological stress also causes physiological changes that can cause and exacerbate somatic illness. Not surprisingly, attempts have been made to develop strategies to minimize the adverse effects of stress. Some of these management strategies are related to cognitive restructuring and other therapeutic approaches within the context of Western psychology; others, such as MEDITATION, are related to older Eastern traditions. This article discusses meditation; its psychological, behavioral, and physiological effects; and how it can be effectively incorporated into the routine care of individuals who require mental and medical interventions.

I. HISTORICAL PERSPECTIVE

The concept of meditation, as well as its therapeutic value, is frequently misunderstood. For centuries meditation has been associated with positive psychological benefits. Although many Eastern cultures have embraced the concept that regular meditation practice

Copyright © 1998 by Academic Press.
All rights of reproduction in any form reserved.

can alter one's state of consciousness or enhance one's perception of reality, the mystical or metaphysical overtones associated with meditation have inhibited Western societies from adopting it more extensively.

Twenty-five years ago, Benson and his colleagues began to examine the psychological and physiological components of meditation within a Western scientific and medical framework. After studying the cultural, religious, philosophical, and scientific underpinnings of meditation, Benson and his colleagues concluded that meditation requires only two specific steps: (1) focusing one's attention on a single repetitive word, sound, prayer, phrase, image, or physical activity; and (2) passively returning to this focus when distracted. When one engages in these two steps, a set of predictable physiological events occurs within and outside the central nervous system (CNS) that promote a sense of calm and behavioral inactivity. Benson labeled this set of physiological events the *relaxation response*. The relaxation response is the biological consequence of a wide variety of mental focusing techniques, one of which is meditation. This widely applicable and beneficial concept should be routinely integrated into psychological, behavioral, and medical treatments.

To appreciate the short- and long-term effects of eliciting the relaxation response and its clinical use it is necessary to understand the physiology of stress.

II. PHYSIOLOGY OF STRESS AND THE RELAXATION RESPONSE

More than 50 years ago, Cannon observed that mammals faced with life-threatening situations respond with predictable physiological arousal of the sympathetic nervous system (SNS) that prepares them to either face the threat or run away from it. He labeled this the now-familiar "*fight-or-flight response*." This response stimulates physiological changes to facilitate vigorous skeletal muscle activity. SNS arousal, mediated by the release of epinephrine and norepinephrine, increases heart rate and blood pressure, which in turn accelerates blood circulation to meet the increased demand for oxygen, nutrients, and waste removal. Platelet activity also increases to enhance coagulation in the event of potential injury with blood loss.

Numerous psychological events (e.g., the perception of physical danger) can automatically elicit the fight-or-flight response. For primitive man, this response was necessary for survival. Today, faced with everyday stresses, such as being kept waiting in line or on the phone, we experience the same response to varying degrees.

The behavioral and physiological opposite of the fight-or-flight response is the relaxation response which is believed to be an integrated hypothalamic response that depresses SNS activity in a generalized manner. Forty years ago, Hess described this effect as the trophotropic response. By electrically stimulating the anterior hypothalamus of cats Hess was able to elicit signs of reduced sympathetic nervous system arousal including decreases in muscle tension, blood pressure, and respiration. This response was the opposite of what he termed "ergotropic" responses, which corresponded to the heightened state of SNS activity described by Cannon as the fight-or-flight response.

The early experimental work of Cannon and Hess, combined with the more recent observations of Benson and his colleagues, suggests that these two responses are actually symmetrical. Although both involve central and peripheral nervous system changes, the fight-or-flight response prepares the organism for action while the relaxation response prepares the organism for rest and calmness, behavioral inactivity, and restorative physiologic changes. Whereas repeated or prolonged elicitation of the fight-or-flight response has been implicated in illness related to stress and SNS arousal, repeated elicitation of the relaxation response appears to prevent or ameliorate stress-related disorders.

III. MEDITATION, THE RELAXATION RESPONSE, AND PHYSIOLOGICAL CHANGES

Benson and his colleagues were among the first to use Western experimental standards to study the physiology of meditation and its potential clinical benefits. In experiments involving Transcendental Meditation conducted at the Harvard Medical School and at the University of California at Irvine, physiological parameters were monitored in subjects in both meditative and nonmeditative states. Measures of blood pressure, heart rate, rectal temperature, and skin resistance as well as electroencephalographic (EEG) events were recorded at 20-minute intervals. During the meditative states oxygen consumption, carbon dioxide elimination, respiratory rates, minute ventilation (the amount of air inhaled and exhaled in a 1-minute period), and arterial blood lactate levels (an indication of anaerobic metabolism) were reduced. These acute changes are all compatible with reduced SNS activity and were not evident when the subjects simply sat quietly. Since these initial demonstrations, others have documented that elicitation of the relaxation response results in important physiological changes that are mediated by reduced SNS activity.

In addition to the SNS effects of the relaxation response, its central nervous system effects have been dramatically illustrated in a controlled study of frontal EEG beta-wave activity. Novice subjects listened to either a tape designed to elicit the relaxation response or a control tape that provided a discussion of the relaxation response and its benefits. Using topographic EEG mapping, researchers found that elicitation of the relaxation response appeared to reduce cortical activation in anterior regions of the brain (see Fig. 1).

Another study has also provided evidence of the effect of the relaxation response on CNS indices of arousal. Jacobs, Benson, and Friedman examined the efficacy of a multifactor behavioral intervention for chronic sleep-onset insomnia. The interventions included education about sleep (e.g., sleep states, sleep architecture) and sleep hygiene (e.g., abstaining from alcohol, caffeine, and nicotine use in the evening), sleep scheduling, and modified stimulus control (restricting use of the bed to sleeping). The subjects were taught relaxation-response techniques and were instructed to practice them at bedtime. Those insomniacs exposed to the intervention exhibited significant reductions in sleep-onset latency and were indistinguishable from

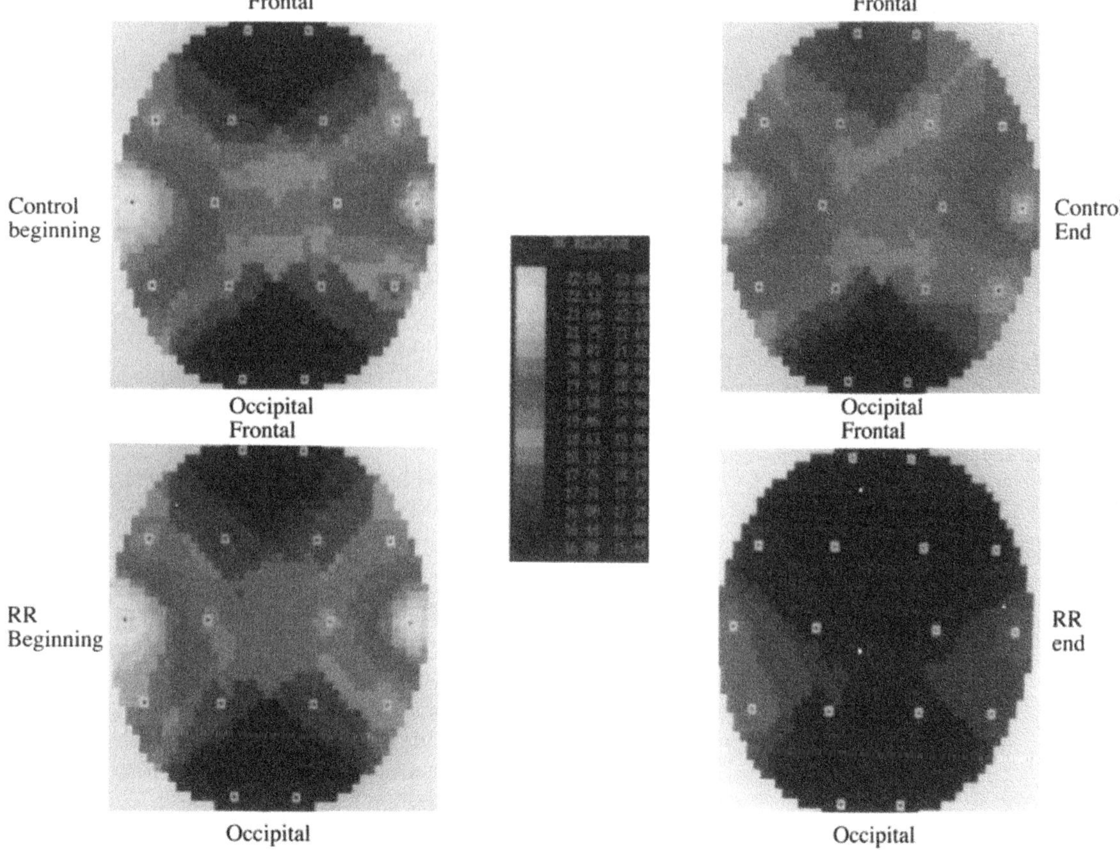

Figure 1 Beta relative power for control and relaxation response (RR) conditions. Vertical color bar indicates beta relative power (white highest, black lowest). Topographic maps are displayed in relative spectral power for greater resolution. *Note:* At RR end (lower right), beta relative power is significantly ($p < .0164$) decreased in frontal areas.

normal sleepers. More importantly, the insomniacs showed a marked reduction in cortical arousal, as assessed EEG power spectra analyses; specifically, the percentages of beta total power decreased from pre- to posttreatment.

The relaxation response training most likely mediated these reductions in cortical arousal and were therefore probably responsible for the dramatic decrease in sleep-onset latency. These findings in insomniacs support the contention that regular elicitation of the relaxation response leads to physiological changes opposite to those seen during the fight-or-flight response (i.e., decreased vs increased cortical arousal, respectively).

Since the physiological changes and therapeutic effects of the regular elicitation of the relaxation response lead to significant beneficial physiological changes and these effects appear to be the same as those associated with rest and sleep, what extra benefits does this practice offer above and beyond those derived from sleeping? Actually, the two activities are quite different. Although oxygen consumption plummets within the first few minutes of eliciting the relaxation response (in this example through meditation), oxygen consumption during sleep decreases appreciably only after several hours (see Fig. 2). The concentration of carbon dioxide in the blood increases significantly during sleep, whereas during meditation it decreases. The electrical conductivity of the skin tends to increase during sleep, indicating reduced sympathetic activity. However, the rate and magnitude of sleep-related increases in skin conductivity are much smaller than those observed during meditation and other relaxation-response techniques. Researchers have demonstrated that CNS effects of the relaxation response also differ from those observed during sleep.

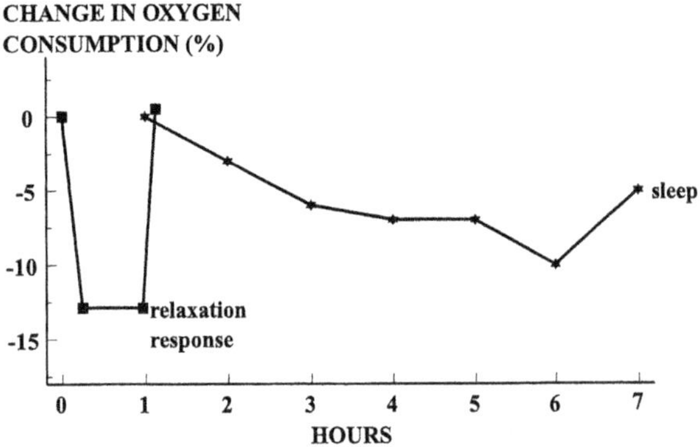

Figure 2 O_2 consumption during sleep and the relaxation response.

IV. RATIONALE AND TECHNIQUE FOR ELICITATION OF THE RELAXATION RESPONSE

A variety of techniques can be used to elicit the relaxation response, including meditation, progressive muscle relaxation, autogenic training, yoga, exercise, repetitive prayer, and the presuggestion phase of hypnosis. Although all of these strategies result in the same physiological response, two components appear to be essential to achieving the relaxation response: mental focusing and adopting a passive attitude toward distracting thoughts.

The following is an instructional set developed by Benson and his colleagues for elicitation of the relaxation response.

Step 1. Pick a focus word or short phrase that's firmly rooted in your belief system.
Step 2. Sit quietly in a comfortable position.
Step 3. Close your eyes.
Step 4. Relax your muscles.
Step 5. Breathe slowly and naturally, and as you do, repeat your focus word, phrase or prayer silently to yourself as you exhale.
Step 6. Assume a passive attitude. Don't worry about how well you're doing. When other thoughts come to mind, simply say to yourself, "Oh, well," and gently return to the repetition.
Step 7. Continue for 10 to 20 minutes.
Step 8. Do not stand up immediately. Continue sitting quietly for a minute or so, allowing other thoughts to return. Then open your eyes and sit for another minute before rising.
Step 9. Practice this technique once or twice daily.

Sample focus words, prayers, phrases include: One, Ocean, Love, Peace, Calm, Relax, "The Lord is my shepherd," "Shalom," "Insha'allah," or "Om."

Regular practice at eliciting the relaxation response has been shown to produce chronic physiological changes by at least two research groups. With repeated practice, patients can experience the benefits of relaxation throughout the day not only during actual practice periods.

It is the clinician's responsibility to help the patient develop a personally relevant and effective technique.

It is important to emphasize that adherence to relaxation regimens will be maximized by selecting a strategy that is compatible with the patient's belief system and customary practices. It is useful to ask patients about their belief systems and to adapt an approach compatible with them. For example, a religious person might be more comfortable focusing on a familiar repetitive prayer, while someone interested in physical exercise might be more comfortable performing a repetitive exercise. The manner in which the response is elicited is immaterial since the psychological and physiological results are the same.

V. THE RELAXATION RESPONSE IN PSYCHOTHERAPY

For many patients with psychological disturbances, who might be hesitant to enter therapy, relaxation-response training is a nonthreatening intervention that can be introduced prior to other more rigorous forms of therapy such as cognitive therapy or medication. Meditation and other modes of eliciting the relaxation response can be a means of preparing for standard psychotherapy by allowing the patient to observe thoughts and mental events.

In 1985, Kutz and colleagues were the first to systematically study the relationship between psychotherapy and meditation. They studied the change in psychological well-being and the impact on psychotherapy of a 10-week meditation program in 20 patients. The intervention consisted of weekly 2-hour group sessions and daily home practice. Patients showed significant decreases in psychological symptoms from pre- to posttreatment as measured by the Symptom Checklist 90 Revised (SCL-90R), a standard psychological inventory, and the POMS. Subjects experienced the largest decrease in depression and anxiety. These results suggested that meditation facilitated the goals of the psychotherapeutic process. It is worth considering why such meditation training may have been helpful.

Patients were instructed in mindfulness meditation and were taught how to become detached observers of their thoughts. This form of meditation helps patients increase their insight regarding how mental categories are developed. With the enhanced awareness patients can detach themselves from their habitual ways of thinking, and through therapy they can progress to greater cognitive flexibility and more adaptive self-images and lifestyle changes. Much of what occurs in psychotherapy is intended to bring about these changes. While meditation alone cannot obviate skilled therapy and is no substitute for a therapeutic alliance, it may be the case that the CNS changes that occur when meditation is used to elicit the relaxation response set the stage for more rapid and persistent psychotherapeutic change.

For many types of disorders such as anxiety and other stress-related disorders, elicitation of the relaxation response via meditation or other techniques can help reduce sympathetic nervous system activity, which can be a part of the treatment. Researchers have examined the effectiveness of meditation-based stress reduction program in a pilot study on patients with anxiety disorders.

Patients participated in an 8-week course in which they attended weekly 2-hour classes. In the sixth week they also attended an intensive 7.5-hour retreat. Patients showed significant reductions in anxiety, panic symptoms, and depression from pre- to posttreatment and results were maintained 3 years later. It has been suggested that, unlike those who participate in cognitive therapy, patients who practice mindfulness meditation are not asked to substitute one thought pattern for another. Instead, patients observe the "inaccuracy, limited nature, and intrinsic impermanence of thoughts in general and anxiety-related thoughts in particular."

While meditation and other techniques used to elicit the relaxation response can play an important role in the treatment of some psychological problems, such interventions might not be recommended for patients with certain personality disorders, dissociative disorders, or schizophrenia.

VI. THE RELAXATION RESPONSE AND BEHAVIOR CHANGE

Relaxation-response training can be used to facilitate behavior modification goals. Most patients who begin a diet or a smoking cessation program are able to stay with the program for short periods of time. When stresses arise, however, it generally becomes more difficult to maintain the new routine. Coping with stress and anxiety has a "psychic cost" that takes the form of a diminished capacity for self-regulation. Presumably, the cause of this "stress disinhibition effect" is a depletion in the cognitive and emotional resources required to maintain self-regulation. Increased stress and anxiety lead to immediately gratifying, but ultimately damaging behaviors, such as dietary indiscretions, alcohol or drug abuse, and an increase in smoking. Relaxation training has proved to be effective as an acute coping strategy to reduce anxiety. [*See* COPING WITH STRESS.]

The extent to which stress-related relapses are prevented is directly related to the degree to which relaxation-response training alleviates stress and anxiety. For example, smoking-cessation programs are unsuccessful in about 60 to 80% of cases and stress has been identified as a major contributor to this high rate of failures. In a recent study, smokers who had completed a smoking-cessation program were assigned to either a relaxation training or a control group each of which met for 3 months. The relaxation-based intervention included audiotapes for home training in guided imagery techniques. The relaxation group was asked to practice 20 minutes a day at least four times a week. Relaxation-trained subjects reduced stress, enhanced imagery effectiveness, and, perhaps most importantly, were more successful in abstaining from smoking compared with control subjects who were not exposed to the training. During a 3-month follow-up only 28% of the relaxation-trained subjects relapsed whereas 49% of the control subjects resumed smoking.

Since relaxation training is often taught as a part of behavior-change programs with multiple components it is difficult to measure to what degree the beneficial effects are attributable to relaxation training alone. The effect of relaxation training was evaluated in one of the most successful behavior-change programs, the Lifestyle Heart program, developed by Ornish. In this program relaxation training is combined with diet and exercise regimens as well as group support to reduce symptoms in patients with coronary heart disease. In a controlled trial patients attended a week-long retreat followed by two 4-hour sessions each week thereafter. They performed 1 hour of aerobic exercise and participated in 1-hour sessions of stress management techniques which consisted of relaxation, yoga, stretching, breathing techniques, meditation, and guided imagery.

Among the participants the mean degree of coronary artery stenosis regressed from 61.1 to 55.8%. These results were compared with those in a group of nonparticipating patients in whom the mean degree of stenosis actually progressed from 61.7 to 64.4%. Analysis also showed that diet alone could not account for the beneficial effects. While almost all the patients maintained a healthier diet, those who practiced stress management more often showed greater stenotic regression.

In another study involving 156 patients who had had a myocardial infarction, relaxation response training augmented the effects of concurrent therapeutic strategies. Patients were randomized into two groups: one was given physical exercise training alone and the other was given both physical exercise and relaxation training. Several questionnaires were administered: the State-Trait Anxiety Inventory (a 40-item standardized anxiety inventory); a sleeping habits questionnaire (a 10-item questionnaire concerning hours of sleep, sleep quality, etc.); a functional complaints questionnaire (a 25-item inventory concerning complaints frequently expressed by cardiac patients); and the Heart Patients Psychological Questionnaire (HPPQ) (including scales on well-being, subjective invalidity, displeasure, social inhibition). Patients in the exercise-only group reported no change in psychological measures, whereas the group who received relaxation training reported less anxiety and subjective invalidity. The two groups also differed on physical outcomes as measured by exercise testing. Improvement was defined as the absence of signs of cardiac dysfunction that required treatment and was greater in the relaxation-training-and-exercise group compared with the exercise-only group.

VII. INTEGRATING THE RELAXATION RESPONSE INTO HEALTH CARE

The relaxation response has been associated with improvements in many medical conditions including: hypertension, cardiac arrhythmias, chronic pain, insomnia, side effects of cancer therapy, side effects of AIDS therapy, infertility, and preparation for surgery and X-ray procedures. It is also important to indicate that more recently, the overall implications of integrating relaxation response in routine clinical treatments has been examined. Some relevant examples will be discussed.

The effect of a behavioral group intervention that included relaxation response training on chronic pain patients. One hundred and nine patients who were members of an HMO participated in the study. The average duration of pain among the patients was 6.5 years. The interventions consisted of 90-minute group sessions, which were held once a week. At the end of the 10-week intervention period, participants in the group showed decreases in negative psychological symptoms including anxiety, depression, and hostility. This study also showed that such an intervention could result in significant cost savings. Group participants showed a 36% decrease in clinic use during the first and second year following the intervention. This latter result is particularly pertinent. There is a growing interest in the use of nonpharmacologic interventions such as elicitation of the relaxation response to not only facilitate psychological and medical goals but to help reduce medical utilization and costs. The above study is simply an example of the way in which such interventions can have this positive economic effect while at the same time have beneficial clinical outcomes.

Relaxation-response training was shown to improve outcomes among a group of patients with peripheral vascular disease who underwent femoral angiography. Forty-five patients participated in the study. Patients listened to either a relaxation tape that included instruction in progressive muscle relaxation and cognitive relaxation involving mental focusing or to a tape of recorded music. A third group of patients listened to a blank tape. Patients who listened to a relaxation-response tape experienced less anxiety and pain during the surgical procedure and requested significantly less medication that those patients who listened to the tape of recorded music or the blank tape. This study also showed that relaxation-response training can be administered very inexpensively and in ways that are practical for staff and patients.

Clearly, there is substantial research that shows that meditation and other relaxation-response techniques can be effective components in psychotherapy, behavior-change programs, and in medical treatment. Resistance to adjunctive use of such treatments, especially elicitation of the relaxation response, appears to be waning. A recent survey of medical schools found that approximately two-thirds now include discussions of relaxation techniques in their medical training. Knowledge of relaxation-response training can be helpful to physicians not only for the physiological benefits to patients but because many patients who present with medical problems really have a psychological disorder. Such patients may feel uncomfortable about seeing a mental health professional or participating in psychotherapy. Relaxation techniques can be a means for the physician to start a dialogue about dealing with psychological disorders.

While the use of relaxation training is unquestioned in psychological treatment, there are still barriers to its use in medical settings. One barrier is a misunderstanding of the relaxation-response interventions and why they are used. Meditation and other introspective procedures bring about important central and peripheral physiological changes because they elicit the relaxation response. These central and peripheral changes are compatible with better mental and physical well-being. However, no single intervention can work for everyone. More research to define under what specific circumstances relaxation-response training would be most beneficial and cost effective for which patients still needs to be completed.

Many practitioners, insurers, and patients remain confused about the differences between the use of such services and psychotherapy. Relaxation training alone and when used with other types of behavioral therapies is more focused than traditional psychotherapy. It is often conducted in groups settings, and sessions are limited to 8 to 10 sessions. The important difference is that while the goal of psychotherapy is to change psychological symptoms, the goal of relaxation-response training with medical conditions is to change somatic manifestations. Relaxation training should be better understood, more routinely used, integrated, as well as paid for in medical settings. Such integration is imperative to the clients/patients and society.

BIBLIOGRAPHY

Benson, H. (1975). *The relaxation response.* New York: Morrow.

Benson, H. (1996). *Timeless healing: the power and biology of belief.* New York: Scribner.

Benson, H., & Stuart, E. M. (1992). *The wellness book.* New York: Simon and Shuster.

Friedman, R., Sobel, D., Myers, P., Caudill, M., & Benson, H. (1995). Behavioral medicine, clinical health psychology, and cost offset. *Health Psychology, 14*(6), 509–518.

Jacobs, G. D., Benson, H., & Friedman, R. (1996). Topographic EEG mapping of the relaxation response. *Biofeedback and Self-Regulation, 21*(2), 121–129.

Kabat-Zinn, J. (1994). *Wherever you go there you are: Mindfulness meditation in everyday life.* New York: Hyperion.

Kutz, I., Borysenko, J. Z., & Benson, H. (1985). Meditation and psychotherapy: A rationale for the integration of dynamic psychotherapy, the relaxation response and mindfulness meditation. *American Journal of Psychiatry, 142,* 1–8.

NIH Technology Assessment Panel on Integration of Behavioral and Relaxation Approaches Into the Treatment of Chronic Pain and Insomnia. (1996). Integration of behavioral and relaxation approaches into the treatment of chronic pain and insomnia. *JAMA, 276(4), 313–318.*

Sakakibara, M., Takeuchi, S., & Hayano, J. (1994). Effect of relaxation training on cardiac parasympathetic tone. *Psychophysiology, 31,* 223–228.

Wallace, R. K., & Benson, H. (1972). The physiology of meditation. *Scientific American, 226,* 84–90.

Personality Assessment

Paul T. Costa, Jr., and Robert R. McCrae

National Institutes of Health

Five-Factor Model An organization of personality traits in terms of the broad factors of neuroticism versus emotional stability, extraversion, openness to experience, agreeableness, and conscientiousness.
Objective Test An assessment device that can be scored clerically, without the need for clinical interpretation.
Projective Technique A method of assessment in which responses to ambiguous stimuli (e.g., inkblots) are thought to reveal aspects of the respondent's personality.
Reliability The consistency with which an assessment instrument gives the same results.
Validity The accuracy with which an assessment instrument measures its intended construct.

The term personality is used by different theorists in widely different ways, and the practice of PERSONALITY ASSESSMENT is correspondingly varied. Nevertheless, most definitions of personality refer to features that characterize an individual and distinguish him or her from others, and most assessment procedures attempt to measure these features, usually in comparison to the average person. Different approaches to personality assessment differ in the variables they measure, in the source of information about the individual, and in the way information is evaluated. This article reviews the most common approaches to personality assessment (projective techniques, self-report questionnaires, observer ratings, and laboratory measures) and their status in contemporary psychological science and practice.

Personality variables are pervasive and enduring, and thus can be expected to have an impact on a variety of areas in the individual's life—for example, the prototypic extrovert has a wide circle of friends, speaks out in class, does well in enterprising occupations, enjoys competitive sports, and has an optimistic outlook in life. In consequence, personality assessment is important in many applied areas. Psychiatrists who need to diagnose psychopathology, counselors who want to suggest meaningful vocational choices, and physicians concerned with behavioral health risk factors may all turn to personality assessment. Personality variables are important in forensic, developmental, educational, social, industrial, and clinical psychology, as well as personality psychology, the discipline which seeks a scientific understanding of personality itself. For all these purposes, accurate assessment of personality is crucial.

Personality is also of great importance to laypersons in everyday life and in such significant decisions as whom to vote for or marry. Lay evaluations of personality are in some respects unscientific and susceptible to many biases; in other respects they are extremely sophisticated interpretations of observed behavior. Much (though not all) of personality assessment consists of knowing how to systematize the information laypersons have about themselves and each other in order to capitalize on the strengths and reduce the limitations of lay perceptions of personality.

The scientific study of individual differences in personality can be traced to the work of Sir Francis Galton in the 1880s, and it has occupied many of the brightest minds in psychology since. During the 1950s and 1960s, personality assessment underwent a period of crisis, based in part on humanistic objections to the depersonalizing labeling that much assessment seemed to foster, and in part on real (although exaggerated) technical problems with assessment instruments. Considerable progress has been made in the past 30 years in both personality theory and test construction, and today personality assessment is once again assuming a central role in psychology.

I. ASSESSMENT METHODS AND INSTRUMENTS

A. Projective Techniques

The single most influential theory of personality is psychoanalysis, a complex system developed by Sigmund Freud and elaborated by a host of his followers. Briefly, psychoanalysis sees human personality as the result of conflict between the individual's sexual and aggressive impulses and society's demand for their control. In the course of early development, people evolve characteristic ways of resolving these conflicts which guide their adult behavior, particularly their interpersonal relationships. Because the underlying conflicts are psychologically painful and threatening, both the impulses and the defenses against them are repressed from consciousness. From this perspective, individuals never really know themselves and hide their most important features from those around them.

Thus, psychoanalytic theory poses formidable problems for personality assessment. The central information is not merely unavailable; it is systematically distorted. The analyst must make elaborate inferences on the basis of free associations, dreams, and slips of the tongue. But patients may not recall dreams or make revealing slips, and psychoanalysts need a dependable source of information that can be gathered as needed. Projective tests were designed to fill this need.

Rorschach's inkblots are a series of 10 cards shown to the patient or subject, who is asked to explain what he or she sees in them. The basic premise is that these abstract blots, having no meaning of their own, will act as a screen onto which the inner conflicts, impulses, and emotions of the patient will be projected. They will of course still be disguised—otherwise they would be censored by the patient's defenses—but they can be interpreted by the knowledgeable analyst just as an X-ray can be read by a skilled radiologist.

The projective technique is an ingenious approach to the problem of assessing unconscious conflicts, and the window it promises into the depths of the mind is extremely appealing. The Rorschach continues to be one of the most widely used instruments in personality assessment, and dozens of variations (including the Holtzman Inkblot Technique) and scoring systems have been developed.

It is therefore more than a little unfortunate that the scientific basis of these instruments—and of psychoanalysis itself—is highly questionable. Different interpreters draw very different conclusions from the same set of responses, and few rigorous studies have demonstrated that inkblot scores predict important external criteria. While clinical psychologists still rely heavily on the Rorschach, academic personality researchers have almost entirely abandoned it. A search of abstracts in the personality research field's most important publication, the *Journal of Personality and Social Psychology,* showed that of over 4000 articles appearing between 1974 and 1992, only four studies employed the Rorschach. (Rorschach studies do still appear regularly in more clinically oriented journals.)

All projective techniques use responses to relatively unstructured, ambiguous stimuli on the assumption that these will elicit spontaneous expressions of psychologically important features. This general approach to assessment is not limited to psychoanalytic theories of personality, but can also be applied to better supported theories about needs, motives, or traits. The Thematic Apperception Test, or TAT, shows a series of drawings about which individuals are asked to tell stories. The responses can be scored in a relatively straightforward fashion—for example, a story about overcoming obstacles in pursuit of a goal is scored as evidence of a need for achievement—and when so scored they typically show somewhat better evidence of scientific validity.

Note that these approaches do not assume that the characteristics they assess are repressed. When asked, people who tell stories about achievement or intimacy often report that they are high in achievement striving or nurturance. These projective tests apparently do not reveal a level of personality from which self-reports are excluded. [*See* PSYCHOANALYSIS.]

B. Objective Tests: Self-Reports

Projective tests are usually contrasted with *objective tests,* typically questionnaires in which subjects are asked to describe themselves by answering a series of questions. For example, a measure of conscientiousness may ask 10 questions such as "Do you always keep your desk clean?" and "Are you devoted to your work?" The test is considered objective because it can be scored directly, without the need for clinical interpretation: The number of conscientiousness items to which an individual responds *true* is that individual's score, and higher scores indicate higher levels of conscientiousness.

That basic paradigm—asking a standard set of questions and scoring responses with a predetermined key—has been used in thousands of assessment applications. Intelligence tests, vocational interest inventories, mood indicators, and measures of psychopathology as well as personality scales have adopted this model. Its scientific appeal lies in the fact that it can be repeated at different times and with different subjects, and consequently its accuracy can be evaluated. A whole branch of statistics, *psychometrics,* has been developed to analyze responses, both for what they tell us about the individual and for what they tell us about the quality of the test. Psychometric analyses provide information that can allow researchers to improve the quality of the test by changing the questions or the response format or the interpretation of the results.

If psychoanalysis formed the theoretical basis of projective tests, then trait psychology must be considered the basis of objective personality tests. Briefly, trait psychologies hold that individuals differ in a number of important ways that are usually thought to be continuously and normally distributed. Just as a few people are short, a few tall, and most average in height, so some people may be very agreeable, some very antagonistic, and most intermediate along this psychological dimension. Unlike moods, traits are enduring dispositions; and unlike specific habits, they are general and pervasive patterns of thoughts, feelings, and actions. Scores on trait measures should therefore be relatively constant, and scale items measuring different aspects of the trait should go together. These theoretical premises are the basis of the psychometric requirements of retest reliability and internal consistency in personality scales.

Among the most important personality questionnaires in current use are the Minnesota Multiphasic Personality Inventory (MMPI), developed in the 1940s to measure aspects of psychopathology; the Sixteen Personality Factor Questionnaire and the Eysenck Personality Questionnaire, representing the personality theories of Raymond B. Cattell and Hans J. Eysenck, respectively; the Myers-Briggs Type Indicator, which is based on C. J. Jung's theory of psychological types; the California Psychological Inventory, a set of scales intended to tap folk concepts, the personality constructs used in everyday life; and the Personality Research Form, a psychometrically sophisticated measure of needs or motives. The NEO Personality Inventory is a more recent addition, based on new discoveries about the basic dimensions of personality. In addition to these omnibus inventories which all measure a variety of traits, there are a number of individual scales that are widely used in personality research, such as the self-monitoring scale and the locus of control scale.

C. Objective Tests: Observer Ratings

The vast majority of personality assessments are made on the basis of either projective tests or self-reports, but observer ratings provide a powerful alternative that is increasingly used in both research and clinical contexts. The clinical interview is a kind of observer rating, because the clinician not only asks questions, but also observes the reactions of the patient to the interview process. With a few exceptions (such as the Structured Interview for the Type A Behavior Pattern), these observations are not standardized, and thus they share with projective tests potential problems of unreliability.

There are, however, assessment methods that are both objective and observer based. These methods apply the same psychometric principles used in self-report questionnaires to ratings from informants. One simple and effective way to do this is by rephrasing questions in the third person. Instead of asking the individual, "Are you devoted to your work?" we could ask her spouse, "Is she devoted to her work?" One advantage of observer ratings is that we are not limited to a single respondent. It is possible to obtain ratings from friends, relatives, and neighbors, and there is evidence that aggregating or averaging several ratings yields better information on the individual.

Ranking methods provide an alternative to observer rating questionnaires. In these methods, all the members of a group rank each other on a series of characteristics. For example, all the members of a fraternity may be asked to decide which fraternity members are most and least *talkative,* and rank order all the other members between them. In the assessment center method, a group of expert raters (typically psychologists) interacts with a group of subjects over a period of a few days, observing them in both standardized and unstructured situations. They then make personality ratings, perhaps by checking descriptive adjectives.

The advantages of these different forms of gathering information from observers are still debated, as are the relative merits of self-reports versus observer ratings. Fortunately, however, many recent studies have shown general agreement between many different objective methods of assessing personality. This consensual validation of observations about personality traits forms an essential basis for scientific personality psychology.

D. Objective Tests: Laboratory Procedures

Researchers dedicated to objectivity have often hoped that personality could be assessed by laboratory tests that did not depend on the judgments of individuals. Quantity of salivation in response to a drop of lemon juice, perspiration as measured by the galvanic skin response, and dilation of the pupil have all been proposed as measures of personality attributes. This approach to personality assessment has been of limited value; physiological responses typically have shown only modest and inconsistent relations to personality variables.

Yet accumulating evidence on the heritability of most personality traits suggests that there is some genetic and presumably physiological basis for many traits. Increasing sophistication in our understanding of the brain and new techniques such as magnetic resonance imaging may one day lead to discoveries about personality/brain relations with implications for assessment. At present, however, our best source of information about personality is the individual and those who know him or her well.

II. EVALUATING ASSESSMENT METHODS

A. Reliability and Validity

Although well-constructed objective measures of personality are valuable scientific tools, it should not be assumed that all objective measures are well-constructed. Psychometricians have, however, established a series of criteria by which scales can be evaluated. It is traditional to divide these into *reliability* criteria and *validity* criteria, although the distinction between the two is somewhat artificial. In essence, both require that the scale perform in ways that are consistent with its intended theoretical interpretation.

The two most common forms of reliability are *internal consistency* and *retest reliability.* If each of the items in a scale is considered to be an indicator of the same underlying trait, it seems reasonable to require that they all agree with each other. Cronbach's coefficient α is a commonly used measure of this internal consistency of scale items. Internal consistency can be increased by discarding items that show limited agreement with other items, or by adding more items of the same kind (longer scales are more reliable because the errors introduced by individual items tend to cancel each other out in the long run).

For narrow constructs, the higher the internal consistency, the better. For broad constructs, however, higher internal consistency is not necessarily better because it may be purchased with a loss of generality. For example, a measure of general psychological distress that consisted of the items, "I am fearful," "I am nervous," and "I am anxious" would probably have high internal consistency, but it would offer a very narrow measure of distress focused exclusively on anxiety. Depression, frustration, shame, and other aspects of psychological distress are omitted. By including items to measure them, we would probably produce a scale with lower internal consistency but higher fidelity to the broad theoretical construct of psychological distress.

Test–retest reliability refers to the reproducibility of scores on different occasions. We would not expect major changes in personality over a 2-week period, so if individuals score very differently when they complete the questionnaire twice over this interval, it suggests that there are problems with the test.

In essence, questions about reliability ask whether the scale elicits responses that are consistent across items and across time. Without some minimum of reliability, it is hard to argue that the scale measures anything meaningful, so reliability is often taken as a prerequisite to validity. *Validity* refers to the degree to which a scale actually measures the construct it is intended to measure. A spelling test might have excellent internal consistency and retest reliability, but no validity at all if it were intended to be used as a measure of extraversion.

The central problem in establishing the validity of a test is that we rarely have completely satisfactory external criteria. A good measure of agreeableness–antagonism would separate agreeable from antagonistic people, but—without giving the test—how do we know who is agreeable and who is antagonistic? No single answer is usually sufficient, so we rely on a pattern of evidence in evaluating the construct validity of a scale. We may correlate it with other scales that measure similar constructs, (e.g., scales measuring trust and altruism), or we may see if it distinguishes between known groups that should differ on the dimension (e.g., social workers versus convicted felons), or we may compare self-reports with ratings on the same scale made by spouses or peers.

All of these studies would give information on the *convergent validity* of the scale, but they would not necessarily speak to its *discriminant validity*. The criterion of discriminant validity requires that scales be *un*related to scales which measure theoretically different constructs. If a test is designed to measure agreeableness, it should not be strongly related to intelligence, because intelligence is theoretically independent of agreeableness. In order to establish discriminant validity, a scale must be related to a series of other measures, especially those with which it is apt to be confounded. The strongest designs for construct validity usually require that multiple methods be used for assessing multiple traits, and that stronger correlations be seen for measures of the same trait obtained from different methods than for measures of different traits obtained from the same method.

Table I gives an example of convergent and discriminant validity across instruments and observers. Five basic dimensions of personality—neuroticism, extroversion, openness to experience, agreeableness, and conscientiousness—are measured by self-reports on adjective rating scales, and by peer ratings on a questionnaire measure, the NEO Personality Inventory. The convergent correlations (given in boldface) show substantial agreement—far greater agreement than would be expected by chance. By contrast, the discriminant correlations (e.g., between peer-rated neuroticism and self-reported openness to experience) are much smaller and generally do not exceed chance. Such data provide evidence that both instruments measure the intended constructs with considerable success.

Table I Convergent and Discriminant Validity of Measures of Five Basic Dimensions of Personality

Mean peer rated NEO personality inventory domains	Self-reported adjective factors				
	N	E	O	A	C
Neuroticism (N)	**.44*****	−.03	.00	−.03	−.15*
Extroversion (E)	.06	**.45*****	.16**	.00	.06
Openness to experience (O)	.07	.08	**.45*****	.13*	−.07
Agreeableness (A)	−.06	−.11	−.15*	**.45*****	−.10
Conscientiousness (C)	−.11	−.05	−.10	−.09	**.39*****

Note. N = 267. Convergent correlations are given in boldface. Adapted from McCrae and Costa (1987). *J. Pers. Soc. Psychol.* **52**, 81–90.

*p <.05. **p <.01. ***p <.001.

B. Sources of Error and Bias; Response Styles

Most personality questionnaires consist of a series of statements that the respondent must answer either *true* or *false* or rate on a scale (e.g., from *strongly disagree* to *strongly agree*). As anyone who has taken such a test knows, the items are often ambiguous and sometimes of dubious relevance. The question, "Are you devoted to your work?" might be interpreted in several ways. Some respondents might compare their devotion to work with their commitment to family. Some might compare their own devotion to that of their co-workers. Retired or unemployed respondents might not know how to respond. Even with the sincerest cooperation, respondents may not give the response the test developer intended.

Further, some respondents may not be sincerely cooperative. They may respond carelessly or at random simply to be finished with the task. Or they may wish to present a flattering picture of themselves to the tester. One of the most troubling discoveries of personality psychology was that laypeople are exquisitely sensitive to the social desirability of items and can, if so instructed, fake most personality tests.

Another common problem is acquiescent responding. It was discovered long ago that individuals differ in the tendency to agree with statements, regardless of content. So-called yea-sayers interpret items in ways that allow them to endorse most of them; nay-sayers find something in most items to which they object. If all the items are keyed in the same direction—that is, if *true* or *agree* responses are always indicative of the trait—then scale scores will confound measurement of the trait with measurement of acquiescent tendencies. Two such scales might show a positive correlation even if they measured very different traits, because both might also measure acquiescent tendencies.

This particular response style can be controlled quite effectively by creating scales with balanced keying: Half the items are scored in the positive direction, half in the negative. For example, we might measure conscientiousness by including the item "I often fail to keep my promises," and giving points for conscientiousness if the respondent *disagrees*. In responses to a balanced scale, acquiescent tendencies cancel themselves out, leaving a purer measure of the trait.

Similar strategies have been developed for dealing with other response styles. For example, random responding can be detected by including a set of items that virtually no one would endorse if they were paying attention and cooperating (e.g., "I keep an elephant in my basement"). Endorsing several such items would suggest random responding, and test results should be considered invalid. Cooperative respondents, however, may find the inclusion of such "trick questions" offensive. An alternative way of detecting one common form of random responding is by looking for a string of identical responses on an answer sheet, which may indicate thoughtless, repetitive responding merely intended to finish the questionnaire. This is an unobtrusive measure of random responding.

The greatest attention has been paid to the problem of socially desirable responding. Many scales have been devised in the hopes that they could identify individuals who responded on the basis of the desirability of an item rather than its accuracy as a description of their personality. Researchers routinely include such scales in construct validity studies to estimate the discriminant validity of the scales of interest from socially desirable response tendencies. Unfortunately, however, no good measure of desirable responding per se has yet been developed, and most research suggests that attempts to correct for social desirability do more harm than good.

The root of the problem is that statements have both substantive and evaluative meanings. Anyone who wished to appear in a good light would endorse the item "I always try to do my best"—but so would highly conscientious individuals who are scrupulously honest in their responses. It is impossible to determine from the response alone whether the individual really has desirable characteristics or is presenting a falsely favorable picture of him- or herself.

Two general strategies appear to be useful for dealing with this problem. First, in most cases it appears that respondents are more truthful than psychologists anticipated. Even though they *can* endorse desirable items when instructed to do so, test takers normally do not, when asked to be honest and accurate. Research volunteers have little incentive to distort their responses, and clients in counseling and psychotherapy should be convinced by the assessor that accurate responding will be in their best interest. Mutual respect and trust between test administrators and test takers is usually the best basis for assuring valid results.

However, in some cases there may be good reasons for mistrusting self-reports. The responses of prison inmates who describe themselves as saints when being evaluated for parole should be regarded with considerable skepticism. In these cases, the most appropriate tactic may be to obtain observer ratings from knowledgeable and impartial informants. The current availability of validated observer-rating questionnaires (such as Form R of the NEO Personality Inventory) makes that approach feasible.

None of these approaches to scale construction or administration eliminates all the limitations of personality assessment by questionnaire. The inevitable ambiguity of items and respondents' imperfect knowledge of themselves or the individuals they rate mean than personality measures lack the precision that we admire in the physical sciences. The data in Table I show that our assessments are on the right track, but they can also be interpreted to show that our measurements are far from perfect. Both self-reports and observer ratings are useful tools that give valuable information about personality, and either is acceptable for use in research on groups. For the intensive understanding of the individual (e.g., in psychotherapy), it is desirable to obtain both self-reports and informant ratings, and all inferences about personality traits should be considered provisional, subject to revision or refinement as new information becomes available.

C. Content and Comprehensiveness in Personality Questionnaires

Psychometric theory gives general guidelines for constructing and evaluating measures of psychological characteristics, but it gives little guidance about *what* should be measured. For decades, one of the central problems in personality psychology was the proliferation of hundreds of scales measuring aspects of personality that some researcher or theorist thought important in understanding human beings. Many of the most eminent personality psychologists were those who offered a system, a model of personality structure that specified the most important aspects of personality and thus brought some kind of order to the chaos of competing ideas.

Factor analysis has frequently been used as the statistical technique for studying personality structure. Factor analysis is a mathematical procedure which condenses the information about intercorrelations among many variables by detecting groups of variables that covary separately from other groups. These groups of variables define a factor, a dimension along which individuals can be ranked. For example, the individual traits of trust, straightforwardness, altruism, compliance, modesty, and tender-mindedness covary to define the broad dimension of agreeableness.

In the days before computers, a factor analysis might consume months of computational labor, and it is not surprising that early factor analysts tended to defend whatever structure they first uncovered. As a result, for many decades disputes raged about whether there were 2 basic factors, or 3, or 5, or 10, or 16. Failure to resolve this issue lowered the credibility of the field, and paralyzed much personality research: How could we study personality and aging, say, unless we knew which aspects of personality we needed to measure as individuals aged?

In 1961 two Air Force psychologists, Ernest Tupes and Raymond Christal, factored data from several different studies and concluded that five, and only five, major factors seemed to recur. Their work was largely ignored during the next 20 years, but around 1980 interest in the five-factor model revived. Initially, these five factors were seen as the basic dimensions underlying trait adjective terms used by laypersons and encoded in the natural language—terms such as *nervous, enthusiastic, original, accommodating,* and *careful.* Questionnaire measures, including the NEO Personality Inventory, were then developed to measure these five factors (see Table I for names of the factors). Subsequent research showed that the same five factors were also found in most of the theoretically based questionnaires that had previously been constructed. For example, the four scales of the Myers-Briggs Type Indicator correspond to four of the five factors (introversion–extroversion to extroversion, sensation–intuition to openness, thinking–feeling to agreeableness, and perception–judgment to conscientiousness).

The same basic dimensions have been recovered in cross-cultural analyses of personality (including studies conducted in Hebrew, German, and Chinese), in self-reports and observer ratings, in men and women, and in young, middle-aged, and older adults. Although disagreements remain over the precise nature and scope of the factors, there is a general consensus that these five represent basic and universal features of personality. (Intelligence, another fundamental dimension of individual differences, is generally considered to be outside the realm of personality proper.) The five-factor model thus provides a general answer to the question of what personality traits should be measured: A comprehensive assessment must include measures of all five factors.

However, the five factors themselves are too broad to give a detailed picture of the individual. Anxiety and depression are both aspects of neuroticism, and in general, people who are anxious also tend to be depressed. But some anxious people are not depressed, and some depressed people are not anxious, and it is extremely important to clinical psychologists to determine whether a patient is anxious, depressed, or both. A global measure of neuroticism would not provide that information; instead, more specific scales are needed to provide the details. The same could be said for all five factors.

While most personality psychologists see the need for assessment of personality at this more specific level, there is no consensus about which specific traits should be measured, or even how to go about identifying the most important specific traits. Advocates of circumflex models suggest that we expand the five-factor model by measuring traits that represent combinations of pairs of factors. For example, friendliness is related to both extraversion and agreeableness, so it might merit separate assessment.

Other researchers believe that there are a large number of important traits—perhaps 100 or more—that should be separately analyzed; the five-factor model could then be used primarily to organize the results. In the Revised NEO Personality Inventory, 30 separate traits identified from an analysis of the psychological literature are measured by facet scales, and global domain scales are formed by summing groups of six of them, as shown in Table II. This scheme encourages hierarchical personality assessment at both the more specific and more general levels.

III. PERSONALITY ASSESSMENT AND PERSONALITY THEORY

Human beings have always tried to understand themselves and the people around them; scientific psychology has made real, if slow, progress in this endeavor over the past century. Theories of test construction and validation and psychometric techniques have provided the technical basis for developing sound measures, and the five-factor model specifies which aspects of personality should be measured. As usual in science, there is a continuing interaction between theory and measurement: The more we know about human personality, the better our techniques for measuring it, and the better we measure it, the more we are able to refine our theories.

Psychoanalysis, behaviorism, and humanistic psychologies in turn dominated personality psychology, and each led to serious problems for personality assessment. Self-reports about thoughts, feelings, and actions were considered trivial by psychoanalysts, who believed that the important psychological variables were unconscious, and unscientific by behaviorists, who preferred observation of behavior in laboratory settings. Humanistic psychologists sometimes opposed assessment on principle, because they believed that rating individuals on a fixed set of dimensions was depersonalizing.

Table II Global Domains and Specific Facets in the Revised NEO Personality Inventory

Neuroticism	Extroversion	Openness	Agreeableness	Conscientiousness
Anxiety	Warmth	Fantasy	Trust	Competence
Angry hostility	Gregariousness	Aesthetics	Straightforwardness	Order
Depression	Assertiveness	Feelings	Altruism	Dutifulness
Self-consciousness	Activity	Actions	Compliance	Achievement striving
Impulsiveness	Excitement seeking	Ideas	Modesty	Self-discipline
Vulnerability	Positive emotions	Values	Tender-mindedness	Deliberation

Trait psychology has always coexisted with these other schools, but has rarely been dominant. But personality assessments based on the principles of trait psychology have shown themselves to be scientifically defensible and useful in applied contexts. For these reasons, trait psychology and the five-factor model appear poised to be the dominant paradigm in personality psychology in the next century.

This article has been reprinted from the *Encyclopedia of Human Behavior, Volume 3.*

BIBLIOGRAPHY

Briggs, S. R. (1992). Assessing the five-factor model of personality description. *J. Pers.* 60, 253–293.

Funder, D. C. (1991). Global traits: A Neo-Allportian approach to personality. *Psychol. Sci.* 2, 31–39.

Kline, P. (1993). "The Handbook of Psychological Testing." Routledge, New York.

McCrae, R. R., & Costa, P. T., Jr. (1990). "Personality in Adulthood." Guilford, New York.

Wiggins, J. S., & Pincus, A. L. (1992). Personality: Structure and assessment. *Annu. Rev. Psychol.* 43, 473–504.

Premenstrual Syndrome Treatment Interventions

Laura Weiss Roberts, Teresita McCarty, and Sally K. Severino
University of New Mexico School of Medicine

Follicular Phase of the Menstrual Cycle The initial portion of the menstrual cycle, starting at the onset of menses until ovulation occurs. The length of the follicular phase is variable.

Hypothalamus and Pituitary Gland Subcortical, midline brain structures that function in the regulation of a number of neuroendocrine systems. Lesions and tumors of the hypothalamus frequently are associated with a broad variety of psychiatric, physical, and behavioral symptoms such as emotional changes (e.g., apathy, sadness, nervousness, irritability, frequent crying), paranoia, abnormal menstrual and thyroid function, and appetite and sleep problems.

Luteal Phase of the Menstrual Cycle The latter portion of the menstrual cycle starting after ovulation until the onset of menses. The phase is about 14 days long and is named after the corpus luteum of the ovary.

Ovaries Paired sexual organs, located in the lower abdomen of women, that serve as the source of ova and secrete a number of steroid hormones necessary for menstruation, ovulation, first trimester pregnancy sustenance, and other aspects of women's sexual health.

Ovulation The point in the menstrual cycle at which the egg, the reproductive germ cell, is released from a mature ovarian follicle.

Premenstrual Dysphoric Disorder (PMDD), formerly Late Luteal Phase Dysphoric Disorder (LLPDD) Terms that refer to that small percentage of women who have premenstrual syndrome with primarily emotional symptoms severe enough to affect their ability to function at home or in the workplace.

Premenstrual Exacerbation Aggravation of such chronic conditions such as asthma, depression, anxiety, eating disorders, substance abuse, headaches, allergies, seizures, or herpes during the premenstrual phase.

Premenstrual Phase, also "Late Luteal Phase" or "Premenstruum" The 5- to 7-day period immediately preceding menses.

Premenstrual Symptoms Those physical, behavioral, or mood changes that appear to change in severity during the late luteal phase of the cycle, do not exist in the same form or severity during the mid or late follicular phase, and disappear or return to their usual level of severity during menses.

Preventive Health Care Clinical care that places an emphasis on the decreased incidence (i.e., number of new cases each year) of disease (primary prevention), the early recognition and eradication of disease (secondary prevention), and the minimization of suffering caused by disease (tertiary prevention).

Uterus The womb, a hollow, muscular organ in women that opens to the vaginal canal and undergoes

Copyright © 1998 by Academic Press.
All rights of reproduction in any form reserved.

sequential and cyclic changes (i.e., proliferative, secretory, menstrual) between menarche and menopause. It is the structure in which the fertilized ovum normally becomes embedded and the developing fetus matures before birth.

PREMENSTRUAL SYNDROME (PMS) refers to a condition that some women experience preceding the onset of their monthly menses. It consists of the cyclic recurrence of physical, psychological, and/or behavioral symptoms of sufficient severity that medical treatment is sought. Optimal care for the physical and psychological well-being of women who suffer from PMS is built on an understanding of the developmental aspects of women's sexual health, including biological, psychological, and social/cultural influences.

I. HISTORICAL BACKGROUND

As far back as the time of Hippocrates, physicians have attempted to describe the relationships between menstruation and the subjective experiences, moods, and behavior changes of women. Over the past 24 centuries, "morbid dispositions of the mind" and "madness" in the form of mania, delusions, "nervous excitement," hallucinations, "unreasonable appetites," and suicidal impulses have been attributed to the cyclic menstrual patterns of women. Although much remains to be understood, our clinical and scientific interest in these relationships has grown in modern times. Robert Frank coined the term "premenstrual tension" and offered this remarkable description of the problem in 1931 (p. 1054):

> A feeling of indescribable tension from 10 to 7 days preceding menstruation which, in most instances, continues until . . . menstrual flow occurs. These patients complain of unrest, irritability, "like jumping out of their skin." . . . [T]heir personal suffering is intense.

Premenstrual tension later became known as premenstrual syndrome or PMS. In particular, the work of Katharina Dalton in England, beginning in the 1950s and ongoing today, established PMS as a legitimate health condition of women, worthy of medical attention and scientific investigation (see Premenstrual Syndrome (PMS) by Katharina Dalton). A conference convened by the National Institute of Mental Health in 1983 established diagnostic guidelines for PMS and affirmed the interest of mental health professionals in the mood symptoms experienced premenstrually by many women. In 1987, Late Luteal Phase Dysphoric Disorder (LLPDD), a more narrowly defined syndrome than PMS, was included as a proposed clinical diagnosis in an appendix of the Diagnostic and Statistical Manual of Mental Disorders (DSM-IIIR). DSM-IV, published in 1994, replaced this terminology and classified Premenstrual Dysphoric Disorder as a clinical diagnosis under the rubric of "Depression Not Otherwise Specified."

After decades of research, PMS remains a puzzle with respect to etiology, physical and psychological correlates, risk and protective factors, and treatment. The true prevalence of PMS remains uncertain, the relative contributions of "nature" and "nurture" to PMS symptomatology have not been determined, and the reasons why only some women develop PMS have not been fully established. We have learned to some extent, however, what PMS is not: PMS is not the result of abnormal menstrual cycles or of abnormal absolute levels of ovarian hormones. It is not solely the result of attributional bias. Moreover, PMS is not a condition relieved uniformly by a single treatment approach such as hormonal therapy or psychiatric medications. After years of inquiry, it appears that PMS is the result of complex interactions among biological, psychological, social, and cultural influences within the lives of women.

For this reason, women's health related to PMS may best be understood from a multidimensional perspective. This article outlines an approach to PMS that focuses on the normal menstrual cycle and the distinct biological, psychological, and social/cultural issues in women's development, and includes a review of the phenomenology of PMS. With this foundation, we describe strategies for restoring mental and physical health related to the menstrual cycle through prevention, accurate diagnosis, and appropriate treatment interventions.

II. NORMAL MENSTRUAL CYCLE

The normal menstrual cycle is an intricately orchestrated, neatly timed physiologic process occurring in women from menarche until menopause. Each cycle revolves around development of an ovarian follicle and the preparation of the uterus, followed by ovula-

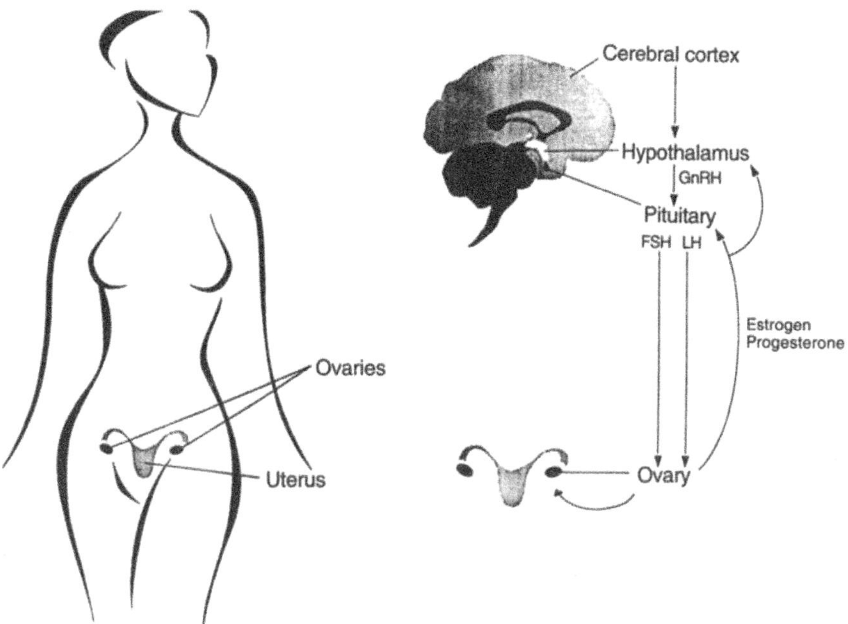

Figure 1 Anatomy and physiology of the menstrual cycle. GnRH, gonadotropin-releasing hormone; FSH, follicle-stimulating hormone; LH, luteinizing hormone. *Illustration by Jim Roberts.*

tion and the transformation of the ovarian follicle into the corpus luteum, which is necessary for sustaining a pregnancy should fertilization and embryo implantation occur. In the absence of pregnancy, the menstrual cycle ordinarily lasts 26 to 32 days (a range of 21 to 36 days), with women between the ages of 20 and 40 having the greatest regularity in cycle length. The menstrual cycle's three distinct phases relate primarily to hormonal changes and events at the hypothalamus and pituitary regions of the brain, the ovary, and the uterus (Figures 1 and 2). The cycle is also influenced by the limbic region of the central nervous system, the adrenal and thyroid glands, the pancreas, and exogenous hormones or medications.

A. Follicular Phase and Ovulation

The follicular phase begins on the first day of menstruation and lasts until approximately Day 14, based on a 28-day cycle. During this phase, a number of ovarian follicles, each typically containing a single ovum, develop under the influence of follicular stimulating hormone (FSH) produced by the anterior pituitary, a deep, midline endocrine organ in the brain. This hormone is produced and delivered in response to the pulsatile release of a neurohormone, gonadotropin releasing hormone (GnRH), which is produced in the medial basal region of a second brain structure, the hypothalamus. The developing follicles, in turn, produce estrogen, which has three main effects: it dampens the further release of FSH by the anterior pituitary; it, along with GnRH, stimulates the production and gradual release of luteinizing hormone (LH) by the anterior pituitary; and it stimulates the growth of the uterine lining or endometrium. Over the course of 2 weeks, one of the ovarian follicles matures more than the others in that it is larger, has evidence of more mitotic and biosynthetic activity, and has greater vascularization. This "dominant" follicle progresses through three phases (preantral, antral, and preovulatory) and manufactures increasing amounts of estrogen and, to a lesser extent, progesterone. The other follicles gradually and irreversibly decline.

Toward the end of the follicular phase, a rise in progesterone and surges of estrogen, LH, and FSH take place, resulting in ovulation. Estrogen peaks 24 to 36 hours prior to ovulation, whereas LH and FSH peak roughly within 10 to 12 hours of ovulation. Luteinizing hormone stimulates the initiation of oocyte meiosis, leutinizes the granulosa cells of the follicle,

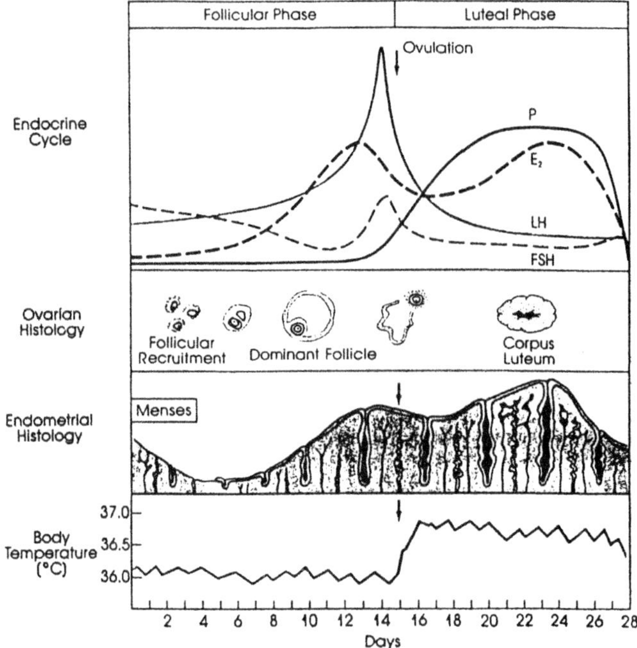

Figure 2 The normal menstrual cycle. Hormonal ovarian, endometrial, and basal body temperature changes throughout the normal menstrual cycle. P, progesterone; E_2, estradiol; LH, luteinizing hormone; FSH, follicle-stimulating hormone. From Carr, B. R., Wilson, J. D. "Disorders of the Ovary and Female Reproductive Tract," in *Harrison's Principles of Internal Medicine*, 13th Edition. Edited by Isselbacher, K. J., Braunwald, E., Wilson, J. D., *et al.*, p. 2022. New York, McGraw-Hill, 1994. Copyright © 1994 McGraw-Hill, Inc. Used with permission.

and promotes progesterone and prostaglandin synthesis within the follicle. Progesterone potentiates estrogen effects and also triggers the FSH surge and activates prostaglandins and enzymes present in the follicle. This allows the follicular wall at the edge of the ovary to rupture. Influenced by hormones and chemicals in the immediate locale, the ovum then detaches from its anchor within the ovarian follicle. The release of the ovum from the ovary, allowing it to travel down one of the two fallopian tubes for possible fertilization, is defined as ovulation.

A number of physical and psychological findings have been noted during the follicular and ovulation phases of the menstrual cycle, including endometrial breakdown and sloughing during the initial 2 to 8 days of the follicular phase (i.e., menses), followed by proliferation, vascularization, and differentiation of the endometrium for implantation; increased production of thin, relatively alkaline cervical and vaginal mucus in response to raising estrogen levels; an initial sustained decrease in basal body temperature, followed by a temperature rise shortly after ovulation; regular alterations of electrolyte composition of urine and saliva; and a heightened sense of personal well-being, enhanced sensory perceptions, and, perhaps, somewhat improved cognitive task performance throughout the follicular phase.

B. Luteal Phase

The luteal phase occurs after ovulation, spanning approximately Days 15 through 28 of the menstrual cycle. Once the ovum has been released, the ruptured follicle becomes the corpus luteum, or "yellow body," named because of the high concentrations of lipids it contains. Its granulosa cells hypertrophy and produce high amounts of progesterone, estrogen, and androgens necessary for sustaining a pregnancy if fertilization and implantation have occurred. At such concentrations, these hormones serve to decrease GnRH secretion by the hypothalamus. They also stimulate the endometrium to become edematous and to undergo glandular proliferation over the 7 days after ovulation. In addition, progesterone reduces some of the pituitary effects of estrogen by decreasing estrogen receptors in this brain structure.

In the absence of pregnancy, approximately 10 to 14 days after ovulation, the corpus luteum regresses and becomes a fibrotic, hyalinized region of the ovary, called the corpus albicans. Progesterone and estrogen concentrations gradually decrease. These events trigger a number of endometrial responses. Local vasomotor reactions within the spiral arterioles of the uterine lining cause endometrial ischemia. Local prostaglandin synthesis increases, augmenting uterine contractility. Menstruation begins as necrotic tissues slough away and blood from interstitial hemorrhaging enters the uterus. The sustained low levels of estrogen and progesterone stimulate the hypothalamus to release GnRH and the pituitary to secrete FSH and LH, triggering the development of another set of ovarian follicles and setting into motion the next menstrual cycle.

The premenstrual phase spans the 5 to 7 days before menstruation, and thus occurs within the luteal phase of the menstrual cycle. A wide range of symptoms, such as increased fluid retention, fatigue, breast tenderness, headaches or other pain syndromes, mood fluctuations, and subjectively increased appetite, have been associated with this segment of the normal menstrual cycle. Only when it is so severe that patients' daily functioning is affected and health care is formally sought for this problem can the diagnosis of PMS be made.

C. Influences on the Normal Menstrual Cycle

Elements that can modify or disrupt the normal menstrual cycle are many and often interrelated. For example, limbic system neurotransmitters (such as dopamine) appear to inhibit GnRH release by the hypothalamus, whereas norepinephrine stimulates GnRH output. In addition, as the ovarian corpus luteum deteriorates, its decrease in estrogen and progesterone production leads to a reduction in hypothalamic endorphin release. This, in turn, triggers greater GnRH, LH, and FSH production and causes follicle maturation early in the next cycle. Psychological and physical stresses may also modify the menstrual cycle through increased secretion of endorphins stimulated by increased corticotropin-releasing hormone (CRH). This leads to a decrease in GnRH release, which interferes with ovulation. Abnormalities in adrenal steroid synthesis or insufficient production of hormones by the thyroid (thyroxin) or the pancreas (insulin) may result in anovulation and infrequent menses, although the mechanisms of action are unknown. Estrogen itself is associated with increased secretion of growth hormone, prolactin, ACTH, and oxytocin controlled in concert by the hypothalamus and the anterior and posterior regions of the pituitary. Genetic syndromes affecting hormone and steroid synthesis or chemical metabolism similarly will influence menstrual cycles. Beyond internal chemical influences, exogenous hormones and medications may induce or prevent ovulation through a number of mechanisms, affecting the length and timing of the menstrual cycle. These richly varied and interconnected processes suggest how women with different central nervous system lesions, life stresses, genetic disorders, endocrine dysfunction, and medical illnesses all may develop interrupted menstrual cycles.

D. Variability in the Normal Menstrual Cycle

The normal menstrual cycle differs between women as well as across an individual woman's lifetime. This variability is shown in many ways: the length of menses (normal range of 2 to 8 days) and the menstrual cycle (normal range of 21 to 36 days); its synchronization with other women in close proximity; symptoms and signs associated with the premenstrual phase and menstruation; the level of interference caused by external factors such as physical illness or extreme exercise; the effects of emotional stress, nutritional deficiencies, medications, and hormonal disruptions; the numbers of follicles that mature during each cycle as a woman ages; and changes that occur at different life stages or with pregnancy and lactation. There is considerable variation that falls within the range of "normal" menstrual cycle experiences. For this reason, recognizing the premenstrual syndrome can be especially challenging.

III. DEVELOPMENTAL VIEW OF WOMEN'S HEALTH AND THE MENSTRUAL CYCLE

Development is an orderly pattern of changes within an individual occurring over time, each stage is built upon and shaped by earlier ones. Development is influenced by the unique relationship between an individual's biology and experiences of the self, of others, and of the world. These factors deeply affect personal attributes such as temperament and personality; cognitive capacities including learning, memory, and intelligence; the meanings given to sensations, relationships, and events in life; and one's sense of the self within a specific familial, social, and cultural setting. With each stage of development, aspects of the individual are reconfigured within the current context. Thus, each moment offers indications of both one's distinct personal history and unique adaptation to the present.

A woman's development begins at conception (Table I). The potential for normal female sexual differentiation is genetically determined by the presence of two X chromosomes and the absence of a Y chromosome in the embryo. The actual course of development, however, is affected by a series of critical periods in the subsequent growth of each individual.

During critical periods in the sequence of development, biology and experience work in concert to organize and delimit the "choices" of an organism. The potential for ovaries and female external genitalia is made possible by the XX genotype. Female fetal tissues will not develop into these anatomic structures, however, unless sex hormones are present in specific proportions in the fetal environment at certain times. Abnormal proportions of fetal hormones or chemical exposures may alter subsequent physical development and sexual behavior, as evidenced by animal experiments in which hermaphroditic external genitalia or male-type sexual behaviors have been induced in genotypic females through fetal androgen exposure. In addition to animal models, patients with anomalous sexual development have clearly demonstrated that aspects of sexual differentiation may be irreversibly "settled" in an individual once a critical period has passed. Analogously, differential androgen production in men and women is implicated in central nervous system sexual differences evident in brain structure, physiology, and vascular patterns. Finally, the clinical observation that mothers, daughters, and sisters often resemble one another with respect to their ages at onset of menarche and at onset of menopause suggests that genetic and other early developmental factors may affect later events of sexual maturation. Further investigation is needed to understand the mechanisms that contribute to critical periods in sexual development.

In infancy and childhood, girls learn through experiencing sensations, through using their muscles, and through relating to others. A girl's sense of herself, her body, and her core gender identity (i.e., the earliest feeling of belonging to one sex) emerges in a familial context of attachment, nurturance, affiliation, intimacy, and identification. Children ideally develop a feeling of fundamental trust through the safety and predictability present in this context; alternatively, they may develop a deep sense of apprehension and vulnerability based on their early experiences. Over time, children become acutely aware of certain social and cultural expectations that may surround gender roles as their bodies grow and mature. Anatomic differences between boys and girls give rise to differences in self-concepts, affirmed or altered by learning and observation. Over time, children also express curiosity and become more comfortable with their anatomic sex. Physical well-being during early childhood may be especially important to later health and illness patterns with respect to recognition of bodily discomfort, interpretations of pain, expression of emotional distress through physical complaints, and external validation or reinforcement of symptomatology.

Puberty marks the beginning of adolescence, bringing with it a number of dramatic physical changes such as breast development, growth of pubic and axillary hair, hip widening, and acne. Menarche normally occurs between the ages of 10 and 16, approximately 2 years after the onset of puberty. Of all of the pubertal changes, the start of menstruation is perhaps the most meaningful event, in that it represents a clear passage into womanhood physically and psychologically. Menarche may be exciting, affirming, frightening, awkward, or all of these and other feelings simultaneously. Although menarche does not itself indicate reproductive maturity, it does signify its future prom-

Table I Menstrual Cycle and Sexual Development of Women throughout the Life Span

Prenatal
- Establishment of sexual genotype (XX or XY) at conception
- Some evidence that genetic factors influence growth, age at menarche, and, possibly, future menstrual characteristics
- Intrauterine environment (e.g., hormones, receptors, timing of exposures) influence anatomical and functional fetal differentiation

Infancy/childhood
- Emergence of core gender identity, i.e., the earliest sense of belonging to one sex, during infancy
- Affiliation, attachment, and identification with parents, other family members, care providers
- Physical growth and development (prepubertal); comfort with one's anatomic sex; emergence of sexual orientation
- Exposure to emotional, familial, cultural, and social expectations related to gender
- Sexual self-stimulation and curiosity, sexual play
- Sense of fundamental safety or vulnerability; potential for sexual abuse and exploitation

Adolescence
- Physical changes associated with puberty, including breast development, growth of pubic and axillary hair, menarche (ages 10–18), hip widening, vaginal discharge, and acne
- Settling into a regular menstrual pattern
- Self-image and body-image changes; for some, risk of eating disorders, other maladaptive patterns
- Gender identity and sexual orientation exploration
- Interest in romantic and sexual relationships and curiosity about sexuality, sexual sensation
- For some, initiation of genital sexual activity, including intercourse
- Learning surrounding emotional and physical intimacy in peer relationships
- Making choices with potentially long-range consequences such as drug use and risky sexual activity
- Forming a value system around personal responsibility, sexuality, relationships, and cultural precepts
- Dealing with potential consequences of initiating sexual relationships, including pregnancy and sexually transmitted diseases
- Making the transition to adulthood and practicing being separate from the family of origin

Young and middle adulthood
- Establishing a regular menstrual pattern
- Active exploration of sexuality in relationships, learning and practicing with enhancement of sexual satisfaction through time
- Coping with physical and emotional risks accompanying sexual activities, including coercion, sexaully transmitted diseases, pelvic inflammatory disease, cervical cancer, domestic violence
- Making committed attachments, marriages, partnerships
- Becoming more comfortable with gender identity and sexual orientation
- Dealing with reproduction issues such as contraception, pregnancy, miscarriage, infertility, premature menopause
- Physiological and psychological changes surrounding pregnancy, lactation, and child-rearing, including alterations in libido, energy, physical comfort, desire, self-image, meaning of relationships
- For some, manifesting psychiatric illness such as anxiety, depression, late luteal phase dysphoric disorder, sexual dysfunction, psychosis, substance abuse

Later adulthood
- Physiologic, anatomic, and self-image changes associated with menopause
- Maintenance of menstruation by means of exogenous hormones
- Facing transitions in relationships, including children moving away, divorce, death of parents
- Dealing with medical illness, medications, and surgery (including hysterectomy) that affect self-image and sexual functioning
- For many, new possibilities and creativity in postreproductive years

Elderly
- Continuing interest in intimate and sexual relationships
- Physical and emotional changes accompanying aging, including the slowing of sexual responsiveness, lessened physical comfort, and embarrassment
- For many, the loss of intimate partner to death and a sense of loss in family, social, and societal roles
- Dealing with medical illness, medications, and surgery that affect sexual health, function, and self-image
- Sense of integrity and wholeness with respect to one's life, including one's sexuality

ise. The temporal pattern of a young woman's menstrual cycle may be inconsistent in adolescence, especially in connection with erratic nutrition and exercise patterns that in some cases are pathological (e.g., anorexia nervosa, bulimia). Within a few years, however, in the absence of severe physical and psychiatric pathology, menses normally tend to fall into a more regular rhythm with predictable ovulation.

The psychological work of adolescence is equally remarkable. A young woman's tasks include making changes in her self-image and body-image, exploring her gender identity and sexual orientation, learning about emotional and physical intimacy in peer relationships, becoming more autonomous and feeling competent in familial and other contexts, and forming a personal value system around relationships, school performance, sexual behavior, and other issues such as drug use and the problems that accompany sexual activity. Through such experiences, a young woman makes the transition from her family of origin to greater independence and prepares for the full responsibilities of adulthood.

During young and middle adulthood, a number of psychological and physical events of development may occur. At this time, women tend to become more comfortable with themselves and begin making committed attachments, marriages, and partnerships. They learn increasingly about their sexuality, sexual orientation, and personal health issues. Their menstrual cycles also become more settled and predictable. Menstruation may be viewed more positively than at other times as a link to desired fertility. Difficult menstrual patterns (e.g., premenstrual magnification, premenstrual exacerbation of other conditions, or premenstrual syndrome) may also become clearer as women gain greater insight into their cyclic symptoms. In addition, much of women's lives during young and middle adulthood may be affected by reproductive issues such as contraception, pregnancy and lactation, miscarriage and termination of pregnancies, infertility, and child-rearing, all of which may affect menstruation patterns and related cyclic mood and behavioral symptoms. A woman's view of her responsibilities in family and professional relationships may become consolidated during her 20s through 40s as she practices these skills as a wife or partner, a parent, a daughter, a sister, a neighbor, a citizen, and a worker. Taken together, such everyday experiences greatly influence a woman's tolerance and perception of physical symptoms, energy level, willingness to seek health care, self-esteem, libido and sexual desire, comfort, and self-understanding.

In later adulthood, women experience physiological, anatomic, and emotional changes throughout their postreproductive years. Menopause ordinarily occurs in women aged 45 to 55, preceded by approximately 2 years of lengthened or missed menstrual cycles and occasional spotting. Premenstrual syndrome, per se, tends to worsen as menopause approaches and to remit after menopause. During this phase of life, women often experience medical illness, undergo surgical interventions, and receive medications that affect menstrual function and general physical well-being such as hormone replacement. During this period, women also face transitions in family relationships, including children moving away, divorce, or the death of a spouse or parent. Over the 20 or more years beyond menopause, many adaptations are required as women experience changes in intimate relationships, social and societal roles, and personal identity. If loneliness was present earlier in life, it may deepen in the postmenopausal years. Despite such difficulties, for many women, this period allows for creativity, generativity, and freedom not possible at a younger age. Ideally, late in life, women will feel a sense of integrity and completeness about all of their experiences in relation to their biological natures, their personal identities, and their familial and societal roles.

IV. PHENOMENOLOGY OF PREMENSTRUAL SYNDROME

A. PMS Symptoms and Their Timing

An immense number of symptoms have been attributed to PMS (Table II). The most common complaints include physical symptoms (breast swelling and tenderness, abdominal bloating, headaches, muscle aches and pains, weight gain, and edema), emotional symptoms (depression, mood swings, anger, irritability, and anxiety), and others (decreased interest in usual activities, fatigue, difficulty concentrating, increased appetite and food cravings, and hypersomnia or insomnia).

Four temporal patterns have been described for PMS. Symptoms can begin during the second week of the luteal phase (about Day 21). Alternatively, they can begin at ovulation and worsen over the entire luteal phase (about Day 14). In both of these patterns, symptoms remit within a few days after the onset of menses. Some women experience a brief episode of symptoms at ovulation, which is followed by symptom-free days and a recurrence of symptoms late in the luteal phase. Women who seem to be most severely affected experience symptoms that begin at ovulation, worsen across the luteal phase, and remit only after menses ceases.

Table II Examples of Premenstrual Symptoms

Abdominal cramps
Aches or pains
Anger
Anxiety
Bloating
Breast tenderness
Clumsiness
Concentration problems
Confusion
Cravings (e.g., carbohydrate, salt)
Depression
Excessive sleepiness
Fatigue
Forgetfulness
Headaches (migraine, tension)
Hot flashes
Insomnia
Impulsivity
Irritability
Moodiness
Rapid shifts in emotions
Swelling (hands, feet)
Weight gain

These women commonly have only 1 week a month that is symptom-free. It is unclear whether these four patterns represent distinct subtypes of PMS or whether they correspond to other conditions. These four patterns of symptoms must be differentiated from underlying illnesses that either are precipitated during the premenstrual phase or demonstrate a cyclic waxing and waning of intensity related to menstruation. They must also be differentiated from other problems associated with menses, including pelvic pain with menstruation (dysmenorrhea), infrequent menses (oligomenorrhea), absent menses (amenorrhea), frequent menses (metrorrhagia), and excessive bleeding with menses (menorrhagia).

The course and stability of PMS over time has not been systematically characterized. It has been observed that PMS can begin any time after menarche, but women most frequently seek treatment for their symptoms in their thirties. Symptoms are believed to remit with conditions, such as pregnancy, that interrupt ovulation. Women generally report that their symptoms worsen with age until menopause, when PMS usually ceases.

B. Prevalence

The true prevalence of PMS is unknown because a prospective, community-based epidemiological study of the syndrome has not yet been conducted. Nevertheless, it is estimated that 20 to 40% of women report some premenstrual symptoms and that 5% of women experience some degree of significant impairment of their work or lifestyle. These figures are consistent with retrospective epidemiological survey data that report the prevalence of PMS to be 6.8% and with two population-based studies that report the prevalence of PMS to be 4.6% and 9.8%, respectively.

The frequency of PMS in different cultures remains undetermined, although at least 24 countries have published studies of PMS. Retrospective surveys of premenstrual symptoms have led to the belief that PMS affects women equally, regardless of socioeconomic status or culture; this belief is a hypothesis that merits further investigation.

C. Etiology and Risk Factors

The etiology of PMS and the factors that place a woman at risk for developing PMS remain uncertain. Etiologic hypotheses that have been proposed include abnormalities in hormonal secretory patterns (ovarian steroids, melatonin, androgens, prolactin, mineralocorticoids, thyroxin, insulin), neurotransmitter levels (biogenic amines such as epinephrine and norepinephrine, endogenous opioids), circadian rhythms (temperature, sleep), prostaglandins, vitamin B6 levels, nutrition, allergic reactions, stress, and other psychological factors. Although investigators may advocate vehemently for one or more of these possibilities, no single, fully explanatory mechanism has been isolated as yet. Furthermore, there are physiological and behavioral correlates of menstrual cycle rhythms such as increases in appetite premenstrually and abdominal discomfort during menstruation that are present in women without PMS. These findings have led to the belief that the etiology of PMS resides in the interaction of many different factors that culminate in symptom expression.

Although not demonstrated conclusively, research suggests that genetic factors may place a woman at a relatively greater risk for the development of PMS or for greater severity of PMS symptoms. In one small study conducted by Dalton and colleagues, the pattern of identical twins both having PMS was found to be significantly higher (93%) than in nonidentical twins (44%) and in nontwin control women (31%). A questionnaire survey of 462 female volunteer twin pairs published by Van den Akker and colleagues further supports the possibility that a genetic predisposition for PMS exists. Similarly, evidence from developmental studies suggests a familial pattern as well. For instance, in a study of 5000 adolescent Finnish girls and their mothers, daughters of mothers with premenstrual "tension" were more likely to complain of PMS than were daughters of mothers who were symptom-free. In addition, 70% of daughters whose mothers had nervous symptoms in this study also had symptoms themselves, whereas only 37% of daughters of unaffected mothers experienced symptoms. These studies represent a crucial step toward clarifying the contributions of nature and nurture to the expression of PMS.

As with all medical illnesses, a number of psychological factors may contribute to PMS symptomatology in women. A young woman's symptoms and signs around menstruation may be interpreted as pathological or as normal according to her internalized sense of sexual health drawn from early family experiences, societal views of gender, and other influences. The ability to cope effectively with severe PMS symptoms may be hampered by the extraordinary stresses (e.g., balancing family and work responsibilities, single-parenting, dealing with financial pressures, or surviving the loss of a spouse) that have become commonplace in women's lives. Sadness and anxiety, vulnerability, and helplessness can become linked to a woman's experience of her menstrual cycle and may be attributed to PMS. Moreover, if a woman has disowned or devalued parts of herself, if she has endured interpersonal violence or other trauma, her suffering may be expressed symbolically through PMS symptoms. In summary, it is likely that the etiology of PMS resides in the interaction of multiple influences from a woman's biology, developmental events, and contemporary life circumstances which find expression in a unique cultural context.

V. RESTORING MENTAL AND PHYSICAL HEALTH RELATED TO THE MENSTRUAL CYCLE

Mild warning signs of the onset of menstruation, as Dalton describes (see Premenstrual Syndrome (PMS)), are a valuable gift of nature. The need to restore mental and physical health related to the menstrual cycle through formal clinical intervention occurs only when

Table III Objectives in Caring for Women's Health: PREVENTION

P	*Prevention*—Prevention of illness, high-risk behaviors, stresses associated with sexuality
R	*Resources*—Provision of resources for safety, learning, and social support
E	*Evaluation*—Evaluation of signs and symptoms, sexual history and practices
V	*Violence*—Exploration of issues surrounding violence and coercive sexuality
E	*Esteem*—Assessment of esteem and well-being associated with sexuality and intimacy
N	*Nonjudgmental*—Communication in a nonjudgmental, open manner
T	*Treatment*—Prompt and appropriate treatment of identified illnesses
I	*Intervention*—Intervention when necessary to ensure physical and emotional safety
O	*Options*—Provision of therapeutic options surrounding sexual health (e.g., contraception)
N	*Nonexploitative*—Establishment of a nonexploitative, ethical relationship with patient

these warning signs, or the experience of menstruation itself, become especially uncomfortable. In such cases, it is essential to take a clinical approach that remains mindful of the objectives in providing clinical care for women's sexual health (Table III) and involves three elements: prevention, accurate diagnosis, and appropriate treatment interventions.

A. Prevention

As evidenced by the virtual elimination of smallpox, polio, and measles in developed countries because of routine immunization practices, primary prevention may offer the greatest promise for many medical conditions that cause tremendous suffering. In the absence of greater clarity and specificity concerning the etiology of PMS, the creation of reliably effective primary, secondary, and tertiary preventive health strategies for this syndrome is difficult. Nevertheless, early work suggests that prevention of PMS hinges on two objectives: the pursuit of overall good health, including sexual health, and the process of unearthing and clarifying patient beliefs that may interfere with personal well-being. Education related to biological or psychological aspects of prenatal care, family patterns and roles, and social/cultural ideas may address these goals and may diminish the likelihood of the initial development of PMS (primary prevention) and increase the chances of recognizing, appropriately treating, and reducing the suffering associated with PMS (secondary and tertiary prevention).

A woman who experiences uncomfortable physical, psychological, and/or behavioral signs and symptoms in relation to her menstrual cycle should thus be understood with respect to her biological nature and the psychological aspects of her life experiences and her contemporary circumstances. In so doing, the clinician can pursue educational interventions that may decrease the incidence (number of new cases each year in a given population) of PMS, improve recognition of PMS, and reduce the morbidity associated with PMS. Three illustrations of preventive educational interventions follow.

1. Early Developmental Experiences and Health

Premenstrual syndrome differs from other endocrine-related mood disorders, such as depression induced by diabetes or hypothyroidism, in that blood hormone levels are essentially normal. These findings suggest that PMS may have special psychobiological features, and these should raise questions about the relationship of PMS to childhood health and nurturing. Early evidence indicates that tactile stimulation before weaning, for example, leads to antibody production, thought to be essential for proper functioning of the immune system in infancy and for immune and pituitary–adrenal activation in adulthood. Research should thus focus on the impact of early development on immunological and neuroendocrinological patterns that may permanently influence the person's susceptibility to or immunity from illness. As these complex issues become clarified, clinical attention should focus on the quality of the caregiver–infant relationship to ensure optimal maturation and enhanced neuroendocrine/immune function later in life. This example of early infant care is a valuable paradigm for exploring the interplay of biological, psychological, and social/cultural factors in preventive health.

2. Women's Development within the Context of the Family

Prevention related to the woman's personal developmental experiences focuses first on family. The family is the predominant institution in which growth and development of each individual member occurs and in which social and cultural values are translated into everyday terms. A girl's identity develops out of a sense of connectedness with others, first as a sense of being like and connected with her first caregiver, and later as a sense of being connected with others. By 18 months, a girl has learned the label, "I am a girl." The process of developing this label into an inner acceptance of herself as a woman—with the accompanying belief that it is *good* to be a woman—is complex. The outcome will depend in part on the convictions of the first caregiver with whom she identifies. It will also depend on the girl's observations of how women are treated in the family and in the world at large and how women's sexuality is understood. If women around her are socially stigmatized, despair and identity confusion may result. Where symptoms of PMS reflect such alienation, attention to these issues rooted in early family experiences may prevent the development of PMS.

Explicit discussion of different kinds of family roles may help women to examine their own family experiences and to reconsider their expectations of themselves. The behavior of each person may be defined by the roles he or she is assigned within a family system. Kinship roles define who is mother, father, daughter, son, sister, or brother. Stereotypical roles define who is nurturer, housekeeper, breadwinner, disciplinarian, and so on, and reflect society's shared beliefs that are passed from generation to generation, constantly reinforcing the structure of a given culture. Unrealistic and irrational role expectations may define the good mother/bad mother, good father/ bad father, good teenager/rebellious teenager, and others, and are generated by unconscious conflicts and shared myths among the family members. To the extent that people can discuss roles and reach an understanding about how roles emerge, the likelihood of role strain diminishes. With this, the likelihood of the expression of role strain through physical symptoms may also decline.

3. Women's Suffering in Relation to Contemporary Circumstances and the Effects of Culture

Prevention related to a woman's contemporary circumstances includes clarification of cultural stereotypes and of implicit social attitudes about women. To the extent that stereotypes and attitudes are applied to women indiscriminantly and without reflection, they can negatively affect the psychological health of women. For example, if early experiences foster the cultural ideal of caretaking as womanly and good, this ideal carries the potential for promoting stereotypes of caring as womanly and a good woman as selfless and self-sacrificing. Thus, self-giving may not be assessed in terms of the intentions of the woman and the consequences of her behavior, but on the basis of whether or not her behavior is viewed as inherently feminine. In other words, the worth of the woman's self-sacrifice may not be acknowledged and rewarded, but instead her behavior is viewed as nothing more than an indication of her fundamental feminine nature. As a result, a woman can believe that no effort she makes in her current situation is of significant value, leaving her feeling unappreciated and unhappy. Alternatively, if a woman insists on recognition for her contributions, is assertive, or expresses personal needs (e.g., through words, behaviors, and/or symptoms), her "request" may be disquieting for men, women, and institutions that equate femininity with self-sacrifice. Those who are threatened may retaliate against the woman rather than reward her. Such role conflicts may be especially likely to occur in cultures or subcultures that are rapidly changing and whose most vulnerable members (often women and children) may bear the brunt of such change.

Similarly, and more specifically, a society's beliefs about menstruation can influence both expectations about the menstrual cycle and the reporting of symptoms. Women with PMS may be greeted with skepticism and invalidation by others because of the cultural taboos that surround menstruation. Moreover, when a woman's complaints of PMS signal that she is not pregnant, her PMS symptoms can be interpreted from a cultural perspective as reproductive inadequacy or "deviance." For these reasons, women may need support as they grapple with how their needs are responded to by others in confusing and negative ways because of cultural stereotypes. Over time, women may learn how to gear their expectations and behaviors so that they can remain true to themselves but also respect others' views and seek appropriate affirmation.

Table IV Diagnostic Evaluation of Premenstrual Syndrome

General medical history
- Overall health
- Current medical and psychological issues
- Medications (prescribed and over-the-counter)
- Past medical and psychiatric history
- Habits (e.g., exercise, sleep, and eating patterns, smoking, alcohol, and drugs)
- Preventative health care (e.g., immunizations, cholesterol levels, pap smears, mammography)
- Developmental and social history
- Family illness history
- Sexual history (e.g., comfort with sexuality, current sexual functioning, past sexual experiences, high-risk behaviors)

Focused medical history
- Overall gynecological health
- Menstrual history (e.g., age at menarche, length of menstrual cycle, quantity and pattern of bleeding)
- Nature, timing, and severity of symptoms around menstruation
- Pattern of menstrual and premenstrual symptoms during adolescence and early adulthood
- Pattern of menstrual and premenstrual symptoms in relation to pregnancy, breast-feeding, and hormonal interventions (e.g., oral contraceptives)
- Unrecognized endocrine problems (e.g., thyroid dysfunction, androgen excess)
- Unrecognized psychiatric illness (e.g., depression, anxiety, posttraumatic stress disorder, somatoform disorder)

Physical examination
- Mental status examination
- Screening physical examination, including examination for signs of
  - endocrine dysfunction
  - gynecologic illness
  - overlooked health problems (e.g., anemia, infection)
- Screening laboratory tests (e.g., thyroid function tests)

Prospective symptom rating

Patient records the timing and severity of physical and psychological symptoms for at least two menstrual cycles. The pattern is evaluated during a subsequent appointment.

B. Diagnosis

Each woman is unique in terms of her physical experience of menstrual cycle events, her cognitive interpretation of sensations related to menstruation, her conscious and unconscious emotional responses to her internal rhythms and timing, and her adaptive behaviors toward menstrual cycle events. When a woman expresses concern about her menstrual cycle or offers complaints suggestive of PMS, the health care provider must attend to the whole person and understand, from a developmental perspective, the complex social context in which the woman lives (Table IV). Such an approach is essential for making an accurate diagnosis of PMS and pursuing appropriate treatment interventions.

As there is no absolute independent, verifiable biological marker (such as a blood test) or physiobehavioral measure (such as increased nocturnal temperature or other signs related to individual circadian rhythms) to identify PMS reliably, the diagnosis of PMS is believed to be a clinical judgment. It is thought to be present when three criteria are met: (1) no other condition is present that accounts for the patient's symptoms, (2) prospective daily symptom ratings demonstrate a marked change in severity of symptoms premenstrually for at least two menstrual cycles, and (3) there is a symptom-free week (usually Days 5 to 10) during the menstrual cycles. It is possible for a woman to have a psychiatric disorder or a physical disorder in addition to PMS as long as the symptoms of PMS are distinct from the other disorder and occur during the luteal phase and remit during menses.

Clinical investigation of PMS thus involves two kinds of information. First, it entails prospective documentation by the woman of symptoms and signs she experiences in clear association with phases of her menstrual cycle. Prospective daily ratings of symptoms with respect to quantity, quality, and severity for a minimum of 2 months are required to confirm a woman's retrospective report of premenstrual symptomatology (Table V). A retrospective history of PMS is not sufficient for a diagnosis because it introduces biases, leading to an overdiagnosis of PMS. Second, other medical conditions that may account for the patient's discomfort must be excluded. Clinicians must therefore perform a careful health history. A complete physical examination must also be conducted, including a mental status examination and a pelvic examination. Psychiatric conditions such as depression, anxiety, somatoform disorders, and others must be considered in the evaluation process. Gynecological conditions such as uterine fibroids, endometriosis, and fibrocystic breast disease, and other physical conditions such as anemia and endocrine dysfunction (e.g., diabetes mellitus, thyroid disease, Cushing's disease) must also be considered and appropriate diagnostic tests performed in the evaluation process. Coexistent medical and psychiatric disorders must be distinguished from disorders that might cause the patient's symptoms and signs.

C. Appropriate Treatment Interventions

Once a diagnosis has been established or refuted, results of the evaluation should be shared with the

Table V Daily Symptoms Calendar

Name: Yolanda Johnson

Choose the symptoms to be monitored and label the columns. Circle the appropriate number for each symptom every day of your cycle.

Symptom severity rating: 1 = Not at all, 2 = Minimal, 3 = Mild, 4 = Moderate, 5 = Severe, 6 = Extreme.

Menses: X = Normal flow, S = Light flow

Date	Menses	Symptom #1 Breast Tenderness	Symptom #2 Irritability	Symptom #3 Food Craving	Symptom #4 Bloating
		(1) 2 3 4 5 6	(1) 2 3 4 5 6	(1) 2 3 4 5 6	(1) 2 3 4 5 6
		(1) 2 3 4 5 6	(1) 2 3 4 5 6	(1) 2 3 4 5 6	(1) 2 3 4 5 6
		(1) 2 3 4 5 6	(1) 2 3 4 5 6	(1) 2 3 4 5 6	(1) 2 3 4 5 6
		(1) 2 3 4 5 6	(1) 2 3 4 5 6	(1) 2 3 4 5 6	(1) 2 3 4 5 6
		(1) 2 3 4 5 6	(1) 2 3 4 5 6	(1) 2 3 4 5 6	(1) 2 3 4 5 6
		(1) 2 3 4 5 6	(1) 2 3 4 5 6	(1) 2 3 4 5 6	(1) 2 3 4 5 6
		(1) 2 3 4 5 6	(1) 2 3 4 5 6	1 (2) 3 4 5 6	1 (2) 3 4 5 6
		1 (2) 3 4 5 6	1 2 (3) 4 5 6	1 2 (3) 4 5 6	1 (2) 3 4 5 6
		1 2 3 (4) 5 6	1 2 3 4 (5) 6	1 2 3 (4) 5 6	1 2 (3) 4 5 6
		1 2 3 4 5 (6)	1 2 3 4 (5) 6	1 2 3 4 (5) 6	1 2 (3) 4 5 6
		1 2 3 4 5 (6)	1 2 3 4 (5) 6	1 2 3 4 (5) 6	1 2 (3) 4 5 6
		1 2 3 4 5 (6)	1 2 3 4 (5) 6	1 2 3 4 5 (6)	1 2 (3) 4 5 6
		1 2 3 4 5 (6)	1 2 3 4 (5) 6	1 2 3 4 5 (6)	1 2 (3) 4 5 6
		1 2 3 4 5 (6)	1 2 3 4 (5) 6	1 2 3 4 5 (6)	1 2 (3) 4 5 6
	X	1 2 3 4 (5) 6	1 2 3 (4) 5 6	1 2 (3) 4 5 6	1 (2) 3 4 5 6
	X	1 2 (3) 4 5 6	1 (2) 3 4 5 6	(1) 2 3 4 5 6	1 (2) 3 4 5 6
	X	(1) 2 3 4 5 6	(1) 2 3 4 5 6	(1) 2 3 4 5 6	(1) 2 3 4 5 6
	X	(1) 2 3 4 5 6	(1) 2 3 4 5 6	(1) 2 3 4 5 6	(1) 2 3 4 5 6
	X	(1) 2 3 4 5 6	(1) 2 3 4 5 6	(1) 2 3 4 5 6	(1) 2 3 4 5 6
	S	(1) 2 3 4 5 6	(1) 2 3 4 5 6	(1) 2 3 4 5 6	(1) 2 3 4 5 6
		(1) 2 3 4 5 6	(1) 2 3 4 5 6	(1) 2 3 4 5 6	(1) 2 3 4 5 6
		(1) 2 3 4 5 6	(1) 2 3 4 5 6	(1) 2 3 4 5 6	(1) 2 3 4 5 6
		(1) 2 3 4 5 6	1 (2) 3 4 5 6	(1) 2 3 4 5 6	(1) 2 3 4 5 6
		(1) 2 3 4 5 6	1 2 (3) 4 5 6	(1) 2 3 4 5 6	(1) 2 3 4 5 6
		(1) 2 3 4 5 6	(1) 2 3 4 5 6	(1) 2 3 4 5 6	(1) 2 3 4 5 6
		(1) 2 3 4 5 6	(1) 2 3 4 5 6	(1) 2 3 4 5 6	(1) 2 3 4 5 6
		(1) 2 3 4 5 6	(1) 2 3 4 5 6	(1) 2 3 4 5 6	(1) 2 3 4 5 6
		(1) 2 3 4 5 6	(1) 2 3 4 5 6	1 (2) 3 4 5 6	(1) 2 3 4 5 6
		(1) 2 3 4 5 6	(1) 2 3 4 5 6	1 (2) 3 4 5 6	1 (2) 3 4 5 6
		(1) 2 3 4 5 6	(1) 2 3 4 5 6	(1) 2 3 4 5 6	(1) 2 3 4 5 6
		(1) 2 3 4 5 6	(1) 2 3 4 5 6	(1) 2 3 4 5 6	(1) 2 3 4 5 6
		(1) 2 3 4 5 6	(1) 2 3 4 5 6	(1) 2 3 4 5 6	(1) 2 3 4 5 6
		(1) 2 3 4 5 6	(1) 2 3 4 5 6	(1) 2 3 4 5 6	(1) 2 3 4 5 6
		(1) 2 3 4 5 6	(1) 2 3 4 5 6	(1) 2 3 4 5 6	(1) 2 3 4 5 6
		(1) 2 3 4 5 6	(1) 2 3 4 5 6	(1) 2 3 4 5 6	(1) 2 3 4 5 6
		(1) 2 3 4 5 6	(1) 2 3 4 5 6	(1) 2 3 4 5 6	(1) 2 3 4 5 6

patient and various treatment strategies should be considered.

1. For Women Thought Not to Have PMS

Women with symptoms caused by another illness, but without demonstrable PMS, should receive reassurance and clarity about possible sources of their discomfort. Accurate information about sexual health, experiences normally associated with the menstrual cycle, and symptom patterns may be tremendously helpful. Treatment of a previously unrecognized or poorly controlled physical illness (e.g., hypothyroidism, diabetes mellitus) may eliminate the premenstrual complaints. New or more intensive treatment of a psychiatric disorder such as depression may lead to improvement in symptoms attributed to the premenstrual phase. Doses of psychotropic medication may need to be increased during the late luteal phase and early follicular phase to control symptoms. It should be made explicit that women who are thought not to have PMS will receive continued health care and will not be abandoned to cope with their symptoms alone.

Women whose evaluations do not yield clear evidence of PMS or of another physical or mental illness should be shown that their daily symptom ratings do not reflect a PMS pattern, that their physical examination and laboratory tests do not suggest another physical illness, and that their psychological evaluation has ruled out a mental disorder. Some time should be spent with women with these experiences to acknowledge the reality of their symptoms, even though the meaning of their symptoms is unclear. For example, these women could be in the incipient phases of developing PMS where their symptomatology is inconsistent or of too low a severity to qualify for the diagnosis of PMS. These women should be encouraged to continue charting their daily symptoms, to return in 3 to 6 months for reevaluation, and to ensure adequate sleep, proper diet, and healthy exercise. Alternatively, other sources of symptoms that are not disclosed early in the evaluative process, such as stressful life situations, can be explored and appropriate supports offered at this time.

2. For Women Diagnosed with PMS

Once PMS is documented, a wide variety of psychosocial and preventive health interventions should be considered. These treatments have not been demonstrated to be helpful to all women and their clinical scientific bases are not proven. Because the etiology of PMS is multifactorial and elusive, single pharmacologic interventions that "target" the causal mechanism of PMS have not been found. This fact should be reviewed carefully with each woman, and it should be understood that the goal of therapy is to find the unique approach that best addresses her specific needs and complaints (Table VI).

- Providing women with accurate information about their sexual health, the menstrual cycle, and PMS in general is crucial in dispelling myths and addressing the sense of helplessness a woman may feel in relation to her symptoms. Explanation of symp-

Table VI Premenstrual Symptom Interventions

Symptoms	Intervention
Psychological	
Anxiety	Biofeedback Benzodiazepines Relaxation training Serotonergic anxiolytic, i.e., buspirone
Depression	Cognitive–behavioral therapy Light therapy Serotonergic antidepressants (e.g., clomipramine, fenfluramine, fluoxetine, nefazadone, paroxetine, sertraline, and venlafaxine) Sleep deprivation
Physical	
Breast tenderness	Tocopherol (vitamin E) Bromocriptine Tamoxifen
Fatigue and/or insomnia	Sleep hygiene Serotonergic antidepressants
Food cravings	High tryptophan (carbohydrate) diet Cognitive–behavioral therapy Serotonergic antidepressants (e.g., fenfluramine)
Headaches	Aspirin (acetylsalicylic acid) Tylenol (acetaminophen) Ibuprofen Exercise
Multiple symptoms	Cognitive–behavioral therapy Group therapy Psychoeducation Serotonergic antidepressants Support group Wellness program (e.g., exercise, nutrition, stress reduction)
Weight gain	Diuretics (e.g., spironolactone) Salt restriction

toms and the natural history of PMS, descriptions of various treatment strategies with anticipated benefits, risks, side effects, and alternatives may prove to be immensely reassuring.

- The temporal pattern of their symptoms should be reviewed with women who experience PMS. Visualizing the type, severity, and timing of her symptoms can bring to the woman a sense of control over her symptoms sufficient enough to relieve distress. Women should be encouraged to develop ways of "planning ahead" for their premenstrual symptoms and signs so that they can prepare their families, close associates, and themselves for their symptomatic times. Efforts to limit external stress as much as possible (e.g., not assuming extra obligations or tasks at certain times) may help some women to navigate their monthly cycles more effectively.
- Consuming large amounts of caffeine or its equivalent (theophylline and theobromine, or methylxanthines) has been associated with women's retrospective reports of more severe premenstrual symptoms. Because caffeine can cause irritability, insomnia, and gastrointestinal distress at any time of the month, it makes sense to limit the consumption of caffeine or related compounds throughout the month.
- Decreasing salt intake is commonly recommended as one way to minimize premenstrual bloating, although many women with this complaint do not actually gain weight premenstrually. As many women consume more salt than necessary and because some women do experience symptom relief from limiting their salt intake, it seems reasonable to recommend limiting salt intake at least prior to and during the usual symptomatic interval each month.
- Some researchers suggest that increased appetite and carbohydrate cravings have been linked to the need to increase sources of tryptophan for serotonin synthesis. A healthy diet of frequent meals including complex carbohydrates may relieve PMS symptoms and may be linked to the steady availability of tryptophan.
- Exercise has been shown to minimize some symptoms associated with fluid retention and to increase self-esteem. Except for women with obvious medical contraindications, women should be encouraged to participate all month in some kind of regular physical exercise. It is the frequency, not the intensity, of exercise that seems to make a difference.

Table VII Menstrual Cycle Interventions

Oral contraceptives
GnRH analogues
Oophorectomy
Danazol
Estradiol implants and patches

If PMS symptoms persist after these measures have been tried, more rigorous pharmacologic and nonpharmacologic interventions may be necessary.

One approach to pharmacologic treatment of PMS is to control the overall menstrual cycle. This approach entails hormonal intervention. Four principal strategies have been used (Table VII):

- Oral contraceptives may minimize physical and psychological symptoms of PMS, as documented in both retrospective and prospective studies. Oral contraceptives may, however, also precipitate symptoms that resemble PMS, such as depression. In addition, risks and side effects of oral contraceptives include cardiovascular complications, migraine headaches, and increases in serum triglycerides. These considerations must be discussed and this strategy undertaken carefully.
- GnRH agonists and oophorectomy (i.e., surgical removal of ovaries) may effectively eliminate PMS symptoms, although this approach is associated with the unwanted effects of low estrogen production. Moreover, surgical risks must be balanced against the severity of PMS symptomatology to justify such an intervention. This strategy is best reserved for very debilitating PMS in older women, and only if less invasive methods have failed.
- Danazol is a synthetic androgen used to suppress the hypothalamic–pituitary–ovarian axis by inhibiting release of gonadotropin. It is superior to placebo when given daily, but many women cannot tolerate the side effects, which include weight gain and an imbalance of estrogen compounds and androgen (e.g., hirsutism, flushing, vaginitis).
- Estradiol implants have also been used successfully to treat PMS. The addition of synthetic progestin has been associated with a return of PMS symptoms but with significantly milder intensity than before hormonal treatment.

A second approach is to manage specific psychological symptoms. With respect to severe psychological symptoms, it is crucial first to verify that the woman, despite her discomfort, is sufficiently safe. A woman who is depressed to the point of being suicidal, or who is so angry that she might harm someone else, should be carefully protected. Four psychiatric medicines that address depression and anxiety have been used effectively in some patients with PMS: Xanax (benzodiazepine anxiolytic, GABA agonist), buspirone (anxiolytic, serotonin 1a agonist), nortryptiline (tricyclic antidepressant, noradrenergic and serotonergic agonist), and fluoxetine, sertraline, and others (antidepressants, selective serotonin reuptake inhibitors). These medications have both proven benefits and numerous side effects, and their use must be dictated by clinical judgment. For example, Xanax is a medication that addresses time-limited, target anxiety symptoms extremely well, but is sedating and highly addicting. Nortryptiline helps depressive symptoms effectively, but it may cause dry mouth, constipation, and sexual dysfunction. The serotonergic medications (e.g., Prozac, Zoloft) alleviate PMS symptoms (even in the absence of depression), but usually are taken daily and, while generally well-tolerated, may have unpleasant side effects (e.g., jitteriness, headaches, nausea). For these reasons, all medication choices must be approached carefully and monitored closely. [*See* PSYCHOPHARMACOLOGY.]

A third approach is to manage the predominantly physical symptoms of women with PMS. Here the interventions will depend on the medical issues and complaints. Diuretics can be helpful if patients have documented weight gain and evidence of fluid retention. Spironolactone has been a preferred diuretic medication because of its potassium-sparing properties. Other diuretics may be used so long as the possibility of hypokalemia is monitored. Vitamin E, bromocriptine (a dopamine agonist that can cause nausea), and tamoxifen (an oral nonsteroidal agent with antiestrogen properties that can cause headaches and fatigue) have all been shown to be beneficial for breast pain. Over-the-counter analgesics may be very valuable and safe in treating PMS-related headaches. In addition to good sleep routines for insomnia and healthy eating routines for food cravings, serotonergic antidepressants may be helpful for addressing fatigue and fostering stable eating patterns.

The choice of treatment should be grounded in the understanding of the woman's needs in terms of which symptoms are most troublesome for her, which treatment interventions are likely to be most effective for these symptoms, and which treatment strategies will be most acceptable to the patient according to her values and way of life.

BIBLIOGRAPHY

Barbieri, R. L. (1993). Physiology of the normal menstrual cycle. In I. Smith & S. Smith (Eds.), *Modern management of premenstrual syndrome* (Ch. 4). New York: Norton Medical Books.

Ferin, M., Jewelewicz, R., & Warren, M. (1993). *The menstrual cycle: Physiology, reproductive disorders, and infertility.* New York: Oxford University Press.

Frank, R. T. (1931). The hormonal basis of premenstrual tension. *Arch. Neurol. Psychiatry 26,* 1053–1057.

Gold, J. H., & Severino, S. K. (Eds.). (1994). *Premenstrual dysphorias: Myths and realities.* Washington, DC: American Psychiatric Press.

Golub, S. (1992). *Periods: From menarche to menopause.* Newbury Park, CA: Sage.

Jensvold, M. F. (1992). Psychiatric aspects of the menstrual cycle. In D. E. Steward & N. L. Stotland (Eds.), *Psychological aspects of women's health care: The interface between psychiatry and obstetrics and gynecology.* Washington, DC: American Psychiatric Press.

Severino, S. K., & Moline, M. L. (1989). *Premenstrual syndrome: A clinician's guide.* New York: Guilford.

Stewart, F., Guest, F., Stewart, G., & Hatcher, R. (1987). Understanding your body: Every woman's guide to gynecology and health. New York: Bantam.

Psychoanalysis

Mardi J. Horowitz
University of California, San Francisco

Abstinence The analyst avoids nonessential advice and reassurance, waiting to hear the patient's usually unspoken wishes and fears.
Dream Interpretation Explaining symbolic meanings behind dream images.
Dynamic Interpretation Explaining the wish-fear-and-defense configurations involved in forming maladaptive patterns of experience and behavior.
Genetic Interpretation Interpretation about situations, memories, and fantasies of infancy, childhood, and adolescence that lead to an understanding of the patient's present patterns.
Interpretation The main tool of the analyst.
Neutrality The analyst does not react as emotionally as he or she might in a personal social situation.
Reconstructive Interpretation Piecing together different topics and inferences to form a plausible story about how possibly significant early experiences account for current beliefs, attitudes, and behaviors.
Resistance Defensive operations that work against authentic emotional expressions and memory recovery thereby obstructing the progress of analysis.
Transference Interpretation Explaining the meaningful configurations of ideas and feelings about the relationship with the analyst.
Transference Neuroses A substitute pathology that reiterates fundamental developmental conflicts based on unconscious schematizations and motives concerning self and other roles in a relationship. In forming such transference-based reactions, the patient regresses to early stages of development, returning to the conceptual source of problems.

PSYCHOANALYSIS is a treatment that aims at a comprehensive exploration and understanding of unconscious conflicts, character, and personality development. Meetings are frequent and often go on for years. The aim of therapy is to alter the interaction of conscious and unconscious processes in the direction of better integration of identity leading to improved adaptation, maturity, and health. The central concepts of theory provide the basis for the treatment. These concepts focus on the interactions of wishes, fears, and defenses against threat, and the influence of enduring but often unconscious motives upon personality structure.

Personality is viewed as a knowledge and procedural structure that is the result of repeated behaviors and decisions for how to reduce or avoid dangerous manifestations of raw wishes, exposures to dreaded situations, and the experience of problems, symptoms, and uncontrolled moods. Thus, a psychoanalytic formulation of personality may include hypotheses about developmental antecedents in terms of how wishes, fears, and immediate defenses lead to more adaptive but still defensive compromises. Although relatively more adaptive compromises may be preferable to problem-filled or symptomatic compromises,

Copyright © 1998 by Academic Press.
All rights of reproduction in any form reserved.

they are not seen as substitutes for new, more optimal solutions that may be achieved through treatment.

I. THE BEGINNING OF PSYCHOANALYSIS: SIGMUND FREUD

Sigmund Freud established psychoanalysis as a combination of theory, mode of investigation, and technique of treatment. Dream work, multiple subpersonalities theory, recognition of unconscious determinants of behavioral patterns, hypnosis, and suggestive techniques were islands of fragmentary knowledge before Freud integrated them, added a developmental approach, described unconscious defensive mechanisms, and recognized transference and resistance.

In initial work, Josef Breuer and Freud emphasized the importance of psychic traumas. Repressed but dynamically active, memories of such traumas might affect conscious thoughts, feelings, and behaviors. Later, Freud added theories of repressed wishes and fears and their elaborations into unconscious but active fantasies.

In his early model, Freud viewed therapy as making the unconscious conscious. He developed one of the most important techniques in psychoanalysis, *free association,* as he gave up hypnosis and yet retained the attention-altering properties of trance and suggestion-induced reveries. No association is, of course, entirely free. The patient is encouraged not to suppress or edit what comes to mind and not to always focus only on one specific topic, instead saying in words all thoughts, images, feelings, and bodily sensations as they occur in the stream-of-conscious representations. Free association has been useful in counteracting unconscious defensiveness in general, in finding linkages between ideas in particular, and in understanding the power of certain symbols.

In order to associate freely, the patient must try to set aside restrictions on thought and reporting that occur because of feelings of embarrassment, shame, guilt, or fear that these emotions bring. A patient can experience such a process as confusing and anxiety provoking, which is why psychoanalysis is not always useful for persons who are vulnerable to conceptual disorganization.

Studying the flow of a patient's associations, therapists look not only at contents but at the sequences that indicate efforts to avoid or distort the communication of meanings. Together, the patient and therapist can observe the derailment of clear expression and elaboration of a topic. Thus, by developing free association as a rule in psychoanalysis, Freud was in a position to describe defense mechanisms.

Early theory dealt with repression as a defense against the repetition of emotionally distressing traumatic memories. Paradoxically, both intrusions into consciousness and omissions from consciousness were seen as the result of defense mechanisms. Omissions of traumatic memories were due to inhibitions; intrusions were due to sudden conscious representation in spite of efforts to inhibit the mental contents. Freud's early observations of both amnesia and excessive intrusion of traumatic memories have stood the test of time. Nonetheless, subsequent research has shown that the repressed memory theory of psychopathology was too limited.

After trauma psychology, Freud began to work on repressed wishes and then on how personality comes to be formed. He proposed that personality developed from the action of two basic drives or instincts, libido and aggression. From biological determinants these drives evolved into structures of learned knowledge during infancy, childhood, and adolescence. Social experiences in interactions with significant others affected the direction and linkages of such drives. Each individual was a complex result of nature and nurture. This was called id psychology.

Freud described the evolution of character in what was one of the first attempts to put psychology into a developmental sequence. He said the libidinal drives proceed in stepwise fashion to invest the oral, anal, and genital zones of evolving sensation, interpersonal communication, and erotism. This is the psychosexual theory of development within id psychology. Some observations of character traits that tended to occur together have been confirmed by subsequent investigations, but the general theory of id psychology has since been modified.

In altering his therapeutic technique from suggestion, hypnosis, and catharsis to free association, Freud simultaneously realized that a "different though not contradictory conception of the therapeutic process" was warranted. With the new emphasis on removal of amnesia and recovery of repressed memories, he observed that the same instinctive forces that brought about repression in order to obliterate pathogenic material from consciousness continued to exert a force—

resistance—against full disclosure through free association; moreover, unexpected feelings toward the analyst—*transference*—was noted.

Freud's view of transference was of ideas and feelings that arose from the past and recapitulated earlier ties with significant persons from childhood. In the case of Dora in 1905, he believed her hostile feelings resulted in her breaking off treatment, which he called "acting out." Just as Fraulein von R. had been the first pivotal failure with hypnosis leading to Freud's major technical shift away from its use, so the case of Dora was the turning point in psychoanalytic technique that highlighted for Freud the necessity to interpret feelings transferred onto the analyst.

II. POST-FREUD: EARLY TWENTIETH CENTURY TO PRESENT

The history and growth of the psychoanalytic movement from classical psychoanalysis to current practices has been marked by repeated revisions by Freud himself, as well as reappraisals and additions by others. From its beginnings, some analysts have argued against nearly all of Freud's basic conceptual premises, from the strictly sexual etiology of the neuroses to his views on feminine psychology. Reacting more directly to their clinical concerns that too few patients are amenable to the rigorous requirements associated with orthodox psychoanalysis, others have attempted to make the treatment more extensively applicable, affordable, and terminable.

Early efforts in the 1920s and 1930s by such analysts as Sandor Ferenczi, Otto Rank, and Wilhelm Stekel were aimed at increasing the applicability of psychoanalyses to a larger clinical spectrum by shortening treatment time (Rank was the first to propose an "endsetting" time limit) and emphasizing a more active, affective, and caretaking approach, particularly the use of the therapist as a substitute primary object in the treatment of young children. However, these therapists soon sparked a major controversy over whether their supportive therapy additions, a departure from a totally neutral-interpretive technique, would compromise treatment.

Karen Horney's rejection of Freud's libido theory of neurosis in favor of a more interpersonal approach in the analysis of neurotic patients also made less distinction between analysis and psychotherapy in that the analyst played a more active role, and dispensed with free association and the couch. Similarly, Harry Stack Sullivan's pioneering work with a population of schizophrenic patients drew attention to their distorted thinking and action patterns in adult interpersonal relationships, and influenced treatment techniques by defining the face-to-face psychiatric interview that examined the role of the analyst as a participant as well as an observer.

Within the framework of existential analysis (e.g., Medard Boss' *Daseinanalysis*), the role of the analyst was further altered by emphasizing the real, here-and-now encounter, as recently updated by Irving Yalom. Others who were engaged in the treatment of patients with character problems began to acknowledge the increasing need to enlarge the scope of treatment by introducing "parameters" (Kurt Eissler's term) that would help such patients in analysis. This technical direction was influenced by the growing effects of ego psychology on the understanding of ego defects and problems wrought by their presence.

Wilhelm Reich's analysis of character armor, as well as Otto Fenichel's investigations of problems of psychoanalytic technique, expanded the analysis of resistances in the form of pathological character traits. As analysts like Merton Gill, Leo Stone, Kurt Eissler, and Wilfred Bibring attempted to define and expand the horizons of psychoanalysis, Anna Freud's delineation of defense mechanisms also placed new emphasis on both their adaptive function and their characterological nature, and George Vaillant has brought this theory into the present.

At the same time, the European influence of the British object relations school, and the theories of Melanie Klein, Wilfred Bion, Donald Winnicott, and Michael Balint, led to modifications in technique to accommodate patients with impoverished or distorted early childhood learning patterns, as embodied in concepts of therapy as a "holding environment," the therapist as "container," and "healing the basic fault."

Elizabeth Zetzel, and later Ralph Greenson, followed Anna Freud's (and others') interests in the real relationship between analyst and patient by developing the now accepted notions of the therapeutic or working alliance that recognized the need to incorporate nontransferential elements into analysis; simultaneously advances were being made on a more theoretical front of interpersonal subjectivities and unconscious resonances as brought up to date by

Evelyne Schwaber, Robert Stolorow, Alan Skolnikoff, Owen Renick, and Morton and Estelle Shane.

Amplifications of ego functions' influence on adaptation were advanced by Heinz Hartmann, Ernst Kris, and Hans Lowenthal. Hartmann especially postulated the existence of a "conflict-free sphere" of the ego, and further defined the concepts of the self as a separate structure within the ego. Edith Jacobson's developmental model as a foundation of comprehensive psychoanalytic theory, which integrated drive theory with ego psychology and object relations theory, was supported by Renee Spitz's and Margaret Mahler's research that directly studied infants and their mothers during development. This work has been brought into current focus by Robert Emde, Fred Pine, and Daniel Stern.

Since the 1970s there has been an increased interest in narcissistic and borderline character disturbances. Heinz Kohut's psychology of the self in the understanding of narcissism and Otto Kernberg's application of psychoanalytic object relations theory to the development of psychoanalytic techniques in the treatment of borderline patients gained center stage. Their observations have profoundly influenced notions of the nature and kind of transference manifestations that appear in treatment.

John Bowlby added new theories having to do with how wishes and fears were incorporated into enduring, usually intrapsychic working models and schematizations of self and other. Like Edith Jacobson, Otto Kernberg, Heinz Kohut, and Mardi Horowitz, he attempted to integrate object relations theory and advances in developmental, cognitive, or ego psychologies. These object relations theorists described a variety of new ways people distort their views of self and others due to discomfort and trauma, including defenses of splitting, projection, and projective identification. Kohut then rejected many aspects of the original Freudian id-ego-superego theory in favor of what he called self-psychology.

Self-psychologists added views of others as extensions of self or self-objects, and of maladaptive patterns of idealization and devaluation to support fragile self-conceptualizations. Rather than real loved personas, with separate wishes and responses to the patient, self-objects are projections onto the other person of what the patient wishes them to be. Of course, these views often are quite at odds with reality and lead to relationship problems.

The control mastery theory of Joseph Weiss and Hal Sampson expanded on previous views of unconscious mental processes. They inferred that each person had unconscious plans at mastery of life. Unconscious calculations appraised the degree of safety or threat in trials of whether or not actions based on these plans could be successfully implemented. If unconscious assessments, based on past and perhaps outmoded developmental experiences nonetheless predicted danger, then processes of control inhibited the plans or led to distorted versions of them.

People like Arnold Cooper and Robert Wallerstein found ways to encompass the divergences in modern theory. Morton Reiser and Mardi Horowitz made efforts to develop a general psychodynamic theory that used modern cognitive neuroscience languages while integrating ego psychological and object relations theories into information processing terminologies. Horowitz developed formulation methods that identified states of mind, each with different schemas of self and models of relationship with other, and differing defensive control processes in each state. He suggested that shifts in control, memories, and person schemas, led to the state cycles of personality based patterns of repetitive but maladaptive interpersonal behaviors.

Table I contrasts the evolving differences between psychoanalysis and psychoanalytic psychotherapy, and Table II outlines the historical development of psychoanalytic psychotherapy.

III. MAJOR METAPSYCHOLOGICAL CONCEPTS

The *dynamic* perspective reflects the notion that all mental phenomena are the result of a continual interaction of forces that oppose one another. It implies that human behavior and motivation are active, goal and plan directed, and slowly changing at all times. It is the basis for such fundamental concepts as *conflict*.

The *topographical* perspective refers to the premise that mental phenomena reveal themselves at different levels of manifestation, from unconscious to the border of awareness or accessibility (preconscious) to conscious representation. This general orientation recognizes a human being's pervasive avoidance of painful feelings or experiences by keeping unpleasant thoughts, wishes, and affect from awareness. It also

Table I Psychoanalysis and Psychoanalytic Psychotherapy Contrasted

Feature	Psychoanalysis	Psychoanalytic psychotherapy	
		Expressive mode	Supportive mode
Frequency	Up to five times per week.	Regular one to three times per week.	Flexible.
Duration	Long term; usually 3 to 5 or more years.	Short or long term; several sessions to months or years.	Short or intermittent long term: single session or lifetime.
Modus operandi	Systematic analysis of all (positive and negative) transference and resistance: primary focus on analyst and intrasession events; transference neurosis facilitated; regression encouraged.	Focus on conflictual topics, interpersonal patterns and transference.	Focus on topics of current concern and increasing skills, reducing tendencies to transference by early interpretations of irrational beliefs.
Sample patient populations	Personality problems and psychosomatic disorders.	Symptom neuroses; personality problems; pathological responses to stressor life events.	Immaturity; severe personality disorders; latent or manifest psychoses; physical illness; ongoing stressor events.
Usual patient requisites	High motivation; psychological-mindedness; good previous relationships; good tolerance for ambiguity.	High to moderate motivation and psychological-mindedness; ability to form therapeutic alliance; frustration tolerance.	Modest degree of motivation and ability to contemplate.
Goals	Reschematization of knowledge structure; resolution of unconscious conflicts; insight into intrapsychic events; improved developmental level and new capacities.	Partial reorganization of personality and defenses; resolution of preconscious and conscious derivatives of conflicts; insight into current interpersonal events; improved relations; symptom relief.	Reintegration of ability to cope; stabilization or restoration of preexisting equilibrium; learning new skills; better adjustment or acceptance of pathology; symptom relief.
Major techniques	Reduced eye contact; free association; full interpretation (including confrontation, clarification, and working through) with emphasis on developmental reconstruction.	Limited free association; confrontation, clarification, working-through, and interpretation.	Expression of feelings and ideas, suggestion, clarification and logical views in the here-and-now, providing a safe relationship.
Treatment with medication	Usually avoided; if used, all negative and positive meanings and implications thoroughly analyzed.	May be used. If applied, negative implications explored and diffused.	May be used. If applied, negative implications explored and diffused.

acknowledges the persistence, resilience, and inaccessibility of underlying conflicts that remain alive and active, but may appear in diverse and disguised forms often unrecognizable by their recipient.

The *structural* perspective refers to the idea that the mental apparatus is organized into functional units of a tripartite nature—the it-like functions of id, the self-like functions of ego, and the over-self-like functions of superego. This basic personality organization forms the theoretical structure of intrapsychic conflict among instincts (*id*), a set of functions integrating identity with external reality demands (*ego*), and one's ideals, moral precepts or standards (*superego*).

The *economic* perspective relates to how psychic intentions are distributed, discharged, and transformed. It has implications for how ideas and affect are expressed (e.g., verbally or somatically), and for how the individual fends off psychic threat through a variety of defense mechanisms (e.g., *sublimation,* whereby unacceptable drives are diverted into socially acceptable forms; *reaction formation,* which turns an impulse into its opposite; or *displacement,* in which feelings belonging to one object are transferred to

Table II Historical Development of Psychoanalytic Psychotherapy

Theorist	Major contributions to psychoanalytic psychotherapy
1920s–1940s	
Rank, Ferenczi	Emphasized supportive as well as expressive technique with emphasis on affective experience: end-setting time limit.
Stekel	Psychoanalytically based brief psychotherapy.
Reich, Fenichel	Expanded analysis of character.
A. Freud, Spitz	Application of ego psychology to psychoanalytic treatment and child analysis, with emphasis on the adaptive function of defense mechanisms.
Alexander, French	Role of analyst to provide corrective emotional experience by being different from parents and offering alternative to early developmental experiences; short-term duration; emphasis on face-to-face interviews.
Horney, Fromm, Sullivan	Closed distinction between analysis and therapy; free association and couch not essential; active therapist role; short-term goals focused on patterns of interpersonal relationships.
1950s–1960s	
Eissler, Bibring, Stone, Gill	Expanded definition, indications, and scope (parameters) of psychoanalysis (Eissler, Bibring, Stone), including broadened analysis of transference (Gill).
Klein, Winnicott, Bion, Balint	Influence of British object relations school on psychoanalytic theory and technique (Klein): concepts of holding environment, good-enough mothering (Winnicott), therapist as container (Bion), healing the basic fault (Balint) addressed patients without adequate mothering in early months of life.
Zetzel, Greenson	Extension of therapeutic relationship to nontransferential aspects: concepts of therapeutic alliance (Zetzel) and working alliance (Greenson) advanced idea that analysis incorporate aspects of reality or real relationship into treatment, utilizing both observing and experiencing ego of patient.
Hartmann, Kris, Lowenstein	Advanced ego psychology in adaptation; postulated conflict-free sphere of ego and defined concept of self as separate structure: concept of regression in the service of the ego emphasized ego's participation in the analytic process.
Jacobson	Developmental model as basis of comprehensive psychoanalytic theory, integrating ego psychology, object relations, and drive theories in terms of multiple layered representations of self and others.
Mahler	Direct observation and research on infants and mothers; delineated separation-individuation subphases of child development, with impact on adult personality and pathology and implications for analytic treatment process.
Arlow, Brenner, Sandler, Stone, Rangell, Wallerstein	Clarified issues of unconscious fantasy and conflicted structures in relation to appraisals of reality. Studied expressive and supportive dimensions of therapy.
Edelson, Peterfreund, Klein, Rosenblatt, Thickstun, Schaeffer	Clarified need for a new theoretical language closer to observation.
1970s–1990s	
Kernberg, Ogden	Extension of object relations theory to psychoanalytic psychotherapy techniques in treatment of borderline disorders; delineation of expressive techniques for analyzing primitive transferences and defenses.
Kohut, Gedo, Goldberg, Basch, Ornstein	Development of self-theory in analytic treatment of narcissistic disorder; delineation of self-object (mirroring and idealizing) transferences; emphasis on empathic atmosphere to facilitate insight and transmuting internalization to crystallize self.
Weiss, Sampson	Developed, in control mastery theory, an enlarged view of unconscious processes as calculating whether life plans could be implemented to achieve mastery or needed to be held in check by processes of control because of dreaded consequences such as harming others.
Horowitz, Luborsky, Singer, Strupp	Integration of ego psychology and object relations theory with cognitive theory to develop coherent case formulations in terms of states of mind, schemas of persons, and habitual processes of control; added research methods.

another). Displacement has direct treatment implications for the phenomenon of *transference,* in which affect meant for early significant figures in the patient's life is placed onto the analyst or therapist.

The *genetic* perspective concerns the historical aspects of personality and its subsequent development. In this view, early experiences are repeated (*repetition compulsion*) until they can be neutralized through consciousness; that regression to infantile modes of behavior is both a manifestation of illness and a technical process facilitated to recreate within analysis the patient's original conflict (*transference neurosis*), whose resolution is the essence of classic analytic cure. It has broader implications for the idea of *psychic determinism,* which illuminates the crucial notion that present behavior is meaningfully related to one's past, and for developmental stages through which the individual evolves from infancy to adult maturity.

IV. FUNDAMENTAL TREATMENT CONCEPTS

A. Transference

Transference is broadly defined as the experience of feelings toward a person that do not befit the intended individual but belong to another person from the past. Intensive analysis of transference is the modus operandi that technically distinguishes psychoanalysis from all other forms of psychotherapy. Since Freud's original serendipitous discovery of the "strange phenomenon" of transference in the psychoanalytic treatment of every neurotic patient, its vicissitudes have been conceptualized in various related ways: (1) as a distinct type of therapeutic relationship, which has since been distinguished from nontransferential therapist–patient bonds (i.e., therapeutic alliance or real relationship); (2) as substitute pathology, expressed in the formation and resolution of a so-called transference neurosis; and (3) as a general phenomenon that transcends the boundaries of analysis into all human relationships.

B. Transference as a Therapeutic Relationship

The typical transference relationship is one in which the patient directs toward the analyst an unusual degree of attachment and affection that is not a realistic response to the relationship between them but can only be traced to wishful fantasies and idealizations that have remained unconscious. These fantasies are repeated in analysis as unresolved childhood attitudes and affects that are anachronistic and inappropriate, in part because repressed material necessarily contains infantile strivings and in part because the analyst may promote their appearance through special methods and analytic rules that intensify reactivation.

The peculiarity of the transference relationship to the analyst lies in its excess, in both character and degree, over what is rational and justifiable. Its major manifestation may include overendowment of the analyst as an idealized image, often including overestimation of the analyst's qualities, adoption of similar interests, and intense jealousy of other persons in the analyst's life. As the transference relationship is based on projection and fantasy on the part of the patient, and the analyst neither responds to the cravings of the patient nor reacts in a reciprocal or personal fashion, it is characterized (and often criticized) as being an artificial and asymmetrical bond. These qualities have been amended in later nontransferential concepts of the therapeutic relationship (e.g., working alliance, real relationship) that have been incorporated into theory and treatment.

Often, what distinguishes a transference from a nontransference reaction is not its content per se, but a group of qualities that tend to characterize transference responses and that may be used as signals to the analyst to denote their occurrence: inappropriateness (which refers to the largely irrational character of the transference response); intensity (which applies to the unusual strength of emotionality); ambivalence (which relates to the contradictions and shifts in affect that occurs toward the therapist); tenacity (which reflects the resilience with which such feelings tend to persist despite the analyst's actual behavior); and capriciousness (which describes the erratic, and sometimes trivial events that evoke the responses).

As transference distortions develop, their manifestations can be either positive or negative, paralleling the ambivalence that underlies all feelings that are in part unconscious. *Positive transference* refers to the expression of good feelings toward the analyst, of love and its many variations, manifested in (albeit excessive) interest, trust, admiration, respect, sympathy, and so on, that can predominate as the motive force behind the wish to change and receive the analyst's approval. In a state of positive transference, the patient overvalues and endows the analyst with some of the same magical powers attributed during infancy to the patient's parents. These feelings may be the basis for benign dependency, utilized by the analyst in gaining the patient's trust and establishing rapport insofar as the patient is well motivated and receptive to the analyst's influence. At the other end of the affective spectrum, *negative transference* refers to equally intense bad feelings toward the analyst—including hate, anger, hostility, mistrust, and rebelliousness—in which the patient undervalues the analyst in ways that also repeat comparable feelings toward parent or parent substitutes of the past. Both types are inevitable aspects of psychoanalysis and must be interpreted. Some analysts have considered positive transference to be libidinal, based on sexual drives, whereas negative transference is regarded predominantly as a function of unresolved aggressive strivings.

For the most part, however, it is negative transference that becomes most problematic and requires analysis if treatment is to proceed because it manifests itself in ways that interrupt treatment, whether through direct attacks on the analyst or by acting out negative feelings instead of exploring them. Nonetheless, very intense positive transference, often expressed in the patient's excessive passionate demands on the analyst, can be misleading in that it too may be manifestation of resistance as the patient defends against further probing into unresolved conflicts. Another obstacle to analytic progress may be the analyst's own strong reactions to the patient, *countertransference,* which can inappropriately enter the treatment if the analyst is not sufficiently aware of personal feelings.

As traditionally understood, transference refers primarily to unrealistic distortions from the past, whether positive or negative; it does not pertain to reactions resulting from reality factors, as when the patient may be legitimately angry. However, transference responses are increasingly recognized as having objective as well as subjective components, relating to significant figures of the past and to real responses of the analyst: "new editions" of old conflicts are exact replicas that are total projections, whereas "revised editions" attach themselves to actual characteristics of the therapist.

C. Transference Neurosis

The most vivid expression of transference is the formation of a *transference neurosis,* a substitute pathology that reiterates fundamental pathology, in which the patient psychologically regresses to early stages of development and returns to the source of personality problems in the past in order to transcend them. Manifestations of the transference neurosis do not arise immediately, but emerge in the so-called middle phase of analysis, when the patient is most subject to the regressive forces induced by the analytic situation and the emergence of infantile needs for gratification. Its appearance may be episodic, or it may never truly appear, although much of the work of the middle phase is spent removing resistances in order to allow the transference neurosis to surface. The transference neurosis was originally regarded as a serious obstacle to analytic work, but it also allows the analyst to observe directly the recapitulation of the patient's childhood responses.

D. Resistance

Resistance is defined as the forces or defensive operations of the mental apparatus that work against the recovery of memories and that obstruct the progress of analysis by opposing the analytic procedure, the analyst, and the patient's reasonable ego. Comparable to transference, analyzing or managing resistances is also central to analytic work, and functions in counterpoint to transference in two ways: (1) as resistance to the transference, which means that the patient fights against the development of a transference and thus prevents the analyst from being able to tap the source of intrapsychic conflict, and (2) as transference resistance, which means that the transference itself is used as a resistance by stubbornly adhering to irrational transference manifestations instead of utilizing the transference as a path to earlier experiences and memories.

Conscious resistance refers to the deliberate withholding of information from the analyst, or the like. Such resistance is transient and usually easily rectified by pointing it out to the patient. Unconscious resistance, however, refers to a much more significant and resilient phenomenon that arises as a defense against emotionality and memory.

The clinical signs and manifestations of resistance

are manifold. Any persistent, stereotyped, or inappropriate interruption of the treatment process may be a clue to resistance. Common examples include the silent patient, who impedes the progress by failure to verbalize, and, at the other end of the spectrum, the compulsive talker, who is ostensibly obeying the fundamental rule to say whatever comes to mind, but whose verbal productions are unconscious barriers to insight. Specific variations of resistant behavior may be undue focus on the past (fixation on a particular point in time) or incessant inclusion of trivia or external events in order to avoid painful or emotionally laden topics. Typical forms of resistance also include lateness, missed hours, and delaying (forgetting) to pay one's bill.

Managing resistances means that the defensive maneuvers of the patient are to be addressed before the material that is fended off can be approached. The analyst must discover how the patient resists, what is being resisted, and why. The immediate cause of resistance (e.g., anxiety, guilt, or shame) may be a superficial or surface indication of what is going on in the patient; repeated uncovering and confronting of resistances should reveal the underlying affects that are unconsciously behind such behaviors.

E. Countertransference

As previously mentioned, and as the name suggests, *countertransference* is transference in the reverse direction—from analyst to patient. It generally refers to unconscious emotional needs, wishes, or conflicts of the analyst evoked by the patient, which are brought into the analytic situation and thus influence the analyst's objective judgment and reason.

Countertransference manifests itself in many ways; it is commonly acute, temporary, superficial, and easily recognized and managed; but it can also be chronic, permanent, deeply rooted, largely unconscious, and out of the analyst's control. The former may occur in response to very specific content that arises or in identification with some concrete aspect of the patient's personality. The latter involves more generalized and ingrained patterns of behavior, often pathological, that pervade the analysis in a way that is untherapeutic and to which the analyst remains blind without external intervention.

The former type of countertransference, fortunately, is more typical and occurs in every analysis. Comparable to the patient's acting out, the analyst brings into the analysis feelings, thoughts, or behavior that do not belong there. Classic countertransferences may manifest themselves in special consideration for an attractive patient, like eagerly making an unavailable hour available, or failing to remember the changed hour of an uninteresting patient. The following are considered common warnings of countertransference in analysis: experiencing uneasy feelings during or after sessions with certain patients; persistently feeling drowsy or actually falling asleep; altering sessions or showing carelessness regarding scheduling (e.g., extending hours or forgetting about them); making special financial arrangements (e.g., overly strict with some patients and underassiduous with others); wishing to help the patient outside the session; dreaming about one's patients or being preoccupied with them in one's leisure time; using the patient as an example to impress a colleague or having the urge to lecture or write about a particular patient; reacting strongly to what the patient thinks of the analyst (i.e., needing a particular patient's approval); not wanting the patient to terminate or wanting the patient to terminate; finding oneself unable to explore certain material or to understand what is going on with the patient; and evincing sudden or excessive feelings, such as anxiety, depression, or boredom.

Countertransference is presumed to relate primarily to unresolved and irrational responses; yet it may also refer to an analyst's relatively reasonable reactions to a patient's behavior, as when feeling aroused by a seductive patient, paternal to a deprived patient, frightened by an aggressive patient, burdened by a demanding patient, or jealous of a successful patient. As such, countertransference feelings are an inevitable part of any treatment. However, when these feelings are not simply situation-specific and evoke strong reactions that belong to former events or persons in the analyst's life, they can become problematic because the analyst is in danger of bringing these unconscious feelings into the analysis in the form of unnecessary, if not actually untherapeutic, behaviors.

Of more serious implication are those forms of countertransference reflecting chronic problems left unsettled in the analyst's own analysis. Some examples may be the analyst with an underlying masochism who accepts abuse from patients without adequately analyzing its reasons; the grandiose analyst who takes on the most difficult patients with promises of cure without recognizing the need for help if the treatment is not going well; the analyst who allows a seductive patient to act out, or reciprocates sexual advances instead of examining the patient's wish to arouse; or the lonely analyst who encourages the patient's dependency and will not terminate treatment for fear of abandonment. When the analysis becomes a source of narcissistic gratification for the analyst who encourages the love or idolatry of the patient without introducing a more realistic appraisal, or prematurely terminates patients who do not improve sufficiently, the analyst's own return to therapy may be indicated.

V. CHARACTEROLOGICAL FORMULATION

The theories of psychoanalysis are an aid to explaining characterological aspects of personality problems and to planning how they may be changed. Therapists combine theory with observation in order to develop a patient-specific set of hypotheses. Typically, in psychoanalytic case formulation, it is assumed that symptoms and problems in living are caused by the interaction of multiple processes at biological, social, and psychological levels. At the level of the individual's psychology, the symptoms and problems might be caused not only by deficits in normal capacity but by conflicts. Active conflicts may lead to the formation of compromises between or among wishes, and their feared consequences. In psychodynamics these compromises are often regarded as defensive mental strategies.

The formation of symptomatic traits is often understood as a compromise between expressive aims and the wish to avoid the threatening consequences of expression. Some traits are learned from identification with others. Because symptomatic character traits are seen as complexly rooted in such multiple causations, psychoanalysts use the term overdetermination or pluralistic determination in making formulations.

For example, an individual may want to both transgress a moral value and also express feelings of guilt over the transgression. He or she fears the distress that could occur and inhibits both the wish and the guilt. Because of the unresolved topic he or she may nonetheless experience anxiety that something dreadful is about to happen. For such a person, anxiety would be a presenting symptom. The topic of the type of transgression might be conflictual or emotionally evocative, but unclear. The warded-off wishes, guilt, and fear can be formulated as the unconscious reasons for forming anxious experiences. The symptoms of anxiety are viewed as the result of the conflict between the impulse to express the guilt and the defensive avoidance of such expressions. Social and biological factors might influence the manner in which the anxiety symptoms are experienced and communicated.

A patient may mysteriously have anxiety symptoms during encounters that are meant to be lovingly erotic. The patient may add descriptions that indicate fears of phenomena that are even worse than the anxiety symptoms, such as horror of becoming enraged upon sexual frustration, guilt about potentially acting on the hostility felt toward a spouse, and/or a warded-off despair on feeling rejected. Avoidance of erotic situations may reduce the frequency or intensity of anxiety symptoms at the expense of diminished opportunities for the satisfaction of sexual wishes. The person might report substitute behaviors such as becoming so interested in morality that he or she is investigating pornography because it is socially bad and ought to be banned.

A patient may present a set of signs and symptoms that are part of a problematic state of mind, but not necessarily the most dreaded. For example, the person may present with moods of tension in which there is preoccupation, diddling with peripheral details, and blockage of work on central aspects of a project. This may be a surface indicator of approach and avoidance conflicts about collaborating on a project or about competing to win a role in a project. The desired state might be one of working well, enjoying mutual effort and, when necessary, competing in a realistic way. A related dreaded state of mind with a work supervisor or rival peer might be guilt over doing so well that the other is harmed or defeated, or doing so poorly that the self is humiliated. Approach and avoidance conflicts can lead to a problematic compromise state, one presenting with symptoms of anxiety and work block. A relatively less symptomatic and so relatively more adaptive compromise state defends against dreaded consequences of working too well by taking a stance of aloofness in regard to work. By procrastinating and isolating the interests of the self from the project, the risks of being one-up or one-down are reduced, but the satisfactions cannot be obtained.

Similarly, on a sexual topic, the presenting state may be a problematic compromise state containing anxiety symptoms and a tense mood. The desire might be for states of sensuous pleasure and closeness. The patient may have even more dreaded states of mind such as a mood of despair over being used and then abandoned. A relatively more adaptive compromise state that the problematic state of anxious tension might be clowning around to ward off states of closeness and intimacy. Just as one does not take the surface symptoms as the whole picture, in making a psychodynamic formulation at the level of observing the states of mind that bring phenomena together into coherent patterns, one does not take the presenting or problematic states of mind as the whole picture.

Psychoanalytic formulations of why states of mind occur focus on unconscious aspects of identity of self and on internalized object relationships. Interpersonal experiences during development leave an enduring inner set of models, comprised of views of self and others, that can cause the styles, moods, and organizations of any particular state of mind. Moreover, these inner schemas about self and the surrounding world may have sequences that can lead to cycles of shifting from one state to another. These sequences can be a part of not only conscious but, very importantly to psychodynamic formulations, unconscious fantasies, plans, or scripts. Once again, the developmental antecedents of various schemas, plans, and scripts are important aspects of formulations, and dynamic formulations change with increased understanding—formed during explorations in treatment sessions—of how the past is influencing, perhaps very irrationally, the present and near future.

Personality is in part a repertoire of schemas of self and others, and of values and plans for how to handle wishes, fears, defenses, and coping. Self-organization is a set of schemas that leads to a conscious sense of identity, of an "I" or "me" that continues over time. Each person's experience of the self varies; this stems from the activity of multiple self-schemas that can lead to different self-images and styles in different states of mind.

Some self-schemas can be activated to ward off the effects of others. An inferior self-schema may organize a potential state of shame. If less inferior and more realistic self-schemas cannot be activated, then grandiose and unrealistic ones might be primed in order to avoid shame by bolstering pride.

Activation of ideal schemas of self, when matched to and discrepant from real or devalued schemas of self, can lead to emotional experiences of shame or guilt. Whether or not such self discrepancies lead to deflation of self-esteem or can be accepted while maintaining emotional equilibrium depends on an individual's level of personality maturity. One way to view maturity is in terms of degree of supraordinate integration of multiple schemas of self. People vary in the degree to which they have or have developed the capacity to develop schemas of schemas. Those who can manage this are said to have an integrated self-conceptualization because they can accept various types of self-discrepancies.

The technique of interpretation and working-through in treatment might differ for patients who do and do not have supraordinate self-schemas to integrate and control subordinate self-schemas. The existence of supraordinate schemas allows a patient to contain in a given state of mind the information relevant to the self-schemas that organized a different state of mind. Patients without this capacity are more vulnerable than others to explosive shifts in state and in how they can view the therapist. These aspects of a formulation can be understood using a tool of inference called *role-relationship models.* Such models contain views of self and other, and self with other, and how transactions may unfold. A role–relationship model, in its simplest diadic form, includes a set of characteristics of self, a set of attributes and roles of others vis à vis the self, and a script of automatically expected transactions between self and other. One example of such a script begins with a wish, goes on to a response of the other, and then to reactions of the self, which may include self-appraisals. This is the aspect that Lester Luborsky called a Core Conflictual Relationship Theme.

Any person may have multiple role–relationship models for internally interpreting any topic, for any relationship, and for any traumatic event. Theories about such unconscious beliefs separate psychoanalytic points of view from cognitive and behavioral approaches to therapy because they add these components to case formulations: (1) there are immature schemas that can influence behavior in some states of mind but not others; (2) there are more mature schemas that can inhibit activity of less mature schemas in some states but not others; and (3) there are defensive layerings so that some schemas may be activated in order to ward off dreaded states of mind that might be organized by other schemas. Psychoanalytic therapies explore this structure of knowledge about self and others, its lack of concordance with real interpersonal opportunities, and its developmental sources. Such insight seeks to achieve a process of working through in order to arrive at new behaviors that can be learned and practiced until new schemas function automatically in organizing behavior and states of mind.

Psychoanalytic formulations include control processes that act beyond full conscious awareness to reduce the expression of ideas and feelings. By uncovering and analyzing such processes the therapist and patient can act to change them if they are resulting in symptoms or obstructions to the patient's life. The idea is not only to increase work on warded-off topics but to modify in an adaptive direction the person's habitual and nonadaptive forms of defensiveness.

Inhibitions of conflicted and potentially emotional topics can lead to the defensive maneuvers known as suppression (conscious avoidance), repression (unconscious avoidance), denial (reducing the impact of the real implications of external stressors), and disavowal or negation (obscuring what has been revealed).

Inhibitions of schemas and facilitations of other schemas, as well as dislocations of roles and attributes, can lead to defensive maneuvers that distort views of self and others. These include such operations as projection (attributing something from self to other), displacement (putting something from one person onto a less dangerous person), and role reversal (exchanging positions to take the role of lesser danger to the self).

Another class of control processes, one that affect the form of expression, can be added to these controls of the topics of thought and communication and their schematic organizers. These are also important to understand because of their implications for technique. A patient may discourse on a conflictual topic in a flat, hyperlogical, or intellectualized, unengaged, or generalized manner. There may be communication only of ideas, without emotion, a defensive mechanism called isolation.

VI. THE GROUND RULES AND CONTEXT OF PSYCHOANALYTIC TREATMENTS

The goal of therapy is to improve the future for the patient. Each party to the treatment has tasks in relation to this goal. The patient is asked to speak truthfully and completely about memories, fantasies, associations, images, dreams, bodily feelings, wishes, and fears that are usually not told to others. The therapist and the patient together observe what it feels like to do this, how it is done, what is communicated, and what the process does to their relationship. The therapist puts this understanding into words in the form of interpretations, which are intended to connect the patient's present feelings with his or her past, giving a broader picture about meanings, including those that have never before been verbalized.

In psychoanalysis, the two people explore private themes, personal dilemmas, conflictual memories, and unsettling feelings of one of them. Most people are not used to speaking openly on such matters. The analyst describes what can be done in the sessions to create this unusual environment of very frank discourse and interpretation. The therapy hour will begin on time and end on time. The patient's feelings about this are often one of the first topics relating to the therapy itself that comes up. Despite the fixed ending of each hour, the patient is not rushed to premature closures. An hour may end but a conflictual topic can be held over until the next session begins. As no one can be sure about interpretations, ambiguity as to meanings will have to be tolerated.

The analyst offers a relationship in which there is respect for the personal attitudes and feelings of the patient. The values of the therapist may be different from the patient and are not imposed on the patient. Clarification of the patient's values and how they may conflict with social norms is, however, an aspect of the dialogue. The therapist also displays more equidistance, abstinence, and neutrality, than one would expect of other relationships as with friends, teachers, parents, or religious counselors.

Equidistance means the therapist is "there" not just for the adult, poised, competent self-schema of the patient, and the states of mind organized by that set of concepts and images, but also "there" for the patient's ideals and values, and also "there" for the childlike self-schemas and immature passions of the patient. The patient may have a conflict among wishes to be taken care of, dangerous wishes to take over the lovers and careers of others, moral injunctions against ruthlessness or dependence, and adult concerns over how to appraise current dangers in the social, political, spiritual, and environmental worlds. The therapist does not side with any sector or any of a variety of self-schematizations of the patient, but remains available as a container for all facets of conflict.

For the therapist, the term abstinence means, at its best, avoiding unessential advice and reassurance while waiting to hear the unspoken and the hitherto unspeakable. The therapist is not there to gratify the patient's wishes but to foster adaptation to life so that the patient can seek constructive gratification in life outside the therapy. A related concept is neutrality, which means that the therapist does not react emotionally as he or she would in a social situation according to his or her own wishes, ideals, and moral standards. Neutrality is not coldness or indifference: warmth, compassion, concern, sympathy, empathy, and understanding are not deflections from neutrality but absolute requirements for the therapist if the treatment is to achieve its full goal.

The major general techniques of psychodynamic treatments are fostering expression, suggestion, clarification, interpretation, and repetition in order to facilitate working through. Working through means the process of revising knowledge structures so that warded-off topics can be confronted, traumatic memories integrated, and conflicts and contradictions resolved or accepted; working through is also the process by which deficiencies are reduced and unconscious fantasies are modified by conscious choices.

A. Fostering Expression

Fostering expression includes helping the patient to assume most of the responsibility for bringing up topics of importance. He or she is encouraged to broaden the topics of discussion beyond the scope of original complaints. The fundamental rule is to try to say everything that comes to mind or is felt in the body.

This fundamental rule of complete disclosure can be expanded to helping the patient to use free associative reveries and to report peripheral and fleeting thoughts and visual images. At times drawings, paintings, poems, letters, and discussions of bodily postures or impulses to move during the hour may be used to widen the modes of representation for initial expression of inchoate feeling states and ambiguous ideas. But while pictures in the mind's eye and bodily enactions are utilized as carriers of meaning, translation into words is emphasized as the clearest form of communication and the beginning of the possibilities for logical and psychological understanding of nonverbal impulses and behavior and through that, the ability to change, if change is desirable.

B. Suggestion

The therapist may suggest that the patient attend to certain topics, follow certain principles of disclosure, or try out certain alternative modes of perceiving, thinking, feeling, or acting. The therapist may ask, for example, "What do you imagine you would feel if it were to happen that . . ." to suggest focusing in a specific direction. The choice about whether or not to follow such suggestions is left to the patient. Firm directions are seldom if ever given, and any type of manipulative or covert suggestion is avoided. This means giving up the use of certain positive effects of suggestion, as in the placebo effect, in favor of fostering a sense of joint exploration in the search for insight and understanding as vehicles to change.

C. Clarification

Clarification includes techniques of questioning or repeating what the patient has told the therapist. Even when the therapist repeats exactly a bit of dialogue spoken by the patient, it sounds different when the patient hears the remark. When the therapist reorganizes information reported by the patient it is usually to convey cause and effect sequences and to show the patient the meaningful relatedness of sequences that have seemed, to the patient, unrelated.

For example, the patient might tell a story like this:

"He really made me mad, implying I had not done my work. I'd like to quit that job. While I hadn't gotten the inventory together, I would have eventually."

The therapist might qualify:

"While you had intended to do it, you had not yet gotten the inventory together. He criticized you for that. Then you got mad and now want to quit."

This intervention is very minor, but it puts the sequence into a temporal order and gives the patient a chance to listen to that and then comment further.

It can be helpful to say how the discourse of the patient is being received. The therapist may say:

"I don't understand this story too well, maybe I haven't got the sequence of events in my mind yet."

Such remarks not only encourage the patient to elaborate on the sequence of events, they clarify the manner in which the patient is telling the story in question.

D. Interpretation

Interpretation is the central tool of the psychoanalyst and dynamic therapist. In an interpretation the therapist says what is important, why it is important, and/or how it comes about. Interpretations are so crucial to psychodynamic techniques that they can be categorized as follows.

Genetic interpretations link current patterns to their developmental antecedents, going back to adolescence, childhood, and infancy as necessary to understand the present. (The word "genetic" here is used to refer to the original or developmental source of current patterns, not to direct action of the genes.) A special form of genetic interpretations is the reconstruction. In a reconstruction the dynamic therapist pieces together different topics and offers a story about what significant early experiences might have been like in order to account for current, clear, important, and maladaptive beliefs, attitudes, wishes, or behavioral problems.

Transference interpretations explain to the patient the meaning of distortions in the relationship with the therapist. A transference interpretation may involve a contrast between the role–relationship models described as transference and the role–relationship model that might describe the current therapeutic alliance of the patient, or the potential for relationship in the treatment setting that takes into account the real opportunities of that setting.

Dynamic interpretations explain to the patient the forces involved in a conflictual constellation. Wishes, fears, and defenses on a given topic are described, and their interaction leading to experiences is also described. The advantage of working with levels of formulation that address phenomena, states of mind, person schemas, and processes of control is that the language of the formulation itself can be used directly in discourse with the patient about desires, threats, and defensiveness.

Dream interpretations explain to the patient the concerns and symbolic meanings that may lie behind the formation of dream images. Some schools of dynamic treatments rely partly on assumed general inclinations such as archetypes or mythic symbols, but most often dream interpretation is delivered in terms of what the therapist actually knows about this specific patient's schemas and role–relationship models. Accurate interpretation of a dream usually requires more knowledge than the description of the manifest content of the dream, and so the patient's free associations to elements in the dream are requested. They suggest the antecedent moods, schemas, and recent experiences that contribute to the dream elements.

Interpretations are tentative and may change over time as understanding deepens. That is why in technique the wording is often put in a tentative way, leading to some jokes about analysts who too invariably repeat "I wonder if perhaps you might be feeling. . . ." Interpretation is not enough to induce psychic change. The change process beyond interpretation is called working through.

E. Repetition and Working Through

The working-through process involves repeated examination of the same topic. If the treatment is progressing, each repetition is perhaps a bit different and contributes to the overall decrease in repression and increase in understanding. Some new aspect of conflict may be identified, and new linkages between topics are established. Realization of developmental antecedents of current conflicts helps the task of differentiating current reality from past fantasy.

Previously warded-off ideas and feelings may be allowed expression and modification during repetitions. Linkages to other domains of meaning may be established. In each repetition there may be a shift in the interaction of wishes, fears, defenses, and beliefs about reality. Should the whole topic again fall under repression, as it characteristically does after the treatment hour, it is in this revised form and can come up again, each time more easily, for further revision until it is completely analyzed.

F. Complications

It has been observed in exploratory psychoanalysis that some patients have an initial period of effective work and then have a deterioration in their condition. This has been called a negative therapeutic reaction. Sometimes character traits of self-punitiveness have been noted in such instances. It is important in such instances for the therapist to be self-observant for feelings of helplessness, guilt, and anger, and to aim instead for understanding with the patient why the condition has gotten worse.

Not to be confused with negative therapeutic reactions are negative transference phenomena. These are a common aspect of treatment. In developmentally immature patients, ones who have unintegrated self-schemas and who are vulnerable to feeling fragmented, empty, worthless, or bad, negative transference reactions can occur and seem to the patient "the whole picture." That is, they are not mitigated by simultaneous schemas of a therapeutic alliance. Early interpretation of the negative transferences and/or very early emphasis on signs of the therapist being helpful in a therapeutic alliance may be needed to prevent the patient from dropping out prematurely in the midst of a negative transference reaction.

VII. RESEARCH AND EVALUATION

Henry Bachrach, Robert Galatzer-Levy, Alan Skolnikoff, and Sherwood Waldron report the following in their review of psychoanalytic efficacy studies: Robert Knight reviewed analytic case outcome research before the late 1930s. The results indicate much improvement or better in 63% of neurotic cases, 57% of character disorder, 78% of psychosomatic conditions, and 25% of psychoses. In a study led by Weber of persons who applied for psychoanalysis and then received either analysis or time-unlimited analytic psychotherapy, the patients in different modalities had a 90% or greater report of being satisfied, and 75 to 90% were rated as improved. In a separate study Jerome Sashin, Stanley Eldred, and Suzanne van Amerowgen reported a 69% agreed-upon completion rather than breaking off of therapy, and a 75% level of achieving at least moderate improvement.

Brief forms of dynamic psychotherapy have been found to be effective in many empirical studies as summarized by Mary Lee Smith, Gene Glass, and Thomas Miller. At outcome the average patient is better than 72% (effect size .59) of subjects in waiting-list control groups. The current questions for research concern which therapy for which type of patient and with what type of emphasis on therapist action.

Different studies led by Robert Wallerstein and by Mardi Horowitz have indicated that therapist actions that are more probing for warded-off contents and more confrontational with respect to control processes may be more helpful for neurotic level cases and less helpful for narcissistically vulnerable, borderline, or psychotic levels of self-organization.

BIBLIOGRAPHY

Brenner, C. (1982). *The mind in conflict.* New York: International Universities Press.

Greenson, R. R. (1967). *The technique and practice of psychoanalysis.* New York: International Universities Press.

Horowitz, M. J. (1988). *Introduction to psychodynamics: A new synthesis.* Northvale, New Jersey: Aronson: masterworks series (first published by Basic Books).

Horowitz, M. J., Kernberg, O., & Weinshel, E. (Eds.) (1993). *Psychic structure and change in psychoanalysis.* New York: International Universities Press.

Pine, F. (1990). *Drive, ego, object, self.* New York: Basic Books.

Shapiro, T., & Emde, R. (1995). *Research in psychoanalysis.* New York: International Universities Press.

Wallerstein, R. F. (1995). *The talking cures: The psychoanalyses and the psychotherapies.* New Haven, CT: Yale University Press.

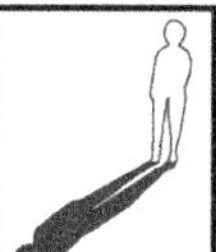

Psychopharmacology

Neil E. Grunberg, Laura Cousino Klein, and Kelly J. Brown
Uniformed Services University of the Health Sciences

Dose A specified amount of a drug.
Drug Any chemical compound that is used medically or recreationally.
Pharmacodynamics Actions of drugs on the body.
Pharmacokinetics Actions of the body on drugs.
Pharmacology The study of drugs.
Toxicity Adverse or untoward effects of a substance.

PSYCHOPHARMACOLOGY refers to the study of drugs as they relate to mind and behavior. This topic includes several different aspects of this relationship. It includes the study, development, and administration of drugs or medications to treat psychological and psychiatric disorders, such as anxiety disorders, mood disorders, and psychoses. It includes the study and development of drugs that affect behaviors in psychologically normal people, such as sleeping, feeding, and sexual functioning. It includes the study and development of drugs that affect cognitions and perceptions, such as attention, memory, learning, hunger, sensory perception, and pain. It includes the study of drugs that are addictive or abused and the study and development of drugs to treat drug addiction, to help alleviate withdrawal from addictive drugs, and to help maintain abstinence from addictive drugs. In addition, psychopharmacology includes the investigation of psychological, pharmacological, biological, neuroscientific, and molecular biologic mechanisms that underlie the actions of psychopharmacologic agents to help understand how these drugs work, underlying particular psychological disorders, and more general aspects of psychology and behavior.

Psychopharmacology can be traced back to the use of botanically derived medicinal agents, particularly alcohol and opium, in Greek culture and throughout the world by shamans or medicine men to achieve particular psychological states and to alter mood, anxiety, hunger, and pain. Psychopharmacology developed markedly in the twentieth century, especially after World War II. Sedative-hypnotics (e.g., barbiturates) and stimulants (e.g., amphetamines) were introduced at the beginning of this century, but it was the dramatic actions of antipsychotic medications (e.g., phenothiazines) that grabbed professional, public, and media attention. The pharmaceutical industry realized the potential market and profitability of psychopharmacologic agents beginning in the middle of this century and the development of psychopharmacologic medications became a major thrust. With cultural changes in the 1960s also came an explosion in popular, recreational use of a wide variety of mind-altering drugs, including marijuana, LSD, amphetamines, and opiates. This societal change also led to debates and discussions about addictive drugs, including drugs used for medicinal and nonmedicinal reasons. Technological and conceptual developments in behavioral sciences, neurosciences, and molecular biology from the 1960s to the present further added to interest

Copyright © 1998 by Academic Press.
All rights of reproduction in any form reserved.

in psychopharmacology. Today, it is taken as a given that drugs can alter mind and behavior, that drugs can be developed to treat psychological problems, that drugs not intended primarily as psychopharmacologic agents also can affect mind and behavior, and that psychopharmacology is a diverse and active discipline to study drugs and to help understand mind and behavior. The present article addresses major issues in psychopharmacology. This article discusses principles and paradigms of psychopharmacology; mechanisms of action of psychopharmacologic agents; clinical psychopharmacology; and issues related to special populations.

I. PRINCIPLES AND PARADIGMS OF PSYCHOPHARMACOLOGY

A. Psychopharmacology versus Behavioral Pharmacology

Within any field different camps develop for a variety of reasons, some historical, some conceptual, some methodologic, and some personal. The study of drugs and psychology is no exception to this truism. Whereas psychopharmacology has come to refer to a broad rubric of issues, methods, and topics, behavioral pharmacology has a narrower focus. This particular subfield is mentioned here because it is so important to the broader topic and it has made so many contributions to knowledge of drugs and behavior. It is singled out because scientists studying drugs and behavior either identify themselves as behavioral pharmacologists or psychopharmacologists. Behavioral pharmacology developed as behaviorists—that is, experimental psychologists who focused on behavior rather than on mind, perception, or motivations—began to study drugs. In addition, behavioral pharmacology refers to a series of techniques (especially operant techniques) that are used to examine drug effects on behavior and the actions of environmental or other variables on behavioral responses to drug actions. The behaviors of interest are operant (responses elicited by the environment) and conditioned behaviors, rather than unconditioned, naturally occurring behaviors. Traditional behavioral pharmacologists are primarily interested in the actions of drugs, the biological and behavioral mechanisms that underlie drug actions, and the identification and development of new drugs that alter behavior.

B. Conditional and Unconditional Behaviors

Conditional behaviors, also called conditioned behaviors, are behaviors that have come under the control of environmental stimuli or under the control of other external stimuli that in and of themselves do not elicit the given response. These conditional behaviors are either classically conditioned (Pavlovian conditioning) or instrumentally conditioned (operant or Skinnerian conditioning). Classical conditioning refers to the phenomenon in which a conditional stimulus (CS) (e.g., tone) is presented with an unconditional stimulus (UCS) (e.g., meat powder to a dog) that leads to an unconditional response (UCR) (e.g., salivation). After repeated pairings of the CS and UCS, the CS comes to elicit a similar response, which is known as the conditional response (CR). Operant conditioning refers to the phenomenon in which the behaviors emitted are shaped by the consequence (e.g., reward or punishment) of the behavior. This approach is typically studied in operant chambers (Skinner boxes). Psychopharmacologists, especially behavioral pharmacologists, use variations of these learning principles and paradigms to study drug actions on behaviors.

Unconditional behaviors refer to innate, or naturally occurring, behaviors. These behaviors include: feeding, drinking, sleeping, moving, exploring, jumping, startling, touching, grabbing, grooming, playing, fighting, nesting, and copulating. Psychopharmacologists examine effects of drugs on these and other unconditional behaviors in order to learn about drug actions, to compare different drugs, and to understand various behaviors.

Together, the study of drugs on unconditional and conditional behaviors offers a more complete picture of behavioral effects of drugs. The conditional behaviors offer the advantage of exquisite control and sensitive measure of drug effects. The unconditional behaviors offer the advantage of information that is of direct clinical relevance as well as information about basic, everyday behaviors.

C. Human and Animal Subjects

Psychopharmacology uses human and animal subjects. Human subjects include patients with particular disorders, conditions, or injuries, and healthy, normal volunteers. It is relevant and important to stipulate and consider the age, gender, race, ethnicity, genotype, and other major demographics of the patients or subjects. Animal subjects are taken from a wide variety of species, including monkeys, rabbits, rats, mice, gerbils, hamsters, and pigeons. Age, sex, and genotype are important variables to consider when examining effects of drugs on animal subjects.

D. Pharmacokinetics and Pharmacodynamics

Pharmacokinetics refers to the actions of the body on drugs (e.g., distribution, metabolism, reabsorption, elimination of a drug). Pharmacodynamics refers to the actions of drugs on the body (e.g., binding to a particular receptor, stimulation of a chemical or electrical response, stimulation of a physiologic or organ response, stimulation of a behavioral or psychological response). Both of these principles are important when studying psychopharmacologic agents. They are relevant to the characterization of the relationship between drugs and the body. In addition, particular situations or stimuli (e.g., stressors, other drugs, history of exposure to the drug of interest, individual difference variables) can alter pharmacokinetics or pharmacodynamics or both types of processes. Identification of the contribution of these mechanisms of action are relevant to the prescription of appropriate drugs and dosages and to elucidate the mechanisms underlying a given drug or condition.

E. Toxicity and Adverse Side Effects

As with all drugs, psychopharmacologic agents have an effective dose range. Outside this range, the drugs either are ineffective or have toxic and adverse side effects. For example, stimulants used to treat attentional problems, to regulate hunger, or to control asthmatic attacks, can cause anxiety, shakiness, dizziness, and panic. Antibiotics used to kill or to control infectious diseases can lead to psychotic-like episodes and hallucinations. Analgesics can result in respiratory distress. The combination of various drugs, especially when used with alcohol, can potentiate these toxic and adverse side effects. It is relevant to consider this issue in the present context because drugs that are not normally considered to be psychopharmacologic agents can cause psychological effects in high dosages or in combination with other drugs. In addition, drugs can have a range of behavioral effects (e.g., discomfort, headache, dizziness, nausea, sedation, altered appetite, sexual impotence) that decrease the likelihood of adherence to prescribed medication regimens. The study of these effects also contributes to psychopharmacologic knowledge.

II. MECHANISMS OF ACTION OF PSYCHOPHARMACOLOGIC AGENTS

A. Neuroanatomy

The brain, central nervous system, and peripheral nervous system all are relevant to the actions of psychopharmacologic agents. The vast array of effects of these drugs is reflected in the range of relevant neuroanatomical sites affected by these drugs. The specific loci of action reveal information about the underlying mechanisms of drug action and also reveal information about the anatomical substrates of specific psychological and behavioral responses. Brain regions that are relevant to the present discussion include the reticular activating system (for arousal and consciousness), pons and medulla (for autonomic control), cerebellum (for motor function and locomotion), pituitary (for hormonal regulation), hypothalamus (for body weight and hunger regulation), amygdala (for aggression), limbic system (for emotions and mood), hippocampus (for memory and learning), ventral tegmental area and nucleus accumbens (for reward), occipital lobe (for vision), parietal lobe (for somatosensory perception), temporal lobe (for audition), and the cortex (for higher cognitive and sensory-motor processing). Increasingly, psychopharmacologists are investigating neuroanatomical structures and loci via electrophysiological (e.g., single cell recording), surgical (e.g., ablation), and pharmacological (e.g., specific agonists and antagonists, radioactively labeled drugs) techniques in conjunction with functional assessment of drug effects. This work can be done on a molecular and cytoarchitectural level in animal subjects. Developments in receptor biology, structure and function, allow for detailed analyses of the cellular bases for psychopharmacologic drug actions. In addition, brain imaging techniques (including positron emission tomography [PET], magnetic resonance imaging [MRI], computed tomography [CT], single photon emission computed tomography [SPECT], and magnetoencephalography [MEG]) allow for the examination of structural and functional information relevant to psychopharmacologic agents in humans.

B. Neurophysiology and Electrophysiology

The function and actions of neurons, nerves, neural tracts, and neural tissue can be evaluated by invasive and noninvasive techniques and are included in psychopharmacologic investigations. In animal subjects, current technology allows for single cell recording of electrical activity relevant to neurophysiologic function. Action potentials, excitatory postsynaptic potentials (EPSPs), inhibitory postsynaptic potentials (IPSPs), long-term potentiation (LTP), and kindling all are studied in response to psychopharmacologic agents. Sensory and motor nerve recording, in animal subjects and in human patients, also provide useful information in this context. Electromyography (EMG) can be used in human patients to evaluate muscular responses, for example, to muscle relaxants and in cases of anxiety and pain. Electrocardiography (ECG or EKG) is used to assess heart function and is relevant in the present context to evaluate side effects of psychopharmacologic agents, as an index of stress responses, and to evaluate effects of psychopharmacologic drugs that may be revealed in cardiovascular arousal (e.g., anxiety, general arousal). Electroencephalography (EEG) is a noninvasive technique used to evaluate electrophysiologic activity of the brain. Detailed analyses of this information (e.g., contingent negative variation [CNV], auditory evoked potentials [AEP], visual evoked potentials [VEP], somatosensory evoked potentials [SEP], and positive or negative deflections in these responses) reveal the relay of information through specific brain regions and, thereby, can be used to evaluate the actions and to suggest mechanisms of psychopharmacologic agents.

C. Neurochemistry

The chemical bases of communication among neurons and the chemical regulation or modulation of this communication are affected by psychopharmacologic agents. These drugs can alter all of the known chemical neurotransmitters, including: amino acid transmitters (e.g., γ-amino-butyric acid [GABA], glycine, taurine, beta-alanine, glutamate, aspartate, cysteic acid), acetylcholine, catecholamines (e.g., norepinephrine, epinephrine, dopamine), indoleamines (e.g., serotonin), histamine, and neuroactive peptides (e.g., pro-opiomelanocortin [POMC], β-endorphin, leucine-enkephalin, methionine-enkephalin, dynorphin, neuropeptide-Y). Psychopharmacologic agents also can alter neuromodulators and chemicals that affect body functions, including: adrenocorticotrophin hormone (ACTH), corticotropin releasing factor (CRF), corticosteroids, and many peptides (e.g., Substance P, galanin, cholecystokinin [CCK], neurotensin, vasopressin, antidiuretic hormone [ADH], thyrotropin releasing hormone [TRH]). In addition to these relatively large molecules, psychopharmacologic agents can affect chemical ions (charged particles, such as Na^+, Ca^{++}, K^+, Mg^{++}, Cl^-) that alter neuronal transmission. Further, psychopharmacologic agents can affect second messengers (e.g., cyclic adenosine monophosphate [cAMP], guanine diphosphate [GDP], nerve growth factor [NGF]) and G-proteins that act to modulate neuronal communication. Genes with altered expression after drug exposure also are under investigation. Evaluations of these actions are active topics of research.

III. CLINICAL PSYCHOPHARMACOLOGY

Psychopharmacologically active agents (e.g., alcohol, opium) have been used for millennia to alter psychological state. Over the past 200 years, specific gases and chemicals have been identified (e.g., nitrous oxide, barbituric acid) that also alter consciousness and psychological state. It was not until the 1950s, however, that use of drugs to treat mental disorders and conditions became formalized and a focus of research and clinical attention. The dramatic reports in the early 1950s of chlorpromazine (Thorazine) to treat psychoses was a breakthrough that allowed previously uncontrollable patients to be cared for in a humane manner. This important development proved to be the genesis of clinical psychopharmacology as a central element in modern psychiatry and as a valuable adjunct to psychotherapy. No single pharmacological class is the panacea for the treatment of mental disorders. In fact, the identification and distinction among mental health disorders continues to be accompanied by the development of many different psychopharmacological agents that either treat the mental health condition or the symptoms associated with the condition. This section addresses the available psychopharmacologic treatments of the major categorizations of mental health disorders presented by the *Diagnostic and Statistical Manual of Mental Disorders* (Fourth Edition; *DSM-IV*) of the American Psychiatric Association and of other important psychological conditions. [*See* DSM-IV.]

A. Anxiety Disorders

Psychopharmacologic treatment of anxiety disorders began with the use of sedative-hypnotics (e.g., bromide salts, alcohol, chlorol hydrate) at the turn of the twentieth century. Barbiturates (e.g., phenobarbital, pentobarbital) were introduced early in the twentieth century but their adverse side effects, including addiction liability and toxic overdose, limited the use of these agents. The development of the benzodiazepines (e.g., chlordiazepoxide, diazepam) in the 1960s as general anxiolytics (separate from the muscle relaxant properties) was a major breakthrough because of the wide effective dose range and the limited adverse side effects. Subsequently, beta-adrenergic receptor antagonists (e.g., propranolol), antihistamines (e.g., hydroxyzine), and anticholinergic agents were used to treat specific cases of anxiety disorders (e.g., speech anxiety, posttraumatic stress disorder [PTSD]). More recently, azapirones (e.g., buspirone) that act via serotonergic antagonism and some dopaminergic antagonism have proven useful for mild forms of generalized anxiety. In the late 1980s, selective serotonin reuptake inhibitors (SSRIs) (e.g., fluoxetine [Prozac], sertraline [Zoloft], paraxetine [Paxil]) were introduced and, in the 1990s, were approved for treatment of specific anxiety disorders (e.g., panic, agoraphobia, PTSD). In addition, tricyclic drugs (e.g., clomipramine, imipramine, amitriptyline) and monoamine oxidase inhibitors (MAOIs) (e.g., phenelzine, tranylcypromine) are used in the treatment of some anxiety disorders (e.g., panic, agoraphobia, PTSD).

B. Eating Disorders

Eating disorders usually are characterized by a morbid fear of becoming fat and a preoccupation with body weight, food, and body image. Eating disorders include anorexia nervosa (restricting type and eating/purging type) and bulimia nervosa (purging and nonpurging type) and occur more commonly among females than among males. Anorexia nervosa is associated with a 5 to 18% premature mortality rate. In addition, these individuals are at risk for comorbid depression, mood disorders, and an increased risk of physical health problems as a result of poor nutrition. Given the serious implications of this illness, hospitalization can become necessary in an effort to restore the patient's nutritional status, electrolyte balance, and hydration. Unfortunately, no psychopharmacologic agent or class of agents cures the primary symptoms of anorexia nervosa. Various drugs are used to treat secondary symptoms associated with these eating disorders. For example, amitriptyline (i.e., the tricyclic antidepressant Elavil) has been used effectively in some patients with this disorder, and cyproheptadine, a drug with antiserotonergic and antihistaminic effects, is effective with some restrictive-type anorexia patients. Some studies suggest that fluoxetine (i.e., an SSRI) administration may result in weight gain, but most studies indicate that antidepressants provide little benefit to these patients. There are risks (e.g., hypotension, cardiac arrhythmias, dehydration) associated with the use of tricyclic antidepressants in these patients and, therefore, it is not recommended that they be used. There are no data on the use of other SSRIs in patients with anorexia nervosa. MAOIs (phenelzine or tranylcypromine) may be useful, but few data are available to establish their value unequivocally. Antidepressant medications seem to be particularly useful with bulimic patients. Imipramine, desipramine, trazodone, fluoxetine, and MAOIs have been successful in treating binge–purge cycles. Antidepressants are effective when used in dosages suggested for the treatment of depressive disorders. However, higher dosages of fluoxetine usually are needed to alleviate binge episodes than those dosages suggested for treating depression. Carbamazepine and lithium are useful in bulimic patients with comorbid mood disorders but are not useful in treating binge episodes alone. Bupropion is contraindicated in patients with a history of anorexia nervosa and bulimia nervosa because it may result in seizures.

Although not usually defined as classical eating disorders, there certainly are many cases of overeating that lead to obesity and excessive body weight. Some people overeat in response to psychological or environmental conditions; others are night-eaters (i.e., they get up and eat excessively after they have gone to bed); and others eat to the point of obesity and excessive body weight as a result of biological variables. Appetite suppressant medications (e.g., dexfenfluramine, diethylpropion, fenfluramine, mazindol, phendimetrazine, phentermine) are useful for some people but the effects are modest. Other appetite suppressant medications (e.g., amphetamines) are not recommended for use because they are addictive. Various antidepressants are used in some cases of overeating.

C. Learning, Memory, Attention, and Related Cognitive Disorders

There is a wide variety of cognitive conditions that deleteriously affect learning, memory, and attention but that do not involve other psychopathology. For example, Attentional Deficit Disorder with and without hyperactivity (ADHD and ADD), senile dementia, and Alzheimer's disease are familiar to the public. Each of these conditions can have profound negative effects on daily living and quality of life. Psychopharmacologic treatment for these conditions is an active, current topic of interest with modest success to date. For example, ADHD is treated with stimulants (including dextroamphetamine, methylphenidate [Ritalin], and pemoline), antidepressants (including imipramine, desipramine, and nortriptyline), and clonidine. Memory deficit-related conditions are an area of great interest and experimental investigations are examining various medications, including drugs that act as: dopaminergic agonists, α-2 adrenergic agonists, cholinergic agonists, general cerebral metabolic enhancers, calcium channel blockers, and serotonergic agents.

D. Mood Disorders

Mood disorders are manifested as either depressive or manic episodes. Among the most serious of the mood disorders are major depressive disorder or unipolar depression, in which a patient only experiences depressive episodes, and bipolar disorder, in which a patient experiences both manic and depressive episodes or only manic episodes. The history and current use of pharmacological agents to treat these separate mood disorders differ. With regard to unipolar depression, amphetamines were first used in the late 1930s. In the 1950s, the tricyclic and tetracyclic antidepressants (TCAs) (e.g., imipramine, amoxapine) and MAOIs (e.g., phenelzine) were serendipitously discovered to elevate depressive moods. These prototypal compounds, however, affect many systems indiscriminately, have a slow action of onset, and produce numerous unwanted side effects that deter patient compliance. The largest new drug class of antidepressants includes SSRIs (e.g., fluoxetine). In general, the SSRIs are no more effective than TCAs but cause limited and more tolerated side effects and have a reduced risk of overdose. Two new antidepressants, with pharmacologic actions and side effects profiles that differ from those of SSRIs, are nefazodone and venlafaxine which inhibit serotonin reuptake and also either exhibit $5\text{-HT}_{2A}/5\text{-HT}_{2C}$ antagonism or inhibit the reuptake of norepinephrine, respectively. Other non-uptake-inhibiting serotonergic drugs that increase serotonin release and function through partial agonism of the 5-HT_{1A} (e.g., buspirone) and 5-HT_{2C} (e.g., *m*-chlorophenylpiperazine) receptors are being investigated. Manipulation of the serotonergic system is the most common, current approach in antidepressant drug therapy, but new selective and reversible MAO-A inhibitors (e.g., moclobemide) are being tested and have been reported as effective to treat unipolar and bipolar patients with no anticholinergic or cardiovascular side effects and minimal dietary restrictions. With regard to bipolar disorder, lithium remains the major pharmacological treatment since its discovery as a calming agent in 1949. Only 60 to 80% of bipolar patients, however, respond to lithium treatment alone. Patients who do not respond to lithium are often given antidepressants in combination with antipsychotics despite the higher risk of developing tardive dyskinesia. Over the past few years, a variety of other drugs, including anticonvulsants (e.g., carbamazepine) and calcium channel blockers (e.g., verapamil), have been used to treat bipolar disorder. Mania also can be treated with benzodiazepines, anticonvulsants, antipsychotics, or calcium channel blockers. In most cases of bipolar disorders, patients receive a combined pharmacotherapeutic treatment during the course of their illness.

E. Pain

Pain is the unpleasant psychological experience associated with actual or potential tissue damage. Pain may be acute, periodic, or continuous; sharp, dull/aching, or burning; annoying, uncomfortable, or unbearable.

Pain occurs in response to readily identifiable accidents, injury, or medical treatments (e.g., surgery); to ambiguous or mixed causes (e.g., weather conditions, disturbed sleep, work environment); and to unknown immediate causes (e.g., undiagnosed pathology, forgotten injury). Pain is treated by a variety of pharmacologic agents including: opiates (e.g., morphine, meperidine, fentanyl, codeine), nonsteroidal anti-inflammatory agents (e.g., salicylic acid derivatives such as aspirin; para-aminophenol derivatives such as acetaminophen; indole and indene acetic acids such as indomethacin) and drugs that are selectively used to treat specific pain-related disorders (e.g., the 5-HT_{1D} agonist, sumatriptan, to treat migraine headaches). With regard to pain of known cause, pharmacologic treatments are relatively effective for the vast majority of people. With regard to pain of ambiguous or unknown origin and with regard to continuous pain, pharmacologic treatments have mixed results. For example, opiate medications alter how chronic pain patients perceive and cope with pain but do not completely alleviate the pain.

Unfortunately, currently available analgesics have many undesirable side effects including sedation, respiratory depression, gastrointestinal upset or constipation, pruritus, and addiction. Ongoing investigations are attempting to develop analgesic medications with greater efficacy and few side effects.

F. Psychoses

Psychotic disorders are characterized by delusions, hallucinations, disorganized speech, or disorganized or catatonic behavior. The major psychotic disorders include schizophrenia, schizophreniform disorder, schizoaffective disorder, or delusional disorder. The most widely prescribed antipsychotic drugs are referred to as neuroleptics. The major antipsychotics are: tricyclic phenothiazines, thioxanthenes, dibenzepines, butyrophenones, benzamides, clozapines, and risperidone. Most drugs of these types block D2 dopaminergic receptors and inactivate dopamine neurotransmitters in the forebrain. Some of these medications also affect D1 dopaminergic, 5-HT_2 serotonergic, and α-adrenergic receptors. Unfortunately, none of these medications cures psychoses, each one helps only some patients, and there are deleterious side effects, including: akathisia, rigidity, tremors, and other neuromuscular effects. In addition to these major drugs, lithium, anticonvulsants, and benzodiazepines are prescribed.

G. Sexual Dysfunction

DSM-IV distinguishes among sexual dysfunctions as: Sexual Desire Disorder, Sexual Arousal Disorder, Orgasmic Disorder, Sexual Pain Disorders, Sexual Dysfunction Due to a General Medical Condition, Substance-Induced Sexual Dysfunction, and Sexual Dysfunction Not Otherwise Specified. These conditions are different from Paraphilias (e.g., intense sexual urges to unusual objects, Exhibitionism, Voyeurism). Psychopharmacology has played a relatively small role in the treatment of these conditions but that role is increasing. Antianxiety agents and antidepressants are helpful in some patients. Other medications (e.g., methohexital sodium) have been used in conjunction with desensitization therapy. Sex hormones (e.g., estrogen, testosterone) have been used in specific cases. With changes in societal attitudes to the discussion of these types of problems also may come increased attention to the development and study of treatment for these conditions. [*See* SEXUAL DYSFUNCTION THERAPY.]

H. Sleep Disorders

Humans spend one-quarter to one-third of their lives sleeping and roughly one-third of all adults experience some type of sleep disorder during their lives. Sleep disorders are categorized by the *DSM-IV* as: Primary Sleep Disorders (including Dyssomnias and Parasomnias), Sleep Disorder Related to Another Mental Disorder, Sleep Disorder Due to a General Medical Condition, and Substance-Induced Sleep Disorder. The most common Sleep Disorder is Insomnia, but other Dyssomnias include: Hypersomnia, Narcolepsy, Breathing-Related Sleep Disorder, and Circadian Rhythm Sleep Disorder. Parasomnias include: Nightmare Disorder, Sleep Terror Disorder, and Sleepwalking Disorder. Primary Insomnia is treated with benzodiazepines or sedative-hypnotics. Primary Hypersomnia is treated with stimulants, such as amphetamines, or SSRIs. Narcolepsy is treated with stimulants, antidepressants, and sometimes with α_1 agonists. Benzodiazepines and other antianxiety medications are used selectively to treat other sleep disorders.

I. Substance-Related Disorders

In the *DSM-IV,* Substance-Related Disorders include taking drugs of abuse, side effects of medication, and toxic exposure. Substance-Related Disorders are categorized as Substance Use Disorders (Substance Dependence and Substance Abuse) or as Substance-Induced Disorders (Substance Intoxication, Substance Withdrawal, any Substance-Induced adverse psychological or behavioral effect). A wide variety of psychopharmacologic agents are used in conjunction with psychological approaches to treat the varied aspects of Substance-Related Disorders. This section provides a brief synopsis of this expansive aspect of psychopharmacology.

Alcohol and nicotine (e.g., in cigarettes, cigars, and other tobacco products) are the most commonly used and abused substances in our culture. Other drugs also are used recreationally and have deleterious effects. Psychopharmacologic treatments can be used to discourage drug use, to decrease withdrawal symptoms, or to treat comorbid psychological conditions. The major Substance-Related Disorders and their Treatments are:

1. Alcohol-Related Disorders

Psychopharmacologic agents used for the treatment of alcohol abuse include disulfiram (i.e., Antabuse). When ingested, disulfiram inhibits the enzyme aldehyde dehydrogenase so that consumption of alcohol results in a toxic reaction to the accumulation of acetaldehyde in the blood. Consumption of alcohol while taking disulfiram leads to flushing, feelings of heat and numbness in the limbs and upper chest, nausea, dizziness, malaise, blurred vision, air hunger, and palpitations. Psychotropic medications that are used to treat anxiety and depressive symptoms in these patients are useful. Recently, these drugs and SSRIs have been used to control craving for alcohol. Specifically, trazodone, serotonin type 3 ($5HT_3$) antagonists, and dopaminergic agonists (e.g., apomorphine, bromocriptine) may be effective in decreasing cravings. Naltrexone, an opioid antagonist, also has shown promise as a possible treatment for alcohol dependence. Benzodiazepines are the primary medications for controlling alcohol withdrawal symptoms (seizures, delirium, anxiety, tachycardia, hypertension). Carbamazepine, β-adrenergic receptor antagonists, and clonidine also have been used to treat sympathetic activity associated with alcohol withdrawal. However, these drugs are not effective in the treatment of seizures or delirium.

2. Amphetamine-Related Disorders

The pharmacologic treatment for amphetamine-induced psychotic disorder and amphetamine-induced anxiety disorder is usually antipsychotics (phenothiazine, haloperidol) and anxiolytics (diazepam), respectively, on a short-term basis. Chronic lithium treatment to attenuate the euphoria associated with amphetamine use, thereby decreasing the likelihood of continued use, is not recommended.

3. Caffeine-Related Disorders

Analgesics such as aspirin, ibuprofen, and acetaminophen usually are sufficient for treating headaches and muscle aches associated with caffeine withdrawal. Benzodiazepines rarely are needed and should only be prescribed for a short period of time (less than 7 days).

4. Cannabis-Related Disorders

Psychopharmacologic treatment for these disorders is less clear, but some patients may respond to anxiolytics for the treatment of withdrawal symptoms. In addition, antidepressants may be useful in treating any underlying depressive disorder associated with cannabis abuse.

5. Cocaine-Related Disorders

Several pharmacologic agents have been used to decrease cocaine craving in cocaine abusers. Dopaminergic agonists, amantadine and bromocriptine, and TCAs such as desipramine and imipramine seem to decrease drug cravings, increase energy, and improve sleep. Carbamazepine also decreases cravings, but not in patients with antisocial personality disorder.

6. Hallucinogen-Related Disorders

Pharmacologic agents such as dopaminergic antagonists are often used to treat psychotic symptoms associated with withdrawal and benzodiazepines can be used to treat anxiety symptoms on a short-term basis.

7. Inhalant-Related Disorders

There are no prescribed methods of psychopharmacologic treatments for these disorders.

8. Nicotine-Related Disorders

Administration of nicotine through a transdermal patch is a useful approach to help individuals quit smoking because it curbs withdrawal symptoms associated with nicotine cessation (e.g., hunger, irritability, inattention). Nicotine also can be administered via chewing gum or in a nasal spray. Clonidine and antidepressants (fluoxetine and buspirone in particular) have been used to help some people who abstain from tobacco use.

9. Opioid-Related Disorders

Methadone, a synthetic opioid agonist that is administered orally, is used as a substitute for heroin to help the patient move away from injectable opiates, maintain a steady job, and reintegrate into a daily lifestyle that is not associated with drug-taking. Levo-α-acetylmethadol (LAMM) is a longer acting opioid agonist that is similar to methadone and only needs to be administered about three times a week. Buprenorphine is a mixed opioid agonist-antagonist that has shown promise as an opioid substitute in the treatment of opioid addiction. Naltrexone can be used to block the pharmacologic actions of opioids, including the subjective high, and, possibly the subsequent drug craving and physical dependence. Clonidine is administered during the initial stages of opiate withdrawal and naltrexone is administered to treat opioid overdose.

10. Phencyclidine (or Phencyclidine-like)-Related Disorders

Benzodiazepines and dopamine receptor antagonists (haloperidol) are used for controlling behavioral disorders associated with phencyclidine intoxication.

11. Sedative-, Hypnotic-, or Anxiolytic-Related Disorders

Carbamazepine may be useful in the treatment of benzodiazepine withdrawal. The treatment for barbiturate abuse is far more complicated than benzodiazepine withdrawal because sudden death can occur during withdrawal. It is recommended that phenobarbital be substituted in the withdrawal procedure and the dosages gradually decreased over a long period of time. Once complete withdrawal has occurred, nonbarbiturate sedative-hypnotics should be used as a substitute for the barbiturate. However, this substitution typically translates the drug dependence to a new substance and does not cure the addiction.

IV. SPECIAL POPULATIONS

A. Pediatric

Age influences pharmacokinetic and pharmacodynamic responses. With regard to psychopharmacology, it is generally assumed that children are small adults and, therefore, adjustments in psychopharmacologic treatments simply need to be made based on body weight. This assumption, however, may be wrong. There are rapid, age-related biological and psychological changes that begin in the newborn and continue throughout childhood and adolescence. These changes demand a psychopharmacologic treatment approach that differs from adults and is sensitive to developmental stages, both physical and psychological. As of now, our understanding of pediatric psychopharmacology is limited and many important investigations of drug actions across developmental periods have yet to be conducted.

B. Geriatric

Aging is a highly individualized process that results in various changes over time that can alter significantly the actions of psychotropic medications in the body and how the body affects the drugs. In elderly patients there are changes in: organ system function, drug distribution, drug action, drug metabolism, and drug elimination. In addition, cumulative drug actions are common among elderly persons who take many prescription medications, over-the-counter medications, and other substances (e.g., alcohol, nicotine, caffeine). Psychopharmacologic treatments in the elderly require coordinated, integrated medical care that captures a complete picture of functioning within each individual. Quality of life in elderly patients can be greatly improved and prolonged by thoughtful use of medications and medical interventions. However, there are several obstacles to compliance that the prescriber should consider, including the expense of medications and treatment, the forgetfulness of some patients, and the deliberate choice by a patient not to take a particular treatment. The same sets of medical advances that offer improved quality of life for some, may represent threats to autonomy if thoughtfulness is not included in the clinical decision-making for each patient.

C. Individual Differences

Besides age, many factors can influence interindividual variability in drug responsivity, susceptibility to negative side effects, and potential drug abuse liability. These factors include biological (e.g, genetics, gender, ethnicity, disease state), environmental (e.g., stress, culture), and behavioral (e.g., diet, drug use, drug history) influences as well as the interactions of any two or more of these variables. The mechanisms by which these variables influence the actions of drugs can be molecular, biological, pharmacokinetic, pharmacodynamic, psychological, or social in nature. The identification of individual difference variables and their contribution to drug action are relevant to the clinical administration of medications as well as to our understanding of the mechanisms underlying drug addiction.

BIBLIOGRAPHY

American Psychiatric Association. (1994). *Diagnostic and Statistical Manual of Mental Disorders* (4th ed.). Washington, DC: Author.

Bloom, F.E., & Kupfer, D.J. (Eds.). (1995). *Psychopharmacology: The fourth generation of progress.* New York: Raven Press.

Cooper, J.R., Bloom, F.E., & Roth, R.H. (1996). *The biochemical basis of neuropharmacology* (7th ed.). New York: Oxford University Press.

Hardman, J.G., Limbird, L.E., Molinoff, P.B., Ruddon, R.W., & Gilman, A.G. (Eds.). (1996). *Goodman & Gilman's The pharmacological basis of therapeutics* (9th ed.). New York: McGraw-Hill, Inc.

Julien, R.M. (1988). *A Primer of Drug Action* (5th ed.). New York: W.H. Freeman and Company.

Kaplan, H.I., Sadock, B.J., & Grebb, J.A. (1994). *Kaplan and Sadock's synopsis of psychiatry: Behavioral sciences, clinical psychiatry* (7th ed.). Baltimore, MD: Williams & Wilkins.

Katzung, B.K. (Ed.). (1992). *Basic & clinical pharmacology* (5th ed.). Norwalk, CT: Appleton & Lange.

Melmon, K.L., Morrelli, H.F., Hoffman, B.B., & Nierenberg, D.W. (Eds.). (1992). *Melmon and Morrelli's clinical pharmacology: Basic principles in therapeutics* (3rd ed.). New York: McGraw-Hill, Inc.

Pirodsky, D.M., & Cohn, J.S. (1992). *Clinical primer of psychopharmacology: A practical guide* (2nd ed.). New York: McGraw-Hill, Inc.

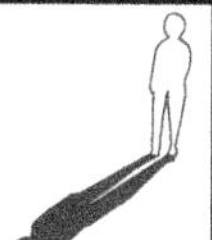

Sexual Dysfunction Therapy

Dinesh Bhugra and Padmal de Silva
University of London

Desire Disorders Problems related to the degree of sexual desire.
Erectile Disorders Problems in obtaining or sustaining a sufficiently strong erection for sex.
Orgasmic Disorders Problems in achieving a climax in sex.
Premature Ejaculation In the male, reaching a climax too soon, thus preventing enjoyable coital activity.
Sexual Dysfunction Difficulties in sexual functioning.

SEXUAL DYSFUNCTION has been classified according to the four phases of sexual activity in both males and females. At each stage the individuals can suffer from high or low levels of activity and additional physical problems and pain at various stages during these phases.

I. INTRODUCTION

Sexual dysfunction and its treatment have been well described in historical, medical and psychiatric texts. The presentation of patients with sexual dysfunction to clinicians is determined by social norms, mores, and expectations. In societies and cultures where sex is seen as a purely procreative process, people are less likely to present with sexual dysfunction—especially if the dysfunction is not interfering with procreation. On the other hand, in societies where sexual satisfaction is seen as a personal pleasure and fulfillment, more people are likely to seek help with the slightest dysfunction. The more severe the problem, the more likely it will be that the individuals seek therapeutic intervention. If there is stigma attached to sexual inadequacy in a society and the individuals believe that they are going to see a mental health professional, it is more likely that their attitudes may well produce a scenario where the pressure is on them and the therapist to do something about the problem furtively and quickly. The decision to seek professional help is very difficult for most people. Under the circumstances, the first impressions of the therapist and his/her response to the problem will be of paramount importance. An additional problem that the individuals may bring with them is an underlying relationship difficulty. A further complication is that the individual's demand may be for physical treatments and not for psychological therapies.

II. CLASSIFICATION OF SEXUAL DYSFUNCTION

The problems of classification in psychiatry are many, and these are reflected in the classification of dysfunction (see Table I). Such a simple division has its advan-

Copyright © 1998 by Academic Press.
All rights of reproduction in any form reserved.

Table I General Classification of Sexual Dysfunction

Phase	Male	Female
Desire/drive/interest	Low interest Excess interest	Low interest Excess interest
Arousal/excitement	Erectile dysfunction	Impaired arousal
Orgasm	Premature ejaculation Retarded ejaculation	Orgasmic dysfunction
Sexual pain/other	Dyspareunia	Vaginismus Dyspareunia
	Sexual phobias	Sexual phobias

tages, but it does not take into account any underlying causative factors that would need to be taken into consideration while planning any therapeutic interventions. Precise labeling of the problem often ignores the relationship, cultural, and physical contexts. In addition, the physical causation of sexual dysfunction may be either central—in the brain, or peripheral—in the genito-urinary system. There may be an underlying biological substrate and there may be biological abnormalities, but on their own these may be insufficient for a full understanding of the disorder in question. The International Classification of Diseases (ICD-10) and the *Diagnostic and Statistical Manual (DSM-IV),* the two principal classificatory systems around the world, use a categorical classification and, apart from minor differences, are broadly similar in their approaches to diagnosis, including a multi-axial approach.

Female sexual dysfunction includes sexual desire disorders along with impaired arousal, orgasmic disorder, and vaginismus. Females may perceive their sexuality differently, and their sexual activity is, in part, culturally defined. This definition impacts upon the way in which women understand their own sexuality and whether they can adjust their expectations of their sexual functioning. Female sexual dysfunction may be due to early childhood experiences, or to later trauma, including sexual abuse, childbirth, and infertility, among others. Myths about sexual activity and sexual functioning may well affect both males and females.

In males, while orgasm and emission are normally linked, they can be separated, because in the latter phase organic muscle contraction and emission are responsible for ejaculation. Male sexual dysfunction includes premature ejaculation, retarded ejaculation, painful ejaculation, and erectile difficulties. The latter could be linked with Peyronie's disease.

Various psychological factors that contribute to sexual dysfunction in both males and females include anxiety, anger, and "spectatoring," and these may result from misunderstandings and ignorance, unsuitable circumstances, bad feelings about oneself, one's partner, or the relationship, as well as poor communication within the relationship. A psychosomatic circle of sex that links cognitions with awareness of response leading on to peripheral arousal and genital response on the one side and activating the limbic system and spinal centers to orgasmic conclusion on the other is often used to describe various etiological points that may contribute to precipitation and perpetuation of sexual anxiety and sexual dysfunction. Thus, a complex set of factors is usually involved.

III. PRINCIPLES OF SEXUAL DYSFUNCTION THERAPY

After assessment of the exact nature of the dysfunction and possible etiological factors, two basic steps mark the early stages of therapy: managing anxiety and education. Quite often, the partners find it difficult to discuss sexual problems with each other or with the therapist, and the underlying lack of sexual education may well contribute to this and to sexual anxiety. Simple reading materials often allow the therapist to discuss problems, offer solutions, and peg the treatment planning. This basic education is often crucial in sex therapy.

Anxiety management is usually carried out in a number of ways—from physical muscle relaxation to yoga training or using tai chi or the Alexander technique. A valuable part of this anxiety management is the process of "despectatoring," which encourages individuals to get away from focusing on the sexual act and instead allowing relaxation in their physical and intimate contact. If the therapist discovers that there are underlying angry or depressive feelings, these may need to be treated medically or with psychological interventions. Bad feelings about sex, oneself, or one's partner need to be aired and discussed at length. If there is any underlying relationship discord, it would need to be assessed and managed. Sometimes this work may need to precede sexual dysfunction therapy.

The principles of managing sexual dysfunction

from a psychological perspective are described in detail below. In the first instance, it is necessary to deal with physical management of sexual dysfunction.

IV. PHYSICAL THERAPIES

There are at least four physical methods—oral medication, intrapenile injections, artificial devices, and surgical procedures. Physical methods are mostly used for treating male patients.

A. Oral Medication

Yohimbine has been shown to be an effective drug in managing erectile difficulties. It works better than placebo and is an α-2 adrenergic receptor blocker. Idazoxan is another selective and specific α-2 adrenoceptor antagonist and works in some cases, although it tends to have more side effects. The heterogeneity in etiology makes the existing clinical trials difficult to interpret.

B. Intracavernosal Injections

Phenoxybenzamine hydrochloride, papaverine hydrochloride, phentolamine mesylate, and prostaglandin-E have been used as intracavernosal injections for erectile difficulties. Phenoxybenzamine usage had led to priapism or painful erections lasting for up to 3 days and has largely fallen into disuse. Papaverine hydrochloride is a smooth muscle relaxant that, when injected intracorporeally, will result in active arterial dilation, corporeal smooth muscle relaxation, and venous outflow restriction—thus producing an erection. It is also less painful to inject, and these injections produce erections that are less painful and last for a few hours generally, at the maximum. A mixture of papaverine and phentolamine has been shown to be superior to papaverine alone.

Such vasoactive substances are also used to diagnose erectile problems, and evaluate indications for surgery of Peyronie's disease. In treatment, they are used for occasional self-injection and for regular self-injection in cases of persistent erectile failure. It has been shown that patients, having obtained erections with injections initially, often go on to have spontaneous erections.

The cases most likely to respond to this form of treatment are: mild cases of arteriogenic etiology, all cases of neurogenic etiology, mild cases of abnormal leakage, and those who have had unsuccessful surgical procedures. Some cases of psychogenic etiology also respond well to it.

The dosage of the drug papaverine should be increased gradually. In the first instance, from 8 to 15mgs should be used and usually this amount is sufficient to produce a slight enlargement of the penis lasting for 15 minutes or so. At subsequent consultations, higher doses may be used until the optimum dose is reached (leading to an erection of good quality (9 out of 10 or better) lasting for perhaps 30 minutes). There is still a lot of variation in individual responses so it is essential that individual doses are determined slowly and carefully. If a mixture of phentolamine and papaverine is used, the first trial dose of papaverine is limited to 15mg. If the response is poor, then a further injection of 0.5 mg phentolamine is given. In subsequent visits, a mixture of 0.5mg phentolamine and 30 mg papaverine is used, going up to a maximum recommended 2 mg phentolamine and 60 mg papaverine. These injections are usually given at the base of the penis at 3 o'clock or 9 o'clock positions (posterolaterally)—away from neurovascular bundle and urethra—using an insulin syringe and a gauge 26 or 27 needle. After cleaning the skin, holding the syringe perpendicular to the penis, the physician on the first occasion, and the patient himself subsequently (or his partner), inserts the needle through the tough tunica albuginea into the left or right corpus cavernosum. As the resistance is overcome and the needle enters the tunica a sensation is experienced at which point the medication is injected. If phentolamine is used first, the injection should be given with the patient lying flat as postural hypotension may occur if there is a leak into the venous system. The patient may then stand and an erection will appear in 10 to 20 minutes. The couple may be taught the technique together, and some patients prefer their partner to do the injecting as part of their foreplay. The patient should be advised not to use injections more than twice a week with a 2-day interval at least. Erectile capability may well return after some months of self-injection treatment. If the injection of papaverine and a combination with phentolamine fails to produce an erection, the possibility of a venous leak must be investigated.

In the United Kingdom in recent years, prostaglandin E has been used in the same way as papaverine and phentolamine but the patient needs to learn to dissolve the powdered compound for injection. The starting dose is 5 to 10 micrograms, with a maximum of from 20 to 40 micrograms. There is some clinical evidence to suggest that this preparation is more effective than papaverine alone and has a lower incidence of priapism or prolonged erections. In some cases, however, the patient may experience pain in the shaft or the glans following the injection.

Cardiovascular problems need to be investigated thoroughly prior to commencing treatment. Severe liver dysfunction, severe substance misuse, allergic reactions, and a history of sexual offending are some of the other contraindications. The most serious side effect is priapism. Other side effects described include painful nodules in the penis, fibrotic nodules, liver damage, pain, infection at the injection site, and bruising. Between 2 and 15% of patients will develop priapism. When this happens, the patient is advised to go to the nearest emergency room to have blood withdrawn from the corpora, and metaraminol (2mgs) or adrenaline (20 micrograms in 0.1 ml) injected at the base of the penis to be repeated half an hour later if indicated. In rare cases, surgical intervention may be indicated.

Using written information sheets and audiovisual aids to inform the patients and their partners, including advice on what to do if priapism occurs, should be encouraged. Written consents are recommended. Ethically, there remain several issues in offering physical treatments where underlying causes may well be psychogenic and the focus of the relationship appears to be on the erection rather than on more general factors. There is no doubt that, in some cases, the quality of the relationship following an improvement in sexual satisfaction due to frequency of intercourse increases intimacy and sexual arousal.

C. Artificial Devices

In 1917 Otto Lederer first patented a vacuum pump that induced erection by creating a vacuum around the penis, and maintained erection by the use of a constriction ring around the base of the penis. The different devices tend to vary according to the use of a pressure-limiting device, the shape of the cylinder, the design of the tension rings, and external versus attached pumps.

The basic mechanism of action is the filling of the corpora cavernosa due to suction and venous stasis, secondary to constriction, which are both passive mechanisms. As the additional volume can only be maintained by the use of the constriction device at the base of the penis, the patient and his partner often find it very difficult to deal with, when compared to papaverine injections. Furthermore, in this method, skin temperature of the penis falls and the erection is often not very strong. The commonest device in use is a rigid tube made of plastic, which is connected to a hand pump at one end and an opening at the other through which the flaccid penis is inserted. Prior to this, the penis and the tube are well lubricated and a rubber constriction band is placed around the open end of the tube. When the pump is used, air is pumped out and the resulting negative pressure draws blood into the corpora, producing an erection. Following this, the constricting rubber band can be slipped off to place it at the base of the penis to limit venous outflow. This band can be left in situ for half an hour. Another appliance—Correctaid—works on the same principle but the condom-shaped device is made of transparent silicon rubber. A tube is passed through at its base to open the inside of the tip of the sheath. The device is worn over the penis. Yet another appliance is the Blakoc suspensory energizer ring, which is rectangular and is made of ebonite, which can be fitted around the base of the penis and under the scrotum. With its small metal plates it can have some stimulatory effect on the erectile mechanism. The success rates using vacuum devices are variable. The side effects include hematoma, pain, ecchymosis, numbness, painful or blocked ejaculation. As in injection therapies, spontaneous erectile activity may return with the use of vacuum devices as increased self-confidence reduces performance anxiety.

D. Surgical Procedures

Surgical revascularization and surgical implants have been tried. Pre-operative counseling, education, and adequate preparation for the surgical procedures and informed consent with some risk/benefit analysis are essential. Originally, arterial bypass was attempted to join the epigastric artery into the side of the corpora cavernosa. Other attempts have included utilizing saphenous vein bypasses from the femoral artery to the corpora, and saphenous vein bypass from the inferior epigastric artery to the corpora cavernosa. The best results are said to be in younger males, although most authorities will agree that the theoretical disadvantages associated with these surgical procedures are genuine. The epigastric artery-dorsal artery revascularization is said to be more advantageous.

The selection of patients for sexual surgery is problematic because of significant areas of disagreement on the indications and the success criteria of various procedures. In spite of surgical intervention, underlying psychological factors often need to be taken into account. Some of these have been identified as poor sexual communication, lack of foreplay, and loss of interest. Preoperative counseling as part of the assessment should help in ruling out some of these problems.

E. Prosthesis

The use of plastic splints for the penis was first described in 1952. Semi-rigid silastic rods result in an almost permanently erect penis which can be bent to different angles. Acceptability of these processes has been improved by using modified appliances. An inflatable penile implant has been used to provide improvements in both girth and rigidity. Such a device works on a fluid-filled system that allows the flaccid and erect penis to appear normal. The choice between semirigid or inflatable devices depends very much on the patient's and his partner's preferences.

The semirigid prosthesis is made of medical grade silicone rubber with a sponge core. The device may be implanted by using perineal approach to insert it in the corporeal bodies. The device is available in lengths of 12 to 22cm, and diameters of 0.9, 1.12, and 1.3 mm. A flexirod prosthesis differs from the above by having a hinged area that enables the phallus to be placed in a dependent position when not being used for intercourse. The diameters here range from 0.9 to 1.2 cm and the length from 7 to 13 cm, and it can be shortened if necessary. Another type of prosthesis (called the "Jonas prosthesis") is used commonly and can be inserted through subcoronal, midshaft, penoscrotal, and suprapubic approaches, as well as through the perineal approach. In addition, it has 3 diameters of 9.5, 11.0, and 13.0 mm, and lengths of 16 to 24 cm. It is malleable and thus the penis can maintain a dependent position as well as an upright one. Variable versions of this prosthesis are now available. A newer prosthesis on the market is made of fabric-wrapped stainless steel that has flexibility of size and positioning.

F. Inflatable Prosthesis

As mentioned above, the inflatable prosthesis in its initial model consisted of an inflate pump, a deflate pump, a reservoir, and paired inflatable penile cylinders. However, the inflate and deflate pumps have been combined into one mechanism, and the original six segments of silicone rubber tubing have been reduced to three. The inflatable prosthesis has the advantage of being cosmetically appealing, it conforms to the patient's own corporal anatomy, and the erosion of the prosthesis through the glans is unlikely. Its side effects include aneurysm formation, high mechanical failure rate, kinking of the tubes, infection, puminosis, and scrotal hematoma. The age of the patient, coexisting medical problems, patient preference, and the risk of complications are some of the factors that need to be taken into account when a decision is being considered.

V. PSYCHOLOGICAL THERAPIES

There is a great deal of literature on the psychological approaches to the treatment of sexual dysfunction. Many authorities consider psychological therapy as the treatment of choice when help is sought for sexual dysfunction, although obviously there are instances where a physical approach might be more appropriate.

Psychological therapies take different forms. Psychodynamic therapy aims to understand the presenting problem as a manifestation of an underlying, unconscious conflict or memory, and it is often assumed that this has its origins in childhood. The therapy takes the form of a verbal, interactive endeavor, which also uses the transference (emotional responses of the patient to the therapist) as a means of resolving problems. Psychodynamic therapy for sexual dysfunction has not been adequately evaluated. There is a practical problem, too, in that such therapy is quite time consuming. However, there are circumstances when such an approach may be appropriate. [*See* PSYCHOANALYSIS.]

The more widely used psychological therapies for sexual dysfunction are best described as behavioral, although in recent years cognitive approaches have also been added.

In the behavioral approach, the treatment is directed toward the sexual problem itself. An important element of this is the reduction of anxiety, as in most cases anxiety acts as a factor that perpetuates the dysfunction. The more one fails in sex, the more anxious one gets. One tends to become a "spectator" of one's own performance, thus inhibiting spontaneous sexual responses and sexual enjoyment. Hence, in therapy the reduction of anxiety becomes a major priority. Early behavior therapists like Joseph Wolpe used this approach in the treatment of sexual problems. He used a method that he called "systematic desensitization," in which the sexual problem was dealt with in graded, nonthreatening stages. As a first step, the couple were asked to refrain from intercourse, but to engage in other intimate behaviors, mainly touching and caressing, in a gentle, step-by-step way. In this fashion, anxiety could be overcome gradually, and full sexual functioning restored. This basic behavioral approach was followed by a more formal, essentially behavioral, treatment package developed by William Masters and Virginia Johnson—universally known as the "Masters and Johnson approach." In this, after the assessment, the couple are asked to agree to a ban on intercourse, and they are then given detailed instructions in graded sexual exercises. The first stage is touching and caressing, excluding the genital area and the woman's breasts; this is called "nongenital sensate focus." After some practice sessions of this, which the couple carry out at home, they move on to the "genital sensate focus" stage, where the genitals and the breasts are not excluded. In these stages, the couple are also encouraged to engage in enhanced communication, both verbal and nonverbal. After the second stage, specific additional behavioral strategies are used, to deal with whichever specific problems the couple have presented with. Examples are the "squeeze" technique for premature ejaculation, "overstimulation" for retarded ejaculation, and the use of graded dilators in the treatment vaginismus. In erectile difficulties, a "teasing" approach may be used, enabling the male to learn to defocus on the erection and to relinquish control. [*See* BEHAVIOR THERAPY.]

The principles of the Masters and Johnson approach can also be used with patients who do not have partners, with certain modifications. In the early stages, they are usually asked to engage in "self-focusing."

Relaxation strategies are often taught to the patients in both couple and individual therapy as an additional technique for reducing anxiety and tension. This is usually done at an early stage.

This basic behavioral approach is often augmented by cognitive interventions. This involves identifying those cognitions that the patient may have that are faulty or dysfunctional. Such dysfunctional cognitions (thoughts, beliefs, attitudes) are often major factors in the etiology and more commonly of the perpetuation of sexual dysfunctions. They include cognition like "I am sure to fail again," "If I do not get an erection, my partner will ridicule me," and "It is going to be painful again." The therapist elicits such cognitions from the patient as part of the assessment, and then works on modifying these, using techniques of cognitive therapy (such as creating situations where they are shown to be false, and pointing out their self-fulfilling nature). [*See* COGNITIVE THERAPY.]

In the practice of psychological therapy, behavioral and cognitive elements are often used in conjunction; hence the term "cognitive-behavior therapy," which many therapists these days use to describe what they do. Cognitive techniques are particularly applicable for those without partners, who tend to avoid developing relationships because of fear of repeated failure.

In recent years, this basic psychological approach has been extended to include a systemic dimension. The sexual dysfunction is viewed in the context of the overall relationship of the couple. Relationship factors such as jealousy, resentment, and dominance often contribute to sexual problems, and the therapist takes these into account and intervenes appropriately. These systemic interventions can be, and often are, undertaken within the context of an overall behavioral framework. There is evidence that this expanded approach is rapidly gaining popularity among therapists who specialize in the psychological treatment of sexual dysfunction.

Group approaches are also used in this field. Therapists sometimes run groups for patients without partners, or even see couples in groups. In these, much cognitive work is done in the group setting, and in addition behavioral exercises are discussed and outlined, which the patients would implement as homework. Sometimes, those in group therapy are given brief individual or couple sessions with the therapist as an additional measure.

The original Masters and Johnson approach always used a team of two therapists, one male and one female, with every couple. In the practice of sexual dysfunction therapy today, this is the exception rather than the rule. In most instances, one therapist sees the couple, or the individual who has no partner, for regular sessions.

It was noted above that a psychodynamic approach is useful in certain circumstances. There are instances where the behaviorally based treatment may lead to some improvement, but progress reaches a plateau. It is considered useful, in these circumstances, to explore intrapsychic factors that may be relevant to the problem. Such exploration is usually undertaken within a psychodynamic framework. Early memories, conflicts, and so on, that may have contributed to the problem, and/or unacknowledged current psychological factors, are explored and, where possible, resolved.

VI. ETHICAL ISSUES

If the couple perceives the male erectile dysfunction as the only problem and the focus is on obtaining erections without looking at underlying problems, ethical dilemmas are raised for the therapist. Equally, if a child molester presents for therapy for sexual dysfunction, there is a clear and serious dilemma for the therapist. It is possible that under these circumstances the patient may not divulge his complete history. The forensic aspects of the underlying problems will need to be taken into account as part of the assessment. When couples are about to break up and the underlying sexual dysfunction tends to take on a greater importance, the couple's energies may be focused on the sexual problem rather than on the relationship itself. Often the patients, their partners, and some therapists may see psychological treatments as time consuming and prolonged, painful experiences, whereas physical treatments may be more appealing. Physical treatments should be offered only after a thorough investigation of the dysfunction, and treatment should not be employed simply to fulfill the patient's or their partner's unrealistic dreams of the "ever-ready potent man."

VII. PROGNOSIS

Prognosis of sexual dysfunction varies according to the type of dysfunction. The literature on sex therapy indicates that prognosis in general depends on a number of factors. One is the motivation of the patient/couple. A good overall relationship is also associated with a good outcome. Concurrent psychiatric disorder is a hindrance to good progress. While the different disorders have varying degrees of success, the prognosis for vaginismus is probably the most positive. In female orgasmic dysfunction, it appears that younger patients do better in treatment.

VIII. SPECIAL GROUPS

A. Gay, Lesbian, and Bisexual Adults

These three groups present with the same varieties of sexual dysfunction discussed above, and the treatment plans, whether physical or psychological, are about the same. However, there are some additional factors that need to be taken into account. The first of these is the fact that, even though a gay or lesbian individual is seeking help, this does not necessarily mean that they are publicly "out" and that everyone knows of their sexual orientation. A second factor is the common use of high-tech sex toys, pornography, and in men, "fist-fucking," sadomasochistic practices, and water sports (urination). Lesbians, on the other hand, may well have feminist views and may have political views on sexual intercourse that may appear to be at odds with those of the therapist. Furthermore, views on pornography, sexual exploitation, and the existence of a patriarchal society may well contribute to models of behavior and expectations of treatment at variance with those of heterosexual women.

Some additional issues in working with these three groups include problems of society's widely held homophobic views and practices, the individual's internalized homophobia, and difficulties inherent in same-sex relationships. On the other hand, same-sex couples have the advantage of not being bound by opposite sexual role expectations, for example, the male must always initiate, and the female must be submissive. Gay men and lesbians tend to have a more varied sexual repertoire, and penetration is not the main focus of the sexual activity. The relationships may be open and nonmonogamous. The therapist's views on nonmonogamy and knowledge of the gay subculture may prove to be of great relevance for the success of therapy. The therapist must inquire closely about the development of sexual identity, detecting discrepancies in sexual orientation in the two partners, identifying the problem areas in the relationship and then setting up appropriate intervention procedures.

Bisexual individuals may feel unable to bring either

partner, and their problems may be with one gender or the other. The nonheterosexual orientation must be seen as equal but different, and the clinician must be familiar with group subcultures. Sexuality carries different meanings for gay men and lesbians and bisexual individuals, and these need to be ascertained and the emphasis on nonpenetrative pleasure encouraged.

B. Older Adults

Both therapists and patients need to question their assumptions about aging adults. There is some truth in the observation that desire for sexual intercourse falls off with age. However, ageist views on the clinician's part do not help the process of therapy. Older adults may change their practices and become more interested in nonpenetrative sexual activity. In addition, the loss of a partner may be more likely and newer relationships may have the additional burden of opprobrium by the extended families. Female and male sexual responses change with aging, usually due to hormonal changes. Whereas a young male may achieve a full erection in a matter of seconds, an older man may require several minutes to achieve the same response. He may also require a lot of physical stimulation to achieve an erection. Seminal fluid may be decreased. In addition, physical debility may contribute to lowered sexual interest and physical functioning. Drugs prescribed for physical conditions may also lead to impaired sexual functioning. Various psychological factors affecting sexuality in the elderly include lack of partners, lack of interest, and social stigma regarding older individuals "indulging" in sex. The therapist needs to be aware of the three fundamental areas of biological changes, attitudinal factors, and the role of life events. Pain, dryness, hot flushes, and physical mobility problems, especially those due to medical conditions like arthritis, are common and the therapist needs to deal with these. In this age group greater care must be taken to exclude physical causes of dysfunction. Psychological and physical therapies can be used in the same way as in younger adults, bearing in mind the essential factors specific to the older adult as highlighted above.

C. Ethnic Minorities

Various ethnic minorities have different cultural values placed on sex and sexual intercourse. As mentioned earlier, if the culture sees sexual intercourse as procreative and not for pleasure, the presenting complaint may be an inability to conceive rather than lack of pleasure. In cultures where semen is considered highly important and valuable, the individual may well have difficulties with suggestions of masturbation, sensate focus activity, and so on, as recommended by the therapist. In some cultures, various sexual taboos may well contribute to the anxiety that the couples experience. Under these circumstances, it would be useful to include this as part of the assessment and to ensure that appropriate therapeutic measures are taken. In some communities, the underlying causation of sexual dysfunction is generally seen as physical rather than psychological, and the patients and their partners may refuse to consider psychological intervention and demand physical treatments only. Under such circumstances, the therapist needs to be innovative in planning and delivering a combination of treatments. Using yohimbine or other physical agents in combination with a psychological approach can be fruitful. The therapist needs to be aware of the cultural nuances and social mores as well as cultural expectations in order to deal with sexual dysfunction problems satisfactorily.

D. Those with Disability/Chronic Physical Illness

Not only do certain chronic physical illnesses such as autonomic neuropathy, damage to nerves, and neurotoxic chemotherapies produce problems with sexual functioning, many drugs that are used for these conditions also contribute to sexual dysfunction. Cardiovascular disease, cancer, arthritis, and so on, increase with aging, and chronic pain may further contribute to low sexual interest and orgasmic dysfunction. A thorough physical assessment must be an integral part of the assessment of sexual functioning. A number of patients may simply be seeking reassurance, education, or permission to carry on with their sexual activity, and a significant proportion may benefit from very simple and focused counseling or intervention. However, in some cases more prolonged therapy may be needed. In a majority of cases, education to change attitudes is a crucial part of therapy. Such an attitude change can be fostered by using a mixture of written and/or audiovisual materials and cognitive methods to combat false beliefs and to deal with inappropriate and handicapping worries. Overcoming physical handicaps along with working on relationship problems may mean that the goals of sex therapy need to be changed and appropriate interventions put in place. Physical treatments need to be combined with sex therapy. The goals of treatment may be limited by the physiological impact of the disease or disability. However, enhancing sexual functioning and enjoyment is generally achievable.

E. HIV/AIDS

The AIDS epidemic has contributed to a change in patterns of sexual activity not only in gay and bisexual communities, but to some degree in the heterosexual community as well. AIDS has also affected how people view their sexuality. In clinics, HIV-positive patients not infrequently present with sexual dysfunction. When dealing with such patients the therapist needs to establish their views on the illness, their knowledge about the illness as well as sexual dysfunction, and their attitudes toward therapy. There is no doubt that HIV-positive individuals can be helped using similar models of therapeutic intervention as those used with others, even though some therapists may find recommending physical interventions like penile prosthesis difficult. A thorough clinical assessment will allow the therapist to deal with some of these difficulties.

F. Paraphiliacs

Those with paraphilias, or variant sexual desires and practices, sometimes present with sexual dysfunction. Paraphiliacs seeking treatment in this way are almost always male, reflecting the vast preponderance of males over females among paraphiliacs. In their presentation, they often complain of difficulties in nonparaphiliac sexual relationships. For example, a man with a strong shoe fetish might seek help for an inability to obtain or maintain an erection in sex without contact with a woman's shoe. These patients need to be assessed carefully, and individually tailored treatment needs to be considered. The aim should be, as far as possible, to incorporate the paraphilia in a limited, controlled way into the person's sexual repertoire. Needless to say, criminal paraphilias such a pedophilia or zoophilia, or any paraphilia that the patient's partner finds intolerable, can not be considered for such incorporation. In such cases, help should be directed toward the control of the person's paraphiliac urges. Various psychological techniques are available for the control of paraphiliac desires and behaviors—for example, orgasmic reconditioning and covert sensitization. At the same time, help should also be given to reduce any anxiety about nonparaphiliac sex, and to build up skills and competencies needed for such activity. In other words, a multifaceted treatment program is often required.

It is also important to note that little can be achieved in the treatment of paraphiliacs unless the patient has motivation and is cooperative.

IX. CONCLUSIONS

Sexual dysfunction therapy is widely practiced today, and many mental health professionals offer this service. Recent years have witnessed several major developments: new physical treatments for males, the use of cognitive therapy principles where needed, the combination of cognitive-behavioral treatment with a systemic approach, and the recognition of cultural differences. The demand for sexual dysfunction therapy is high, and more training is needed in this area within the mental health professions. Where competently used, on the basis of careful assessment, the therapy helps many patients and couples make significant improvements. Needless to say, further research is needed into the treatment techniques as well as into the dysfunctions themselves. One can expect further major progress in several areas in the next few decades.

BIBLIOGRAPHY

Bancroft, J. (1989). *Human sexuality and its problems* (2d ed.). Edinburgh: Churchill Livingstone.

Hawton, K. (1992). Sex therapy: For whom is it likely to be effective? In: K. Hawton & P. Cowen (Eds.), *Practical problems in clinical psychiatry*. Oxford: Oxford University Press.

Kaplan, H. S. (1995). *The sexual desire disorders: Dysfunctional regulation of sexual motivation*. New York: Brumner/Mazel.

Rosen, R. C., & Leiblum, S. R. (1992). *Erectile disorders: Assessment and treatment*. New York: Guilford Press.

Wince, J. P., & Carey, M. P. (1991). *Sexual dysfunction: A guide for assessment and treatment*. New York: Guilford Press.

Standards for Psychotherapy

Robyn M. Dawes
Carnegie Mellon University

Hortatory Rules Those that mandate what should be done.
Meta-Analysis A statistical technique for combining studies with different outcome measures in order to test the generality of their results.
Minatory Rules Those that mandate what should not be done.
Psychotherapy The attempt to use psychology—through some form of conversation—to alleviate distressing or debilitating symptoms or hypothesized conditions leading to them.
Randomized Trials Experiments Investigations in which subjects are randomly assigned to an experimental versus a control group, as in evaluating vaccines.
Regression Effects The statistical fact that when two variables are not perfectly correlated, the standardized value of the one predicted will on the average be closer to its standardized mean than is the standardized value of the one from which the prediction is made.

STANDARDS OF PSYCHOTHERAPY practice refer to what psychotherapists actually do, not to their education or their credentials or experience—although these factors might be precursors for practicing in a way that meets standard of ethics and efficacy. To understand these standards, it is first necessary to know what has been established about the effectiveness of psychotherapy. Randomized control studies indicate the existence of particular "protocol" therapies that are effective for specific conditions, and otherwise all types of therapies appear to work equally well (the "Dodo Bird" finding), perhaps due to the quality of the "therapeutic alliance." It follows that standard dictate what should be done ("hortatory rules") when conducting a protocol therapy, but do not provide explicit rules about what to do in other types of therapies, which constitute the vast majority. Instead, the standards for these require that therapists not behave in ways inconsistent with what is known from scientific research, or at least what is believed to be known on the basis of empirical investigations interpreted in a rational manner. Thus, standards are minatory ones that prohibit "out of bounds" behavior. Such behavior occurs, often justified on the grounds that "we do not know," or that something might or could be true (e.g., recovered repressed memories), or may be shown in the future to be true to at least some extent or other. Standards of practice require, however, behavior consistent with what is currently known.

I. INTRODUCTION

Standards of practice refer to principles governing effective and ethical practice of psychology—whether in a private setting, clinic, or a nonprofit institution. The standards refer to the actual behavior of the individual alleging to apply psychological principles, or

Copyright © 1998 by Academic Press.
All rights of reproduction in any form reserved.

experience, or even "intuition" for the purpose of helping other individuals or groups or organizations, most usually for monetary remuneration. The standards refer to what people do—or should do—not to their training, or knowledge, or "consideration" prior to acting. There are also standards of training (often assessed by educational record) and knowledge (often assessed by testing), but they are secondary to practice standards. First, meeting these standards in no way guarantees meeting standards of practice; second, the very existence of these secondary requirements is based on the belief that satisfying them will enhance the probability of high quality and ethical practice. These secondary standards (e.g., "credentialing") can not substitute for standards of practice.

In order to justify these standards of actual practice, it is first necessary to understand what we know about the practices of psychology. Here, I will concentrate on what we know about psychotherapy for mental health problems. Moreover, I will concentrate on knowledge that can be justified by current empirical evidence assessed in a rational manner. A particular practitioner, for example, may have some ideas about psychotherapy and mental health that under later close examination turn out to be valid, or at least useful. If, however, there is no systematic evidence at the time the practitioner applies these ideas, then they cannot be categorized and part of "what is known" in the area of mental health. As will be argued later, the fact that these ideas are not yet validated (and might never be) may not *prohibit* their use, although it may. The conditions of such potential prohibition will be considered later. What is important at this point is to understand that practice standards must be based on current knowledge, which can be equated with current belief justified on an empirical and rational basis—even though some later time such belief may turn out to be incomplete, flawed, or even downright wrong. People claiming to apply psychological knowledge, however much individual skill may be involved in the application, are bound by the nature of the knowledge at the time they apply it.

II. FINDINGS ON PSYCHOTHERAPY EFFECTIVENESS

A. Standard Randomized Trials

There are two basic findings in the area of psychotherapy, the subject of this article. Both of these findings are based on standard randomized trials investigations, where subjects are randomly assigned to experimental group versus comparison group and outcomes are assessed using as "blind" a method as possible. The comparison group can consist of a no-treatment control group, of a wait list control group, or of a commonly accepted treatment to which the experimental one is to be compared. The reason for random assignment is that the *expectation* of the effect of variables not manipulated by the assignment itself is the same for both groups (or for all groups in multiple assessments), and we have greater reason to believe that this expectation will approach reality the larger the sample. The mathematical result is that (critics might argue somewhat circularly) the expectation of deviations from these expectations becomes smaller the larger the sample, so that we can have greater and greater confidence with larger samples that "nuisance" and "confounding" variables do not affect the outcome of the investigation.

B. Quasi Experiments

The alternatives to standard randomized trials often involve matching or some type of quasi-experiment that can lead to plausible but not "highly justifiable" results. Consider, for example, a study using a matching strategy to attempt to assess the effect of having an abortion. We might have two groups of women experiencing unwanted pregnancy who are alike in many of the respects we think may be relevant to how an abortion will affect them (e.g., religion, social class, education, political orientation) and observe how the women in these two groups are different some years later—after most in one group have freely chosen to get an abortion and in the other group have freely chosen not to do so. The problem, however, is that there must be *some* variable or variables on which the women in these two groups are radically different, given that they made different choices. In fact, this variable or variables must be very powerful given that we have "controlled" for the important variables that we believe are relevant to the choice and its effects. This "unobserved variable problem" is an extremely important one that makes matching studies suspect.

In contrast, true quasi-experiments tend to be valid to the degree in which they approach true randomized ones. For example, consider the "interrupted time series" assessment of providing a psychoactive drug. Individual or individuals are assessed prior to the time the drug is administered on a regular basis and then assessed afterwards. But in the actual clinic setting, the introduction of the drug is often in response to some particular problem or problems that lead the clinician to believe that drug treatment is desirable or necessary. For example, a woman who is raped at a halfway house by a counselor may enter an inpatient treatment facility and—due to her condition—be immediately given Prozac. Now she is calmer. Is this calmness the effect of getting away from the halfway house? Due to the more relaxed inpatient environment itself (which people do not learn to hate immediately)? Due to the Prozac?

C. Regression Effects

A *regression* effect refers to the fact that if two variables are not perfectly correlated, the one we predict will on the average be closer to its standardized mean than the one from which we make the prediction. (In the linear prediction equation for standard scores, the predicted value of y is equal to r times actual value of x, and conversely the predicted value of x is equal to r times the actual value of y.) Moreover, we have no way of assessing regression independent of other factors, because regression *includes* "real world" variables responsible for the lack of a perfect correlation. Now if instead the drug is introduced at a randomly determined time, we do not have to worry about such systematic regression effects or confounds. (But we may be justified in worrying about unsystematic ones.) What we are doing when we introduce the manipulation at a randomly determined time, however, is to approximate a truly randomized experiment.

D. Rationale for Randomization

The basic rationale for randomization is that we ideally want to know what *would* have happened to subjects had they not been assigned to the experimental treatment, a hypothetical counterfactual. Of course, because we cannot both assign and not assign at the same time, a direct assessment of this counterfactual is impossible. Randomly assigning people so that the expectation is that they are equivalent on variables that might affect outcome but in which we are not interested is the best justified substitute for actual knowledge of the hypothetical counterfactual. There are, of course, problems, particularly in the psychotherapy area. For example, it is impossible for the subject to be "blind" to receiving therapy, and often it is impossible for those evaluating its effects to be blind as well. Experiments in this area contrast quite sharply with many experiments in medicine, where subjects are given placebos without being told if they are given the actual drug or placebos (or one of two drugs) and those evaluating their status are also ignorant of the assignment. Another problem is that randomized control experimentation can (should) be conducted only with subjects who agree to be randomly assigned. Perhaps such subjects—or even those who agree to be evaluated in a setting that does not use random assignment—are different from those who will receive or not receive the treatments evaluated. But that problem arises in any evaluation, not just random ones. (While there is the possibility of using "phony" therapy as a "placebo control," such a procedure raises severe ethical problems.) Thus, not because it is perfect, but because it yields the best knowledge available, we must turn to randomized trials to understand psychotherapy. As the eminent statistician Frederick Mosteller vigorously argued in 1981, while we should strive to appreciate the strengths and weaknesses of different approaches instead of being dogmatic about statistical purity, we must be aware that "the alternative to randomized controlled experiments is fooling around with peoples' lives."

E. Conclusion of Randomized Trials

Randomized trials of psychotherapy effectiveness yield two rather simple conclusions. The first is that there exists a set of problems for which carefully constructed ("protocol") therapies are effective—according to the criteria that at least one randomized trials study has "validated" these forms of psychotherapy. These therapies are listed in a 1995 report from the Task Force on Promotion and Dissemination of Psychological Procedures, division of clinical psychology, American Psychological Association. As the critic Garfield pointed out that same year, these results could not be used as a basis for justifying all—or even most—psychotherapy, or for setting standards. First, the number of conditions and the number of therapies is quite limited, hardly representative of the practice of "psychotherapy." In fact, the task force itself noted that these types of validated therapies are often not even taught in programs that are listed as good ones in various sources for training graduate students in clinical psychology. The constrained nature of the types of therapy provided overlooks, to quote Garfield (pg. 218): "the importance of client and therapist variability, the role of the common factors in psychotherapy, and the need to adapt therapeutic procedures for the problems of the individual client or patient." In a highly influential report of a Consumers' Union study he published that same year of 1995, Seligman refers to such studies as "efficacy" ones. He writes (pp. 965–966) "In spite of how expensive and time-consuming they are, hundreds of efficacy studies of both psychotherapy and drugs now exist—many of them well done. These studies show, among many other things, that cognitive therapy, interpersonal therapy, and medications all provide moderate relief from unipolar depressive disorder; that exposure and clomipramine both relieve the symptoms of obsessive-compulsive disorder moderately well, but that exposure has more lasting benefits; that cognitive therapy works very well in panic disorders; that systematic desensitization relieves specific phobias; that "applied tension" virtually cures blood and injury phobia, that transcendental meditation relieves anxiety; that aversion therapy produces only marginal improvement with sexual offenders; that disulfram (Antabuse) does not provide lasting relief from alcoholism; that flooding plus medication does better in the treatment of agoraphobia than either alone; and that cognitive therapy provides significant relief of bulimia, outperforming medications alone." [*See* COGNITIVE THERAPY; PSYCHOPHARMACOLOGY.]

But then Seligman compares such studies to what he terms "effectiveness" studies, that is, those of "how patients fare under the actual conditions of treatment in the field" (p. 966)—and finally reaches a conclusion with which few of his critics agree: "The upshot of this is that random assignment, the prettiest of the methodological niceties in efficacy studies, may turn out to be worse than useless for the investigation of the actual treatment of mental illnesses in the field" (p. 974).

F. SUMMARIES AND META ANALYSES

There are, despite the claims of Seligman, a multitude of studies involving random assignment that attempt to assess what is actually done in the field—without limiting the practitioner to following a carefully crafted protocol. See, for example, the article of Laneman and Dawes—discussed in greater detail later—for a description of the diversity of the studies involving random assignment.

These diverse studies have been either summarized qualitatively, analyzed by "vote counts" based on their outcomes, or subjected to meta-analysis to reach general conclusions, because each in fact concerns one type of distress in one setting, often with a single or only a few therapists implementing the procedure under investigation. (Note that the same limitation applies to the "validated efficacy studies" as well.) Most summaries and meta-analyses consider reductions in symptoms that the people entering therapy find distressing or debilitating. Some measure of these symptoms' severity is then obtained after the random assignment to treatment versus control, and the degree to which the people in the randomly assigned experimental group differ from those in the control group on the symptoms is assessed, and averaged across studies. (Occasionally, difference scores are assessed as well.) The summaries and meta-analyses concentrates on symptoms, which can be justified because it is the symptoms that lead people to come to psychotherapists. The summaries and meta-analyses involves "combining applies and oranges," which can be justified by the fact that the types of nonprotocol therapies are extraordinary diverse (fruits). For example, simply providing information on a random basis to heart attack victims in an intensive care unit can be considered to be psychotherapy.

The "classic" meta-analysis of psychotherapy outcomes was published by Smith and Glass in 1977, and there has been little reason since that time to modify its conclusions. In general, psychotherapy is effective in reducing symptoms—to the point that the average severity of symptoms experienced by the people in the experimental group after completion of therapy is at the 25th percentile of the control group (i.e. less severe than the symptoms experienced by 75% of the people in the control group after the same period of time). That translates *roughly* (assuming normality and equal variance of the two groups) into the statement that if we chose a person at random from the experimental group and one at random from the control group, the one from the experimental group has a .67 probability of having less severe symptoms than the one from the control group. The other major conclusions were that the type of therapy did not seem to make a difference overall, the type of therapist did not seem to make a difference, and even the length of psychotherapy did not seem to make a difference. These conclusions are based both on evaluating the consistency of results and evaluating their average effect sizes. These conclusions have survived two main challenges.

The first is that while Smith and Glass included an overall evaluation of the "quality" of the study, they did not specifically look at whether the assignment was *really* random. To address that problem, Landman and Dawes published a paper in 1982 reporting an examination of every fifth study selected from the Smith and Glass list (which had increased to 435 studies by the time it was given to Landman and Dawes); these researchers concluded—with a very high degree of inter-rater reliability based on independent judgments—that fully a third of the studies did not involve true random assignment. A particularly egregious example involved recruiting students in a psychology department with posters urging group psychotherapy to address underachievement; the authors then compared the students who self-selected for this treatment with some students with similar GPAs "randomly" chosen from the registrar's list, who for all the experimenters knew have given up and left town. A more subtle example may be found in comparing people who persist in group psychotherapy with people in an *entire* randomly selected control group. Yes, the two groups were originally randomly constructed, but the problem is that we do not know which people in the control group *would* have stayed with the group psychotherapy *had* they been assigned the experimental group—thereby invalidating the control group as a comparison to the experimental one. While it is possible to maintain that it seems bizarre to include in an evaluation of group psychotherapy those who did not actually participate in the groups, if there is really an effect of a particular treatment and assignment is random, then it will exist—albeit in attenuated form—when the *entire* experimental group is compared to the control group. (A mixture of salt and fresh water is still salt water.) The way to deal with selective completion is to study enough subjects to have a study powerful enough to test the effects based on "subsets" of the people's assigned to experimental manipulation (e.g., those who completed). Landman and Dawes deleted the 35% of their studies that they believed not to be truly random ones from their meta-analysis, and reached exactly the same conclusion Smith and Glass had earlier.

A second problem is the "file-drawer" one. Perhaps there are a number of studies showing that psychotherapy does not work, or even having results that indicated that it might be harmful, which simply are not published in standard journals—either because their results do not reach standard results of "statistical significance" or because flaws are noted as a result of their unpopular conclusions that might be (often unconsciously) overlooked had the conclusions been more popular. The problem has been addressed in two ways. First, the number of such studies would have to be so large that it appears to be unreasonable to hypothesize their existence in such file drawers. Second, it is possible to develop a distribution of the statistics of statistical significance actually presented in the literature and show that their values exceed (actually quite radically) those that would be predicted from randomly sampling above some criterion level that leads to publication of the results.

Another problem concerns the identity of the psychotherapists. Here, there is some ambiguity, because the studies attempting to "refute" the conclusion of Smith and Glass are generally conceived poorly, in that the psychotherapy subject rather than the psychotherapists themselves are sampled and used as the unit of measurement—especially for statistical test. But if we want to generalize about psychotherapists, then it is necessary to sample psychotherapists. For example, if a standard analysis of variance design is used where therapists are the "treatment" effect, then generalization to therapists—or to various types of therapists—requires a "random effects" analysis rather than a "fixed effects" one. One study did in fact follow this prescription, but then concluded on the basis of a post hoc analysis how more successful therapists were different from less successful ones after finding no evidence for a therapist effect overall!

The results of studies treating each psychotherapist as a separate sample observation generally conclude that beyond a very rudimentary level of training, credentials and experience do not correlate (positively) with efficacy, as summarized by Dawes in his 1994 book, Chapter 4. There is some slight evidence that people who are considered "empathetic" tend to achieve better outcomes (where this characteristic is assessed by colleagues—not in a circular manner by clients who themselves improve); also there is some evidence that when therapists agree to engage in different types of therapy, they do best applying ones in which they have the greatest belief. (It is possible to question the importance of the latter finding, given that outside of randomized control studies, therapists tend to provide only the type of psychotherapy that they believe to be the most helpful to their clients.)

III. WHAT FINDINGS IMPLY ABOUT STANDARDS

The overall conclusion supports the importance of "nonspecific" factors in therapeutic effectiveness. This general result about the quality of the "therapeutic alliance" as opposed to the specific type of therapy has been somewhat derogatorily referred to as the "Dodo bird finding" in that "all win and all must have prizes." (For the latest explication see the 1994 paper of Stubbs and Bozarth.) The problem is that findings hypothesizing the "quality of relationship" generally lack independent definitions of "quality" or evaluation of exactly *which* nonspecific factors are responsible for success or failure.

Now let us consider what these two findings—about specific protocol therapies and about nonspecific factors—imply about standards. In a 1996 report from the Hasting Center entitled "The Goals of Medicine," a panel of international group leaders sponsored by the Institute wrote: "On necessity, good caring demands technical excellence as a crucial ingredient" (p. s12). The protocol therapies clearly demand technically correct implementation as a crucial ingredient; failing to be technically correct completely violates standards of practice.

But what about the other types of therapies? It is very difficult to require technical excellence of "relationship" therapies—which, again, constitute the majority.

What then can be demanded as a standard? Therapists often point out that the research in psychology does not imply exactly what they should do. True, except for the protocol therapies. Conversely, however, research does imply what should *not be done,* what is "out of bounds." Thus, research in psychology and related areas implies minatory ("thou shalt not") as oppose to hortatory ("thou shalt") directives and standards for much of therapy. Of course, it is possible to rephrase minatory statements to become hortatory (e.g., "thou shalt avoid doing this thing," such as committing murder), but most people recognize the distinction between two types of statements. For example, laws are based on violation of minatory rules, not hortatory ones, and even outside of the legal context we often make the distinction between the morality of simply not breaking rules versus that of doing something positive for our fellow humans. Moreover, people are often willing to engage in compensation between differing hortatory goals, but not "weight" various violations of minatory rules, unless explicitly decided in advance—such as killing in wartime or lying when a spy or carrying messages for Refusniks. We do not, however, talk about "trade-offs" between murder versus achieving some valuable goal (for example, saving the lives of 10 people by slaughtering a homeless man whose body can provide 10 organs to be transplanted in these people who would otherwise die).

Of course, when the boundaries of "thou shalt not" are sufficiently narrow, then minatory directives can become hortatory ones, but that is not common in psychological practice. We find, for example, a positive correlation between *peer* evaluations of therapist empathy and therapist effectiveness—as mentioned earlier—but we cannot demand a therapist be empathetic all the time: in particular, not that therapists be empathetic "types" of people, which are what their peers are evaluating.

IV. SPECIFYING UNACCEPTABLE BEHAVIOR

Is there really the possibility of specifying such "out of bounds" behavior? Does it occur? Or does "anything go?" There is a possibility, it does occur, and anything does not go. Such behavior clearly violates standards of psychotherapy—whether the standards are based on our views of ethics or of effectiveness. For example, psychology research shows memory to be "reconstructive" and hence prone to errors that "make sense" of what happened, considered either by itself or in broader contexts such as one's "life story." Further, there has never been any research evidence for the concept of "repression." That absence does not mean it is impossible for someone to "recover a repressed memory," or that such reconstructed memories are necessarily historically inaccurate. What it does mean is that as *professionals* practicing their trade—which means applying psychological knowledge as we now know it—therapists should not be involved in attempting to do something that current research evidence indicates can easily create illusion, and needless suffering.

Nevertheless some are. For example, in a survey of licensed U.S. doctoral-level psychologists randomly sampled from the *National Register of Health Service Providers in Psychology* by Poole, Lindsay, Memon, and Bull in 1995, 70% indicated that they used various techniques (e.g., hypnosis, interpretation of dreams) to "help" clients recover memories of child sexual abuse; moreover, combining the sample from the register with a British sample from the *Register of Chartered Clinical Psychologist,* the authors conclude: "Across samples, 25% of the respondents reported a constellation of beliefs and practices suggestive of focus on memory recovery, and these psychologists reported relatively high rates of memory recovery in their clients" (pg. 426). The study asked about the use of eight techniques that cognitive psychologists have found to involve bias and create errors. Hypnosis, age regression, dream interpretation, guided imagery related to abuse situations, instructions to give free reign to the imagination, use of family photographs as memory cues, instructions for remembering/journaling, and interpreting physical symptoms. Remarkably, with the exception of the last three techniques, the proportion of survey respondents who reported using them was overshadowed by similar or higher proportions of respondents who "disapproved" of using them.

In addition, failure to disapprove of interpreting physical symptoms as evidence of unusual events can be traced to a failure to understand the base rate problem in interpreting diagnostic signs—a failure that has been decried ever since Meehl and Rosen first discussed it in detail in 1955, but which is remarkably robust—as experimental studies in the area of behavioral decision making indicate that people equate inverse probabilities without equating simple ones, even in the face of evidence that these simple probabilities are quite discrepant. It takes one step to move from the definition of a conditional probability to the ratio rule, which states that $P(a \text{ given } b)/P(b \text{ given } a) = P(a)/P(b)$. For example, the probability of being a hard drug user given one smokes pot divided by the probability of smoking pot given one is a hard drug user is exactly equal to the simple probability of being a hard drug user divided by the probability of smoking pot. Exactly. To maintain that because (it is believed that) a very low base rate event (e.g., being brought up in a satanic cult, an event that may have probability zero) can imply high base rate distress (e.g., poor self-image and an eating disorder) it therefore follows that the distress implies the event is just flat-out irrational. Doing so violates the standard of practice proposed, which is that it be based on empirical knowledge interpreted in a rational manner.

Unfortunately, however, the debate about recovered repressed memories has degenerated into claims and counter claims about whether they *can* exist, or the—totally unknown—frequency with which they are accurate or invented, rather than around the question of whether attempting to recover them is justified by what is known. In fact it is not; the real question is whether doing so is "out of bounds" behavior, and given we do know a lot about the reconstructive nature of memory, but very little about whether memory of trauma differs from other memories—and if so in exactly what way—such recovery must be categorized as out of bounds, that is, practice that violates standards.

V. PURPOSE OF STANDARDS

The purpose of standards of psychological practice is to aid the client with knowledge-based skills; ignoring knowledge is no more appropriate than having sexual contact with a client. Standards must be extended in a minatory way to prohibit application of ignorance, just as there are minatory standards about the behavior of the therapist that may both harm the client and degrade the profession (e.g., sexual contact). Moreover, a minatory standard can be enforced, and in the current author's experience on the American Psychological Association Ethics Committee, such standards were indeed the ones enforced. People were kicked out of the American Psychological Association or lost their license to practice (in one order or another) primarily on the basis of sexual contact with the clients, on the basis of having been found guilty of a felony involved in their practice (e.g., cheating on insurance), or on the basis of practicing beyond their area of competence.

VI. CHANGING DEFINITION OF COMPETENCE

The last reason for kicking people out of the association brings up a specific distinction between the standards proposed in the current chapter versus those proposed by the American Psychological Association. (See its Ethics Code published in 1992.) The latter *defines* "competence" in terms of education, training, or experience. Specifically, principle 1.04 (a) reads that: "psychologists provide services, teach, and conduct research only within the boundary of their competence, *based on their education, training, supervised experience, or appropriate professional experience*" (italics added). The problem with this definition of competence is that it does not indicate that training must be in something for which there is some scientific knowledge. For example, training in the alleviation of posttraumatic stress disorder (PTSD) could involve people whose trauma was supposedly that of being kidnapped by aliens. In fact, (see Dawes, 1994, Chapter 5) there is a set of psychotherapists who have exactly this specialty, and one of them mentions the others in the back of her book, others who are licensed and can receive third-party payment for treatment of this type of PTSD.

The other problem with this definition is that it allows a very specific characterization of what is relevant "training," a characterization that could even *exclude* generalizations based on scientific studies. For example, Courtois criticized in 1995 those who criticize recovered repressed memory psychotherapists, on the grounds that these critics themselves have not been involved with recovering repressed memory. She writes: "Unfortunately, a number of memory researchers are erring in the same way that they allege therapists to be erring; they are practicing outside of their areas of competence and/or applying findings from memory analogues without regard to the ecological validity and making misrepresentations, overgeneralizations, and unsubstantiated claims regarding therapeutic practice" (p. 297). The criticized claims are, of course generalizations that are based on what is known about *memory in general,* and the claim that a specific type of memory is inadequately or incorrectly characterized by such generalizations requires assuming a "burden of proof." Exceptions to rules require evidence that they are indeed exceptions. No evidence is presented. Instead, a statement is made that people who based generalizations on well-established principles derived from empirical research are themselves behaving unethically because they have not been immersed in the context in which these exceptions are *claimed* to occur. It is a circular argument that can equally well be made against those of us who believe that PTSD researchers who help people recover the memory of being kidnapped by aliens should not be reimbursed from government or insurance funds. Since we ourselves would not even think of conducting such therapy, how can we evaluate it?

The Ethics Code of the American Psychological Association also emphasizes "consideration of" what is known, but it does not mandate applying it. More specifically, for the type of relationship therapy, it does not mandate that psychotherapists should definitely not do what careful consideration indicates they should not. Certainly, training and consideration are precursors to practicing well and ethically, but as pointed out earlier, they cannot be substitutes. The reason that they cannot be substitutes is that the training must be training in that which works, which is then applied. "Consideration" must be consideration of valid knowledge, which is then applied. Again, I'm not claiming that knowledge will not change in the future, or that everything psychologists currently believe to be true is necessarily true. The point is that good practice must be based on the best available knowledge and evidence—not on what *might* be, *could* be, or what *may* turn out to be true after years of subsequent investigation. Moreover, what is believed to be true *does* provide bounds—minatory standards.

The philosophy espoused in this standards of practice chapter is close to that of the National Association for Consumer Protection in Mental Health Practices. (See its goals as enunciated in 1996 by its President Christopher Barden.) The major difference, if there is one, involves how much emphasis is placed on the clients' explicit recognition that when the type of therapy is a "relationship" one, there is really no hard evidence that the *particular* type offered works better than any other. Relationship therapies do work overall, and it is very tricky to obtain "informed consent" about a whole huge category of therapy, while at the same time indicating that particular members of it may not have empirical justification. The additional problem is that by emphasizing that lack for particular members, whatever placebo effects can account for the efficacy of the entire class may be diminished. Avoiding such emphasis in obtaining informed consent is clearly self-serving for the psychotherapist. The question is whether it also serves the client. Rather than just assuming that it does, we could put this question to an empirical test—through randomized trials.

VII. CONCLUSION

The final point of this article is part minatory, part hortatory. The purpose of psychological practice is to provide *incremental validity,* that is, to help in ways that the clients could not help themselves (at least to increase the probability of such help). The fact, for example, that a flashbulb memory may be corroborated by others does not imply that the practitioner should encourage or interpret such memory, because corroboration by others involves historical accuracy, and the psychologist provides no incremental validity about how such corroboration may be obtained, or what sort of corroboration may validate or invalidate the conclusion that the memory is historically accurate. Incremental validity, however, is both desirable and required, especially in a society that demands "truth in advertising."

A note at the end. This article has been devoted to the questions of standards of practice in psychotherapy. It has not dealt with forensic psychology and the subsequent standards of expert testimony in courts and other legal settings. Everything argued here applies to such settings. Because testimony in courts can result in loss of freedom, it is urgent that psychotherapists who do testify meet the standards enunciated in this article.

BIBLIOGRAPHY

American Psychological Association. (1992). Ethical principles of psychologist and code of conduct. *American Psychologist, 47,* 1597–1611.

Barden, R. C. (1996). The National Associations for Consumer Protection in Mental Health Practices: Office of the President. Plymouth, MN: Copies available from R. Christopher Barden, PhD., J.D. 4025 Quaker Lane North, Plymouth, MN 55441.

Courtois, C. A. (1995). Scientist-practitioners and the delayed memory controversy: Scientific standards and the need for collaboration. *The Consulting Psychologist, 23,* 294–299.

Dawes, R. M. (1994). *House of cards: Psychology and psychotherapy built on myth.* New York: The Free Press.

Garfield, S. A. (1996). Some problems associated with "validated" forms of psychotherapy. *Clinical Psychology: Science and Practice, 3,* 218–229.

The Hasting Center. (1996). The goals of medicine: setting new priority. Briarcliff Manor, NY: Publication Department, The Hasting Center.

Landman, J. T., & Dawes, R. M. (1982). Psychotherapy outcome: Smith and Glass' conclusions stand up under scrutiny. *American Psychologist, 37,* 504–516.

Meehl, P. E., Rosen, A. (1955). Antecedent probability and the efficiency of psychometric signs, patterns, or cutting score. *Psychological Bulletin, 52,* 194–216.

Mosteller, F. (1981). Innovation and evaluation. *Science, 211,* 881–886.

Poole, D. A., Lindsay, D. S., Memon, A., & Bull, R. (1995). Psychotherapy and the recovery of memories of childhood sexual abuse, U.S. and British practitioners' opinions, practices, and experiences. *Journal of Consulting and Clinical Psychology, 63,* 426–437.

Seligman, M. E. P. (1995). The effectiveness of psychotherapy: The consumer reports study. *American Psychologist, 50,* 965–974.

Smith, M. L., & Glass, G. V. (1977). Meta-analysis of psychotherapy outcome studies. *American Psychologist, 32,* 752–760.

Stubbs, J. T., & Bozarth, J. D. (1994). The Dodo bird revisited: a qualitative study of psychotherapy efficacy research. *Applied and Preventative Psychology, 3,* 109–120.

Task Force on Promotion and Dissemination of Psychological Procedures. Division of Clinical Psychology, American Psychological Association (1995). Training in and dissemination of empirically-validated psychological treatments. Report and recommendations. *The Clinical Psychologist, 48,* 3–23.

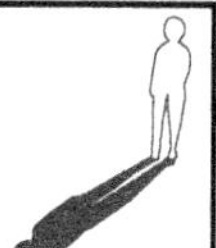

Support Groups

Benjamin H. Gottlieb
University of Guelph

Social Comparison The process of comparing one's own actions, beliefs, abilities, feelings, or other personal characteristics to other people's in order to see how well or poorly one is doing.

Social Support A process of interaction in relationships that can improve coping, esteem, belonging, and competence through actual exchanges of practical or psychosocial resources or through their perceived availability.

A SUPPORT GROUP is composed of from 6 to 10 people who share a similar life stressor, transition, affliction, or noxious habit, and who receive expert information and training, and exchange mutual aid for a predetermined period of time in order to foster improved coping and adjustment. This article will present the rationales for and core characteristics of support groups, it will review evidence concerning their impacts on participants, and it will discuss the varied ways in which the groups' structures and formats affect the support process.

I. INTRODUCTION

Jimmy Armstrong's Mom knows that every Tuesday she is to pack a double dessert in Jimmy's lunch pail because that's the day he attends his K.O.P.S. group in Pioneer Elementary School. The acronym stands for Kids of Parental Separation, but none of the eight sixth-grade students who attend this weekly support group would recall that. All they know is that, halfway through the hour, they get to dump the extra desserts in a pile on the table, and then pick numbers from a hat to determine the order of choosing the desserts. On this, the fifth of eight meetings, the hat will do extra duty because each of the children is supposed to deposit a question, an upset, or a happiness in it, and then, one by one, each child will choose a slip of paper, read it aloud, and discuss it with the group. Ms. James, the social worker from the local community mental health center, and Todd Williams, a high school senior whose parents separated when he was in grade six, will help lead the discussion of each note. They have a way of getting the group to talk about the things they feel angry, sad, and glad about without anyone getting too upset. Last Tuesday, when Jimmy's Mom picked him up from school, she was amazed because, for the first time, Jimmy told her how much he missed Dad, but not the fights she and Dad always had after he went to bed.

Carol Swenson, 48-year-old mother of two active teenagers, and daughter of Sylvia, who was recently pronounced to have Alzheimer's Disease, attends a support group called "Coping with Caregiving." So far, the best thing that has happened in the group is that the leader taught the members some very practi-

Copyright © 1998 by Academic Press.
All rights of reproduction in any form reserved.

cal techniques of managing their anger toward their relative and of relaxing by using their imagination and their muscle control. The worst thing that has happened is that, 2 weeks ago, one group member's demented relative actually died from the disease. What made the death so hard to understand is that the deceased was only 63 years old and in perfect physical health. Carol knew this because the group members bring pictures of their relatives to each meeting, and this relative's picture displayed a vital gentleman wearing a pair of shorts that showed off his muscular legs. But as Dr. Morton, the group facilitator, pointed out, there was nothing that could have been done to prevent or postpone the death, and it surely was softened by the love and compassion of a dutiful wife. In fact, although frightening, the death seemed to draw the group members closer together, and some members were beginning to call one another and even get together between meetings. It looked like more lasting friendships were being formed.

At 7:30 A.M., in the Hotel Excelsior's fitness center, 10 middle-aged men sit around a treadmill, 8 of them sitting in pairs while pouring over the results of their latest stress tests. One of the men is their physician and another is an occupational therapist. The members of this "Heart Club" have met together on a biweekly basis for the past 6 months. After the first few meetings in the cardiac rehabilitation unit of the hospital, the group's venue changed to the hotel's fitness center because it was located within easy striking distance of each member's workplace. They had also formed a buddy system so that each of them had a partner to call if he wanted to work out with someone or just talk about how to deal with a boss who had forgotten to ease up on the pressure or with a spouse who was afraid of the exertion required by lovemaking and lawn mowing. Today, the topic was called "Stress: Body and Soul." The format was always the same, beginning with a lecturette by the doctor on the body's response to stress, followed by a half hour of experience swapping among the participants. After the hour meeting, the Heart Club adjourned to the bagelry downstairs to enjoy the food and camaraderie.

II. DEFINITION AND OVERVIEW

These are only three examples of a vast and growing number of support groups that have been organized by virtually every health and human service organization in North America. As the examples reveal, support groups have been convened on behalf of people of all ages who face a wide range of adaptive challenges that call for more specialized or intensive support than is naturally available to them. The groups are typically led or co-led by professionals who meet with from 6 to 10 people who are facing similar stressful events, transitions, or circumstances, or who have in common an affliction, disability, noxious habit, or problem in living. Typically, once composed, the support group is closed to new members, and meets on a regularly scheduled basis for a predetermined period of time and number of sessions. Although there are innumerable variations, the standard format involves the transmission of information and skills by one or more professionals, and exchanges of information and mutual aid among the participants. In principle, the combination of expert and experiential knowledge in the context of a supportive peer culture creates optimal conditions for improved coping and adaptation.

This chapter sets out the distinguishing characteristics of support groups, including their basic structural properties and formats. It explains the theoretical justification for this type of psychosocial intervention, and delves into the social influence processes that arise during the course of the intervention. Drawing on recent reviews of support groups for cancer patients and family caregivers of elderly persons, it weighs the empirical evidence concerning the mental health impact of such groups, spotlighting aspects of their design, composition, and process that deserve greater attention in the future.

III. RATIONALES FOR THE IMPLEMENTATION OF SUPPORT GROUPS

The theoretical rationale that usually introduces studies on the use of support groups to maintain and promote mental health is based on the broad fabric of evidence, reviewed by Cohen and Wills in 1985, revealing that the support of one's personal community of associates has health protective effects. They concluded that it is largely perceived support that cushions the impact of a wide range of stressful life events and transitions. In addition, in 1988, House, Landis, and Umberson reviewed a number of epidemiological studies that showed that social integration was prospectively linked to lower morbidity and mortality. That is, the stress moderating function of social support appears to rest on people's belief that they are reliably allied with certain associates who are prepared to provide needed practical assistance and emotional support. From an epidemiological perspective, the advantage that social support confers on health and survival stems from more abundant contact with family members and friends, as well as from participation in voluntary associations. Support groups therefore cannot be justified on the basis of either the stress-related or epidemiological findings. Such groups do not concentrate on conditioning a psychological sense of support, nor do they intensify or enlarge contact with natural network members.

Instead, support groups are artificial and temporary systems of mutual aid. In large part, they involve the disclosure of personal problems, fears, and doubts to a set of strangers, collective problem solving, and the sharing of coping strategies. Yet evidence for the protective effect of actually receiving support is mixed, with null or negative effects resulting from the damaging psychological implications of seeking help from others or from a miscarried support process. In short, the weight of the empirical evidence suggests that the adaptive value of support derives largely from the perception that one has worth and importance to others and can count on them when needed, rather than from actual exchanges of help and support.

This distinction between perceived and received support generally has not been recognized by those who have mounted support groups. Since the stress-buffering effect of social support is mainly predicated on perceived rather than received support, the most appropriate intervention would be to persuade people that they can gain the support they need from others rather than involving them in a process of mutual aid. On the other hand, it is possible that involvement in the process of mutual aid is a precondition of perceived support, giving rise to perceptions of caring and belonging. In fact, whatever beneficial effects of support groups may occur could result from the psychological sense of support that the group instills rather than from its helping processes. This is why it is particularly important to compose the group in a way that will enable the members to perceive one another as similar peers who are "in the same boat" since this will magnify feelings of connection and mutual responsiveness. This may also help to explain why support group members generally agree that the most beneficial aspects of their group experience were that they felt less emotionally alone, and gained comfort from learning that their thoughts, feelings, and behaviors were normal and validated by others.

A second rationale for introducing support groups is based on the supposition that certain stressful events and transitions create rends in the affected parties' natural networks or overtax the resources or tolerance of network members. In circumstances that call for prolonged help from family members and friends, when stigma and embarrassment surround the affected parties, or when the victims of life events express threatening emotions, close associates are often incapable of providing needed support. In addition, there are instances when the stressor is so severe or pervasive that it restricts social participation, such as when family caregivers withdraw from employment and become homebound in order to supervise a demented relative. Similarly, people with certain medical conditions, diseases, or disabilities must often limit or surrender their social activities, with the attendant loss of valued relationships. [*See* Coping with Stress.]

Short of losing touch with their natural network, people may feel that their associates simply do not understand what they are experiencing or that their difficulties are compounded by their associates' own efforts to cope with the difficulty or by their misguided helping efforts. For example, there is evidence that a spiral of conflict can occur when spouses clash with one another in their ways of coping with a shared stressor, such as a child's serious illness. In 1988, Coyne, Wortman, and Lehman identified several other ways in which support can miscarry and undermine close relationships.

Hence, support groups have been introduced to compensate for absent, insufficient, or irrelevant support from the members' natural networks. For example, based on the findings of their survey of 667 cancer patients, Taylor, Falke, Shoptaw, and Lichtman found in 1986 that 55% wished "very much or somewhat" that they could talk more openly to family members, and 50% said the same thing about friends. More than a third agreed with the sentiment that family members did not truly understand their experience of cancer. However, it is important to note that those patients who had participated in a support group did not differ from those who had not with respect to their network's support, suggesting that other factors come into play in spurring support group participation. In fact, Taylor and colleagues discovered that support group users generally disclosed their cancer-related concerns to a larger number of informal and professional resources than the nonusers, and also had a more extensive help-seeking history than the nonusers. Support group users, or perhaps those who benefit most from such groups, may therefore be particularly disposed to cope by seeking information and feedback, a point that is discussed in greater detail later.

Another rationale for introducing support groups has more to do with the transmission of information, education, and skills to the participants than with the emotional support provided by the group. There are several reasons why a support group is a desirable context for learning new information and skills. First, there may be a significant amount of technical information that all participants want and need to know to improve their comprehension and handling of their situations. The sheer volume of information may require it to be divided into consumable chunks that can be disseminated more efficiently en masse than individually. For example, support groups for cancer patients typically cover the following topics: the causes of cancer; explanation of the diagnoses, tests, and prognoses of the various subtypes of the disease; explanation of the various components of the treatment plan, such as surgery and chemotherapy, and their side effects; discussion of the personal and social impacts of treatment, such as changes in body image and sexuality; education about diet, exercise, and any other life-style changes; explanation and demonstration of the use of prostheses; instruction about relaxation and visualizing techniques; and discussion of issues that arise in communicating needs and problems to both health care providers and network members.

Second, it is widely understood that discussion facilitates the learning of new information, an advantage that is offered by the group context. Moreover, since the group meets over a period of several weeks, the information can be divided into manageable units and time can be set aside to practice, review, and reinforce any skills that are taught. For example, in 1994, Gallagher-Thompson described two different cognitive-behavioral group programs for the family caregivers of persons with dementia, one focused on the alleviation of depression and the other on anger management. In each case, she has planned eight sessions plus two additional booster sessions at 3-month intervals, beginning with an overview of the model, progressing to the acquisition and practice of component skills in the group and at home, and culminating with continued implementation and monitoring of outcomes.

Third, aside from their cost-effectiveness compared to individual education and skill training, support groups offer other advantages over individual counseling. The group members can serve as role models for each other, sharing methods of solving problems and coping. In these ways, they are at once being helped and helping others, the latter counteracting feelings of helplessness and enhancing feelings of self-worth and usefulness to others. In addition, the support group can lead to the formation of friendships that endure beyond the formal group sessions, helping to populate the participants' natural networks with similar peers.

IV. CORE CHARACTERISTICS OF SUPPORT GROUPS

A support group can be defined as a small group of from 6 to 10 people who are in similar circumstances that pose an adaptive challenge, and who are convened and led by a professional who provides education and/or training over a period of several weeks, and who facilitates a process of mutual aid among the participants for the purpose of fostering their health and well-being. Support groups differ from self-help groups by virtue of three characteristics: the direct involvement of professionals in the group sessions, their time-limited nature, and the tendency of support groups to look inward rather than outward, generally eschewing advocacy and social action. Support groups differ from conventional group therapy as well. In support groups, professionals do not make psychological interpretations or keep case records, and the members come for information, guidance, emotional validation, and skill training, not for psychotherapy.

While acknowledging the differences between support groups and other similar vehicles of social influence, it is also necessary to highlight the similarities. Like self-help groups, support groups aim to animate a process of mutual aid from similar peers and thereby to temporarily enrich and specialize, if not compensate for deficiencies in the support available from the participants' natural networks. Like psychoeducational groups, support groups provide extra information and training that professionals believe will shore up the participants' coping efforts. Like therapy groups, support groups provide a context that promotes emotional catharsis, social comparison, and mutual identification.

The structural properties of support groups are highlighted in Table I. These properties can be altered in accordance with practical or logistical constraints, and to meet the adaptive challenges faced by the group members. More important, since the support process is likely to be affected by the ways in which the group is structured, practitioners should consider these properties carefully when they design the group. For example, in planning the group's membership (see criteria for matching in Table I), they must consider how the support process would be affected by including spouses in a group for men who are recovering from heart attacks. Would their inclusion preclude discussion of interspousal conflict about the timing of the husbands' return to work? Would the wives express emotions that might threaten the men? Similarly, in designing the individual sessions (see format in Table I), would it be better to adopt a fixed format involving a predetermined series of didactic presentations during the first half of each meeting, followed by experience swapping on any topics during the second half? Or would the members' needs be served better by opening each session with a free-floating discussion and introducing the educational or skill-training component only if and when its subject matter is raised by the group members?

The group's composition should be of paramount importance to those planning support groups since members have to be chosen in a way that will optimize their identification with one another and their participation in the group process. If they do not perceive one another as similar along certain valued dimensions, and if they do not have a common basis for comparing the feelings, actions, and thoughts that arise out of their circumstances, then the group will have little appeal to them and could actually intensify the stress they experience. For example, in composing a support group for the family caregivers of persons with dementia, practitioners must carefully weigh the importance of similarity with respect to the stage and severity of the disease (e.g., early- versus late-stage Alzheimer's), the relationship between the caregiver and relative (e.g., spouses versus daughters and daughters-in-law), and the two parties' living arrangement (e.g., living in the same or different households). Other stressor related, demographic, and contextual variables may also affect the members' rapport and ease of communication, such as their education, ethnicity,

Table I The Design and Processes of Support Groups

Design Features: The Structural Properties of the Support Group

Venue or setting
- Geographic proximity to participants
- Informal or agency/institutional setting
- Total number, length, and duration of sessions
- Interval between sessions

Leadership and facilitation
- One or more professionals only
- Co-led by a participant and a professional
- Rotating professional leaders

Composition
- Number of participants
- Open or closed membership
- Geographic proximity of participants to one another

Criteria for matching, including
- Gender, age, socioeconomic, ethnic, racial, and verbal skill factors
- Severity of the stressor
- Stage of coping with stressor
- Intensity of distress and emotional expression
- Extent of mobilization of personal coping skills

Format
- Structured vs. unstructured agenda and allocation of time
- Balance between expert input and experience swapping
- Rotating or continuous leadership
- Use of contracts vs. no contract
- Homework assignments (e.g., skill practice) vs. none
- Prescribed extra-group contacts among participants or not
- Instructions regarding extra-group exchanges of support or not
- Occasional participation of network associates or not

Mechanisms of Action: Processes Linking Support to Outcomes
- Catharsis: emotional ventilation
- Normalization of emotions
- Validation: affirmation of valued role and identity
- Helper-therapy: helping others helps oneself
- Reduction of uncertainty in novel circumstances
- Modeling of coping strategies
- Hope and a positive outlook
- Making meaning of the adversity and consolidating a new or changed identity
- Predictability and anticipatory coping
- Social comparisons

income, and gender, their family and occupational contexts, and their level of physical and emotional functioning at the time they join the group.

To date, there has been little experimentation with alternative ways of composing groups and virtually no follow-ups of people who have dropped out of groups in order to determine the social dimensions that impede and facilitate communication and exchanges of information and support. Nor have prospective group members been canvassed about who they would and would not prefer to meet with. Consequently, there is no empirical basis for deciding how to compose a support group to optimize members' attraction, active participation, and social learning and support.

As for a theoretical rationale for the group's composition, social comparison theory offers abundant but inconsistent predictions about the benefits and risks of both downward and upward comparison processes, leaving considerable ambiguity about how to engineer a social milieu that will lower distress, and maintain or increase self-esteem as well as other bases of self-evaluation. Specifically, as Gibbons and Gerrard pointed out in 1991, there is a vast literature testifying to the esteem-enhancing functions of downward social comparison or comparisons to people or even imaginary targets perceived to be worse off than oneself on certain dimensions. There is also an extensive list of papers documenting that self-esteem is bolstered when people assimilate their status to that of upward targets, and that they gain useful information from their observations of superior others. As Collins observed on the basis of her 1996 review of the social comparison literature, "Ultimately, positive self-regard depends on striking the proper balance between the number of people who are better than oneself and the number who are worse" (p. 65). Unfortunately, her conclusion provides little guidance regarding the optimal composition of a support group.

Even if the literature yielded more consistent propositions about the dimensions of comparison that enhance self-appraisals and mood, it contains no information about how the social comparison process might affect group cohesion and the exchange of support. For example, it is conceivable that exposure to a target who is perceived to be coping less effectively than oneself might raise one's self-esteem, but it may also result in rejection of the target due to the distressing affect that he or she is displaying. Indeed, most people who refuse invitations to join a support group or who drop out explain that they do not want to expose themselves to others' distress and complaints.

A second factor that militates against systematic experimentation with group composition is logistical. Those who convene support groups usually do not have the luxury of selecting the optimal membership because there are too few candidates for the groups to match people on the relevant dimensions, and most agencies do not have the resources or know-how to screen prospective participants in advance. For example, if the local chapter of the Alzheimer Disease Association attracts only 10 caregivers who are interested in attending a support group, half of whom are elderly spouses and half middle-aged daughters, and their demented relatives range from mild to severe cases, then the organization is ethically bound to offer them a group despite these apparent differences. Moreover, even when a large number of prospective group participants is available for group assignment, if a formal evaluation is in the offing, then random allocation of participants to experimental and control or comparison conditions may preclude appropriate matching within groups.

In sum, although there is little doubt that the social comparisons that occur both overtly through discussion and covertly through observation constitute a fundamental process whereby support groups influence adaptation, there exist no guidelines regarding ways of structuring the group's membership to optimize the support process and beneficial outcomes arising from it. Short of exploring how the support process and its outcomes are affected by systematically varying certain dimensions of comparison, such as the stage and severity of the members' stressful experience or their apparent mastery of their circumstances, researchers can gather information directly from members about their preferences for and reactions to their fellow sufferers. If an individual with a mild case of Multiple Sclerosis does not wish to see and hear from someone who is confined to a wheelchair due to the disease's progression, then they can report this before or after their first group session. Similarly, if a teenager who is acutely distressed by his parents' recent separation finds it reassuring to talk to youths who are calmer now that their parents have concluded the divorce and each has established a new household, then they can report this. Such information can be immensely helpful to other practitioners by informing their decisions about the composition of subsequent support groups, and it can enrich social comparison theory by adding knowledge based on intervention.

V. THE IMPACTS OF SUPPORT GROUPS

To properly assess the impacts of support groups, it is necessary to adhere to the requisites of a scientific evaluation. This means that ideally, a reasonably large number of participants should be randomly assigned to support and control or comparison groups, and outcomes should be standardized and examined well after the formal intervention concludes. In addition, it is desirable to carefully document the actual substance of the intervention so that any observed effects can be appropriately attributed to the intervention maneuvers. For example, if the process of experience swapping consumes virtually all the group's time, then any effects can be reliably attributed to this component of the intervention. However, few investigators have been able to devote the resources and develop the tools needed to gauge the differential impact of the several components that typically comprise support groups. These components may include educational input from expert sources, skill training, supportive contact among members within and between group sessions, homework assignments, and more general group discussion and problem solving. Hence, to date, evaluations of this multifaceted social intervention have not isolated the effects of its components.

As one might expect, it is impossible to offer any general conclusions about the mental health impact of support groups because of the sheer volume of studies that have been completed and the many differences in the characteristics of the participants and their stressful predicaments, the structure, format, and content of the group sessions, the "dosage" (number, length, and duration of the group sessions), as well as the measures used to tap outcomes. Although there are many individual reports of support groups that have had impressive and relatively lasting desirable mental health effects, there are also many articles reporting marginal or null effects.

There have been three critical reviews of the literature on the effects of support groups for family caregivers of elderly relatives (Bourgeois, Schulz, and Burgio in 1996, Lavoie in 1995, and Toseland and Rossiter in 1989), and two concerning their effects on cancer patients (Fawzy, Fawzy, Arndt, and Pasnau in 1995, and Helgeson and Cohen in 1996). Generally, the evidence strongly suggests that the typical, short-term support group that meets on a weekly basis for 6 to 10 sessions does not have a comparative edge in terms of its mental health effects. The impact of longer term groups, specifically, groups that meet for at least 6 months, shows more promise. However, as discussed later, the group's duration is not the only factor that affects its success.

A. Support Groups for Caregivers of Elderly Relatives

Although the evidence is mixed, the general consensus is that groups for the caregivers of elderly family members have a negligible impact on mental health outcomes, measured by widely accepted psychiatric symptom, general distress, and burden scales, and by indices of socioemotional functioning. Toseland and Rossiter's careful review of this literature led them to conclude that the groups should be composed of more homogeneous subgroups of caregivers, such as separate groups for spouses and adult children, and that they should last longer, gauge more specific behavioral changes, and experiment with alternative formats and curricula. Finally, both Lavoie and Bourgeois, Schulz, and Burgio suggest that support groups may not address the unique circumstances and needs of individual caregivers, and therefore in many cases the outcomes that are measured are not relevant.

Generally, family caregivers report high levels of satisfaction with their group experience, and deeply regret the fact that the group must terminate after the prescribed number of sessions. This suggests that a short-term model of practice is inappropriate for a population that is dealing with a host of chronically stressful demands that change over time. Most family caregivers require continuing support, training, and guidance, in addition to a range of community services that can alleviate the objective burdens they shoulder. As Lavoie observed in 1995, "To expect to change well-established behaviors such as personal coping styles, or deep-seated dynamics such as anxiety or depression over the illness of a loved one and the need to care for that person, by means of a limited number of group meetings with peers could seem like wishful thinking" (p. 589).

Even more fundamental questions can be raised

about the nature and meaningfulness of the mental health outcomes that have been gauged. Is it appropriate to reduce feelings of sadness and loss when such feelings are to be expected under the harsh circumstances imposed by dementia? Should a statistically significant reduction in anxiety or depressive affect be considered meaningful apart from its clinical significance? Are there other mental-health-related variables that may be more important to the subjective well-being of family caregivers, and more amenable to the influence of a support group? For example, through group discussion and social comparisons, the members may come to adopt a more sanguine perspective on their situation, normalize their feelings of frustration and loss, and even rid themselves of the guilt they anticipate experiencing if they were to avail themselves of respite programs and solicit more help from other family members. These are important potential contributions of the support group, yet they have not been systematically addressed in evaluations of its effects.

B. Support Groups for Cancer Patients

Reviews of the mental health effects of support groups for cancer patients have also yielded mixed results. In 1995, Fawzy, Fawzy, Arndt, and Pasnau identified 15 "group interventions" for cancer patients, the majority of whom were women who participated in heterogeneous groups composed of patients with mixed diagnoses and with both initial and recurrent/metasticized disease. With one exception, the groups met from 4 to 11 times over a period of from 2 to 8 weeks, and typically included education, stress management (coping; relaxation) training, and mutual aid. In 1996, Helgeson and Cohen identified seven evaluations of support groups that involved various degrees of peer discussion and education from expert leaders, as well as four studies that compared the effects of group discussion only to the effects of education only or combined education and group discussion. Both reviews underscore the fact that many of the studies did not meet the requirements of a formal randomized controlled trial (RCT).

Fawzy and colleagues concluded that separate support groups should be convened for cancer patients who are newly diagnosed or in the early stage of treatment versus those who have advanced metastatic disease. They suggest that the former population benefits most from a structured, multifaceted, short-term program that combines didactic education, skill training, problem solving, and mutual support, whereas the latter population benefits most from a long-term, weekly support group that concentrates on shoring up the participants' daily coping and pain management skills, while offering the empathic understanding and emotional validation of peers. Both reviews cite the support groups for metastatic breast cancer patients that Spiegel, Bloom, and Yalom organized in 1981, as exemplary of the kind of long-term program of support that appears to be needed by and of benefit to patients with advanced disease. It consisted of weekly, 90-minute sessions that lasted for 1 year and focused on ". . . the problems of terminal illness, including improving relationships with family, friends, and physicians and living as fully as possible in the face of death" (p. 527). Each of the three groups they organized was co-led by a psychiatrist or a social worker and a counselor whose breast cancer was in remission. The group's main emphasis was on the development of an emotionally sustaining culture, not on educational material supplied by the leaders. Finally, participants also had supportive contact with one another outside the formal group sessions, and after the 1-year mark of data collection, the survivors continued to meet as a group for a second year and informally thereafter.

The findings of this RCT underscore the importance of offering a relatively long-term program of support, and of measuring various intervention effects at several points in time. Specifically, compared to the control group, those in the three support groups reported better adjustment after a year but not at the 4-month or 8-month time points. That is, the effects of the intervention on total mood disturbance, and on the subscales of tension-anxiety, vigor, fatigue, and confusion appear to have been cumulative in nature. Moreover, in 1989, Spiegel, Bloom, Kraemer, and Gottheil presented a 10-year follow-up of the study participants that revealed that the intervention increased survival by 18 months.

In comparing the effects of short-term groups that concentrate on discussion and support with the effects of groups that concentrate on education, Helgeson and Cohen tentatively conclude that the latter demonstrate superior adjustment benefits. This is not to say that the support and discussion component is superfluous, but that the education component is necessary to achieve desired effects. It may be that people who have been diagnosed with cancer need the technical information that professionals provide, and gain a stronger sense of security from the professional's presence and special interest in the group members. It is also possible that feelings of control and predictability are uniquely predicated on the authoritative information and skill training professionals provide. In contrast, Helgeson and Cohen suggest that groups that concentrate strictly on peer support may undermine feelings of control if they disrupt denial or other emotionally avoidant modes of coping. In addition, they may adversely affect participants' reactions to their illness by exposing them to peers who are losing their battle with cancer, or who raise frightening topics that are not worked through with professional guidance, or whose cancer site and stage are so different that they cannot validate one another's emotional experience. In the future, more careful measurement will be needed to identify these and other potential mediating processes associated with the peer and professional sources of influence in the group.

VI. LINKING GROUP STRUCTURE, PROCESSES, AND COMPOSITION TO OUTCOMES

There is a tight interdependence among the structure, composition, and process of support groups. Leaders can place varying emphases on the experience-swapping, behavioral-training, and information-dissemination functions of the group, thereby affecting the group's cohesion, intimacy, and overall social climate. Leaders can concentrate on either the emotional or the instrumental coping assistance offered by the group, and establish norms governing the extent and style of disclosure, confrontation, and affective release. There are also vast differences in the training and orientation of leaders themselves, a factor that is rarely taken into account in interpreting and comparing the effects of the groups. Moreover, the credentials and style of the leaders can play a critical role in recruiting and retaining group participants. For example, experience shows that support groups for male cardiac patients are more successful when the leader is a staff member with medical training in heart disease, the group is introduced as a routine aspect of medical care, and is called a rehabilitation group rather than a support or therapy group, and when wives are not included in the same group because they would interfere with their husbands' tendency to resist discussing their feelings about the threatening aspects of their condition. Hence, the group's composition can powerfully affect its process.

A. Documenting Support Group Processes

There is no dearth of hypotheses about the mediating processes or mechanisms at work in support groups. Biological pathways include alterations in immune system function, blood pressure, and urinary cortisol, whereas behavioral changes range from improved adherence to recommended dietary and drug regimens to changes in modes of coping, including the use of community services. The psychological factors that have been cited most frequently as potential mediators include the 10 listed at the bottom of Table I. At present, little is understood about the complex ways in which psychological, biological, and behavioral changes interact to produce durable and important outcomes such as the improvements in mood and survival of the cancer patients who were involved in the support groups organized by Spiegel, Bloom, Kraemer, and Gottheil in 1989.

It is therefore necessary to begin documenting aspects of the process of support groups, and systematically varying their structure and emphasis to determine how the process is altered and how it affects the observed outcomes. In addition to varying the proportion of time that is devoted to education and peer discussion, group planners can vary the emphasis they place on various goals. For example, Lavoie maintains that those who have organized support groups for family caregivers have aimed to reduce the participants' stress, whereas the participants themselves have typically aimed to improve and gain confidence in their caregiving skills. Obviously, some attention should be paid to participants' goals at the outset of the intervention, and different groups can be formed to address different goals. Even when support groups are designed to blanket all the principal sources of stress and to foster improved coping, as is the case in groups for children whose parents are divorcing or for recently bereaved people, large differences among individuals in the salience of certain stressors and in their need for supplemental coping resources may call for more specialized groups. It is also important to acknowledge that even when groups are initially structured along the same lines, each will develop its own culture and participants who are in the same group will experience the support process differently (J.-P. Lavoie, personal communication, August 19, 1996).

In addition, as Lavoie and Bourgeois, Schulz, and Burgio observe, implementation evaluation that involves assessment of the intervention process and structure is so rare that the details regarding the psychoeducational maneuvers, the leadership, the balance between mutual aid, skill training, and education, and the group's composition are not available for the purpose of replication or verification that the intervention is faithful to its blueprint. Without knowing what actually transpired over the life of the group, it is impossible to determine whether the process accurately reflected the theory that links the intervention's content to its intended outcomes. For example, if support groups for the family caregivers of persons with dementia concentrate on the acquisition of anger management skills, then it is necessary to adopt outcome criteria that reflect this specific goal, and to ensure that the requisite amount of time is spent on effectively teaching these skills and proficiently applying them at home. Similarly, if the intervention aims mainly to decrease stress and uncertainty by disseminating authoritative information about the nature and typical course of dementia, and by introducing the specialized support of similar peers, then measures of knowledge and of global stress or subjective burden should be adopted as outcomes, and members' perceptions of their similarity, the support they exchange, and the information they receive should be tapped through formative evaluation.

B. Support as a Means or as an End

When program planners consider participants' needs for supplemental coping resources, they must assess not only the kind of resources that are needed, but also how long they will be needed. Earlier, evidence was presented in favor of the efficacy of longer term groups for patients with advanced cancer and for family caregivers. It stands to reason that the duration of the support group should be matched to the duration of the adjustment demands faced by the participants. Chronic disorders, disease, and life difficulties may require ongoing or prolonged support, whereas time-limited acute life events and transitions may be addressed through a short-term group. Moreover, those designing support groups may wish to use the group as a way of permanently adding similar peers to people's natural social networks. This may be called for when existing network members are unable or unwilling to extend the kinds of practical help and emotional support that are needed because they feel helpless, drained or threatened, or because they have become critical, emotionally overinvolved, or overprotective. Among the techniques that can be used to accomplish this is to explicitly state this goal at the outset of the group, informing members that they can choose to continue to meet on their own following the final formal group meeting, and that a resource person can be made available to them when needed. In addition, members can be encouraged to have contact with one another between the group sessions, either informally or by setting up a rotating or permanent buddy system with or without a specific agenda. For example, buddies can be encouraged to simply call one another when they need extra support and dialogue, or to practice together the skills they have learned in the group. Naturally, to examine the impact of such supplemental support, records must be kept of the kind and amount of extra-group contact. Evaluation researchers should also keep in mind that social support may be an end in itself, rather than a means to an end. That is, the goal of some groups may be to combat social isolation by establishing durable and intimate dyadic or group ties among the members, as in the case of support groups for chronically mentally ill persons or teenaged, sole-support parents. Other groups may concentrate on mobilizing support as a resource for resisting stress-induced disease, illness, or maladjustment, or for promoting more positive functioning.

C. Group Composition and the Bases of Similarity

As discussed earlier, as long as the members perceive one another as similar peers, social comparison will be an ongoing covert process throughout the course of the group. Ideally, in composing the group, some thought should go into ways of exploiting this psychological process to the best advantage of the participants. For example, in most self-help groups there is a "veteran sufferer" who serves as a model of effective coping and thereby instills hope and motivation to comply with the group's behavioral prescriptions. Social comparison theory also postulates that, to accomplish its stress-reducing effect, the companions must be perceived to be reacting relatively calmly to their situation, suggesting that support groups are not appropriate during periods when people are feeling emotionally overwhelmed. It is therefore advisable to recruit participants only after they have recovered from the initial shock of a crisis, and are ready to commence a structured and paced social support program.

Once it is conceded that experiential similarity serves as a stronger basis for mutual identification and empathic understanding than structural similarity based on age or marital status, for example, questions arise concerning how similar the common experience must be in order for the participants to attend and compare themselves to one another, and to develop bonds of affection and belonging. For example, for a group of recent widows, their bereavement is probably not sufficient to level differences based on the cause and age of their partner's death. It is unlikely that widows whose husbands had died of heart attacks would perceive themselves to be "in the same boat" as widows whose husbands had been murdered or killed in a traffic accident or who had died in the line of wartime fire or by taking their own lives. The same careful consideration of the bases of similarity is warranted in planning the composition of virtually every group for people who have undergone stressful life events and transitions, such as parental death or divorce, retirement, new parenthood, job loss, serious accidents, and illness diagnoses. Three factors in particular warrant consideration: (1) the contextual or situational parameters that are likely to be most salient to the participants; (2) factors that are known to affect people's risk status; and (3) the probable trajectory the participants will experience. For example, in composing support groups for the family caregivers of elderly relatives, program planners should recognize that caring for a relative afflicted with dementia poses greater risk to the mental health of the caregiver than caring for a frail but cognitively intact relative, and that the future course of dementia is distinctly different from other disabilities and conditions. Hence, it would not be advisable to compose a group that combines caregivers in these contrasting situations. Of course, if the prospective participants are children or youth, it is necessary to ensure that the group content and composition is developmentally appropriate.

Finally, the similarity of the participants not only bears on their ability to relate and compare themselves to one another, but it also affects the substantive content of the educational component and ultimately, the impact of the intervention. As noted earlier, reviews of the support group literature have been consistent in their criticism of the heterogeneity of groups, arguing that interventions will impact differently on various subgroups of participants and suggesting that null results may mask differential effectiveness for such subgroups. In addition to structural and experiential differences among participants, they may also differ on the basis of the stage of the condition or problem they face, their use of both informal and formal supports in the community, and a number of personality and coping factors that affect their receptiveness to and benefit from this type of intervention.

D. Adapting the Group to Personal Coping Styles

This brings us to the larger question concerning the personal characteristics that distinguish those who gravitate toward support groups from those who decline participation, and those who are most likely to benefit from those who do not benefit or who may be adversely affected by joining such a group. Although only rarely reported, refusal rates for support groups are quite high, and to a lesser extent, attrition is a problem as well. Aside from the standard psychological (e.g., stigma and fear of disapproval or rejection) and logistical (e.g., access, scheduling, and coverage of competing demands such as childcare) impediments to participation in any social program, support groups pose some unique threats and offer a particular way of coping with one's difficulties that does not have universal appeal or benefit.

The threats posed by support groups include a fear of becoming overwhelmed by attending to and disclosing one's difficulties, and by exposing oneself to the more severe difficulties faced by other group members, especially if those difficulties preview one's own possible fate. Although some members may benefit from this because of the anticipatory coping and sense of control such advance information may promote, others may cope most effectively by keeping such information out of conscious awareness. In short, differences in people's coping styles may powerfully affect their interest in and the value they gain from participating in support groups. Specifically, differences in information and help seeking, and more generally, avoidant versus approach-oriented coping styles under threat, may distinguish between those who are attracted to and make good use of the group experience and those who do not. In plain language, some people deal with threat by seeking as much information about it as they can and by venting their fears and emotional distress, whereas others maintain their equilibrium best by avoiding threatening information and blunting their emotions. In their 1996 review of psychosocial interventions for patients with chronic physical illnesses, Devins and Binik cite numerous studies revealing that social programs that concentrate on imparting information are more effective when they are matched to the participants' information processing style. Hence, "blunters" may fare better with more structured, task-centered, behavioral intervention protocols, whereas "monitors" may respond best to formats that provide plentiful details about the stressful context, and that allow them to discuss their feelings and experiences, and to ask questions.

Depending on how they are marketed and actually run, support groups may be more or less threatening or attractive to people with contrasting information- and support-seeking coping styles. As noted earlier, if they smack of group therapy with all of its emotional trappings and disclosure requirements, or if their advertisements promise to deliver detailed information about the more threatening aspects of the present and future, then they are likely to be shunned by and maladaptive for those who tend to regulate their emotions by avoidance and distraction. Indeed, the combination of unbridled emotional expression among peers and abundant information from experts is likely to drive the blunters away, while appealing to the monitors whose emotional self-regulation and sense of control are augmented by these two components. It follows that, in both advertising and implementing groups, the format, emotional climate, and type of information supplied should be pitched differently, depending on the prospective participants' coping styles. Where feasible, a measure of their information-processing style can be used as a screening and group placement tool. If this is not possible and people with different styles are assigned to the same group, then potential moderating effects of these coping styles can be tested to determine whether they have influenced intervention outcomes.

VII. POTENTIAL RISKS AND SHORTCOMINGS OF SUPPORT GROUPS

If prospective participants are geographically dispersed, as is the case for people who reside in rural areas, then logistical difficulties may prevent them from attending a support group. Alternatives that have recently been initiated are to create telephone and electronic mail support groups. By means of teleconferencing and occasional face-to-face visits, much of the experiential knowledge and a substantial amount of emotional and esteem-relevant support can still be exchanged in such groups. A second shortcoming is that support groups do not allow for the individualization of helping. Thus, what is gained in cost efficiency through the group format is lost in personalized attention. However, in many instances, support groups are designed to supplement rather than to substitute for the individual counseling or treatment offered by mental health or medical practitioners, and so members' unique needs are addressed. Moreover, when individual counseling precedes support group participation, the counselor may be able to make more judicious judgments about group assignments. As Gottlieb pointed out in 1988, there are also several types of one-to-one formats for marshaling support that may be better suited to people's needs and preferences than a group intervention. Hence, practitioners should consider and even compare the effectiveness of alternative support strategies.

Third, support groups can have adverse social repercussions. They can threaten natural network members who perceive the group as an affront to the support they offer instead of recognizing that the support of similarly stressed peers is a vital complementary coping resource. The group leaders can guard against such resentment, injury, or backlash from the participants' network members by not only advising the participants to explain the special value of the support group, but also by inviting key network members to attend a meeting of their own in which they can ask questions, air their concerns, and learn how they can optimize the group's impact on their associate. A related social and ethical concern that has not received sufficient attention from group planners is the potential negative effect of withdrawing the peer support when the final group session has ended. In virtually every published report of support groups, the members lament the group's termination. This suggests that many groups do, in fact, terminate prematurely and ought to have a longer course or at least offer the members the option of continuing to meet on their own as a mutual aid group or at least to socialize with one another. Naturally, this will not be possible if the participants are minors or if they are dealing with such sensitive or technical matters that they require professional guidance. In any case, it behooves the group leaders to carefully plan for the group's termination, and to monitor any rebound effects that may result therefrom.

Finally, as is the case for all group interventions, there is the possibility that a negative emotional contagion will spread through the group, especially if the members face circumstances that are known to deteriorate over time or suffer from a condition that has a poor prognosis. Many practitioners question the wisdom of bringing together people with terminal diseases such as cancer because they fear that they will only exacerbate their distress and further demoralize them. Although this adverse development is certainly possible, its likelihood can be minimized by leaders who carefully monitor and control the group's affective tone. Moreover, those who clinicians worry about most are usually people who suffer from both social and emotional isolation, and who therefore are most likely to benefit from the empathic understanding, companionship, and solidarity that a support group can offer. It is also important to keep in mind that people want to be well and that the support group can teach participants how to reinforce one another's wellness rather than their distress.

VIII. CONCLUSION

If there is a single message that deserves emphasis it is that practitioners need to attend more closely to the composition and duration of support groups, and apportion the time allotted to expert information and peer interaction in a way that suits the participants' needs and coping styles. Where possible, the group's composition should be determined by taking into account at least three sets of similarity factors, namely, experiential similarity, structural similarity, and similarity in the members' information-processing style of coping. Sustained rather than brief groups are called for and have proved more effective for chronic life difficulties, role strain, and other circumstances of unremitting demand, whereas short-term groups are called for during periods of crisis and transition.

Support groups have broad, although not universal, appeal. For people who tend to cope by seeking information and affiliation with similar peers, such groups can reduce distress and promote adjustment. Yet the processes implicated in the group's ameliorative psychosocial impact are not well understood. For this reason, more careful documentation is needed of the physiological, behavioral, and psychological mechanisms that underlie this mode of intervention. In addition, there is a need for comparative studies that systematically vary the group's structure, composition, and emphases, in order to discern how the process and outcomes are affected. Although mental health ranks among the most important of these outcomes, the support group may also give the participants a sense of reliable alliance and belonging that can dispel their feelings of emotional isolation. At bottom, the support group is a highly specialized personal community that gives full expression to the human impulse to care for others and to be cared for by them.

BIBLIOGRAPHY

Bourgeois, M. S., Schulz, R., & Burgio, L. (1996). Interventions for caregivers of patients with Alzheimer's Disease: A review and analysis of content, process, and outcomes. *International Journal of Aging and Human Development, 43,* 35–92.

Cohen, S., & Wills, T. A. (1985). Stress, social support, and the buffering hypothesis. *Psychological Bulletin, 98,* 310–357.

Collins. R. L. (1996). For better or worse: The impact of upward social comparison on self-evaluations. *Psychological Bulletin, 119,* 51–69.

Coyne, J. C., Wortman, C.B., & Lehman, D. R. (1988). The other side of support: Emotional overinvolvement and miscarried helping. In B. H. Gottlieb (Ed.), *Marshaling social support* (pp. 305–330).

Devins, G. M., & Binik, Y. M. (1996). Facilitating coping with chronic physical illness. In M. Zeidner & N. Endler (Eds.), *Handbook of coping* (pp. 640–696). New York: John Wiley & Sons.

Fawzy, F. I., Fawzy, N. W., Arndt, L. A., & Pasnau, R. O. (1995). Critical review of psychosocial interventions in cancer care. *Archives of General Psychiatry, 52,* 100–113.

Gallagher-Thompson, D. (1994). Clinical intervention strategies for distressed caregivers: Rationale and development of psychoeducational approaches. In E. Light, G. Niederehe, & B. D.

Lebowitz (Eds.), *Stress effects on family caregivers of Alzheimer's patients* (pp. 260–277). New York: Springer.

Gibbons, F. X., & Gerrard, M. (1991). Downward comparison and coping with threat. In J. Suls and T. Wills (Eds.), *Social comparison: Contemporary theory and research* (pp. 317–346). Hillsdale, NJ: Erlbaum.

Gottlieb, B. H. (1988). Support interventions: A typology and agenda for research. In S. Duck (Ed.), *Handbook of personal relationships: Theory, research and interventions* (pp. 519–542). Chichester, England: John Wiley & Sons.

Helgeson, V. S., & Cohen, S. (1996). Social support and adjustment to cancer: Reconciling descriptive, correlational, and intervention research. *Health Psychology, 15,* 135–148.

House, J. S., Landis, K. R., & Umberson, D. (1988). Social relationships and health. *Science, 241,* 540–545.

Lavoie, J.-P. (1995). Support groups for informal caregivers don't work! Refocus the groups or the evaluations? *Canadian Journal on Aging, 14,* 580–595.

Spiegel, D., Bloom, J., & Yalom, I. D. (1981). Group support for patients with metastatic breast cancer. *Archives of General Psychiatry, 38,* 527–533.

Spiegel, D., Bloom, J., Kraemer, H. C., & Gottheil, E. (1989, October 14). Effect of psychosocial treatment on survival of patients with metastatic breast cancer. *Lancet,* pp. 888–891.

Taylor, S. E., Falke, R. L., Shoptaw, S. J., & Lichtman, P. R. (1986). Social support, support groups, and the cancer patient. *Journal of Consulting and Clinical Psychology, 54,* 608–615.

Toseland, R. W., & Rossiter, C. M. (1989). Group interventions to support family caregivers: A review and analysis. *The Gerontologist, 29*(4), 438–448.

Encyclopedia of Mental Health

Editor-in-Chief

Howard S. Friedman
University of California, Riverside

Executive Advisory Board

Nancy E. Adler
University of California, San Francisco

Ross D. Parke
University of California, Riverside

Christopher Peterson
University of Michigan, Ann Arbor

Robert Rosenthal
Harvard University

Ralf Schwarzer
Freie Universität Berlin

Roxane Cohen Silver
University of California, Irvine

David Spiegel
Stanford University School of Medicine

Contributors

Carolyn M. Aldwin
Assessment of Mental Health in Older Adults
Department of Human and Community Development
University of California, Davis
Davis, California 95616

John J. B. Allen
DSM-IV
Department of Psychology
University of Arizona
Tucson, Arizona 85721

Philip Barker
Family Therapy
Departments of Pediatrics and Medicine
University of Calgary Mental Health Program
and Alberta Children's Hospital
Calgary, Alberta T2T 5C7, Canada

Herbert Benson
Meditation and the Relaxation Response
Mind/Body Medical Institute
Harvard Medical School
Beth Israel Deaconess Medical Center
Boston, Massachusetts 02215

Dinesh Bhugra
Sexual Dysfunction Therapy
Institute of Psychiatry
London SE5 8AF, United Kingdom

Kelly J. Brown
Psychopharmacology
Portland V.A. Medical Center
Portland, Oregon 97201

Andrew Christensen
Couples Therapy
Department of Psychology
University of California, Los Angeles
Los Angeles, California 90095

Paul T. Costa, Jr.
Personality Assessment
Laboratory of Personality and Cognition
Gerontology Research Center
National Institute on Aging
National Institutes of Health
Bethesda, Maryland 21224

Robyn M. Dawes
Standards for Psychotherapy
Department of Social and Decision Sciences
Carnegie Mellon University
Pittsburgh, Pennsylvania 15213

Anita DeLongis
Coping with Stress
Department of Psychology
University of British Columbia
Vancouver, British Columbia V6T 1Z4, Canada

Padmal de Silva
Sexual Dysfunction Therapy
Department of Psychology
Institute of Psychiatry
London SE5 8AF, United Kingdom

Kathleen Coulborn Faller
Child Sexual Abuse
University of Michigan School of Social Work
Ann Arbor, Michigan 48104

Sabine Elizabeth French
Community Mental Health
Department of Psychology
New York University
New York, New York 10003

Richard Friedman
Meditation and the Relaxation Response
Mind/Body Medical Institute
Harvard Medical School
Beth Israel Deaconess Medical Center
Boston, Massachusetts 02215

Eileen Gambrill
Clinical Assessment
School of Social Welfare
University of California, Berkeley
Berkeley, California 94720

Benjamin H. Gottlieb
Support Groups
Department of Psychology
University of Guelph
Guelph, Ontario N1G 2W1, Canada

Sandra A. Graham-Bermann
Domestic Violence Intervention
Department of Psychology
University of Michigan, Ann Arbor
Ann Arbor, Michigan 48109

Neil E. Grunberg
Psychopharmacology
Medical and Clinical Psychology
Uniformed Services University of the Health Sciences
Bethesda, Maryland 20814

Richard J. Haier
Brain Scanning/Neuroimaging
Department of Pediatrics
University of California, Irvine, Medical School
Irvine, California 92717

Mardi J. Horowitz
Psychoanalysis
Department of Psychiatry
University of California, San Francisco
San Francisco, California 94143

Robert M. Kaplan
Behavioral Medicine
University of California, San Diego, School of Medicine
La Jolla, California 92093

Ernest Keen
Classifying Mental Disorders: Nontraditional Approaches
Bucknell University
Lewisburg, Pennsylvania 17837

David N. Kerner
Behavioral Medicine
University of California, San Diego, School of Medicine
La Jolla, California 92093

John F. Kihlstrom
Hypnosis and the Psychological Unconscious
Department of Psychology
University of California, Berkeley
Berkeley, California 94720

Laura Cousino Klein
Psychopharmacology
Department of Psychology and Social Behavior
School of Social Ecology
University of California, Irvine
Irvine, California 92697

Elise E. Labbé
Biofeedback
Department of Psychology
University of South Alabama
Mobile, Alabama 36688

Michael R. Levenson
Assessment of Mental Health in Older Adults
Department of Human and Community Development
University of California, Davis
Davis, California 95616

Maxie C. Maultsby, Jr.
Behavior Therapy
Department of Psychiatry
Howard University College of Medicine
Washington, District of Columbia 20060

Teresita McCarty
Premenstrual Syndrome Treatment Interventions
Department of Psychiatry
University of New Mexico
School of Medicine
Albuquerque, New Mexico 87131

Robert R. McCrae
Personality Assessment
Laboratory of Personality and Cognition
Gerontology Research Center
National Institute on Aging
National Institutes of Health
Bethesda, Maryland 21224

Ricardo F. Muñoz
Depression—Applied Aspects
Department of Psychiatry
San Francisco General Hospital
University of California, San Francisco
San Francisco, California 94110

Patricia Myers
Meditation and the Relaxation Response
Mind/Body Medical Institute
Harvard Medical School
Beth Israel Deaconess Medical Center
Boston, Massachusetts 02215

Robert A. Neimeyer
Constructivist Psychotherapies
Department of Psychology
University of Memphis
Memphis, Tennessee 38152

Sarah Newth
Coping with Stress
Department of Psychology
University of British Columbia
Vancouver, British Columbia V6T 1Z4, Canada

Laura Weiss Roberts
Premenstrual Syndrome Treatment Interventions
Department of Psychiatry
University of New Mexico
School of Medicine
Albuquerque, New Mexico 87131

Theodore R. Sarbin
Classifying Mental Disorders: Nontraditional Approaches
University of California, Santa Cruz
Santa Cruz, California 95064

Edward Seidman
Community Mental Health
Department of Psychology
New York University
New York, New York 10003

Sally K. Severino
Premenstrual Syndrome Treatment Interventions
Department of Psychiatry
University of New Mexico School of Medicine
Albuquerque, New Mexico 87131

Alan E. Stewart
Constructivist Psychotherapies
Department of Psychology
University of Florida
Gainesville, Florida 32611

Kieran T. Sullivan
Couples Therapy
Department of Psychology
Santa Clara University
Santa Clara, California 95053

Marjorie E. Weishaar
Cognitive Therapy
Department of Psychiatry and Human Behavior
Brown University School of Medicine
Providence, Rhode Island 02912

Mariusz Wirga
Behavior Therapy
Las Vegas Medical Center
Las Vegas, New Mexico 87701

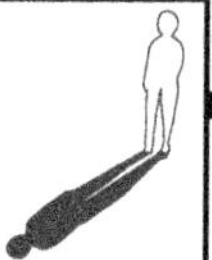

Index

C

D

F

G

H

I

L

M

N

O

P

R

S

T

U

V

W

Printed and bound by CPI Group (UK) Ltd, Croydon, CR0 4YY

03/10/2024

01040315-0013